FERTILITY AND JEWISH LAW

BRANDEIS SERIES ON GENDER, CULTURE, RELIGION, AND LAW

Lisa Fishbayn Joffe and Sylvia Neil, *Series Editors*

This series focuses on the conflict between women's claims to gender equality and legal norms justified in terms of religious and cultural traditions. It seeks work that develops new theoretical tools for conceptualizing feminist projects for transforming the interpretation and justification of religious law, examines the interaction or application of civil law or remedies to gender issues in a religious context, and engages in analysis of conflicts over gender and culture/religion in a particular religious legal tradition, cultural community, or nation. Created under the auspices of the Hadassah-Brandeis Institute in conjunction with its Project on Gender, Culture, Religion, and the Law, this series emphasizes cross-cultural and interdisciplinary scholarship concerning Judaism, Islam, Christianity, and other religious traditions.

For a complete list of books that are available in the series, visit www.upne.com

Ronit Irshai, *Fertility and Jewish Law: Feminist Perspectives on Orthodox Responsa Literature*

Janet Bennion, *Polygamy in Primetime: Media, Gender, and Politics in Mormon Fundamentalism*

Jan Feldman, *Citizenship, Faith, and Feminism: Jewish and Muslim Women Reclaim Their Rights*

HBI SERIES ON JEWISH WOMEN

Shulamit Reinharz, *General Editor*

Sylvia Barack Fishman, Associate Editor

The HBI Series on Jewish Women, created by the Hadassah-Brandeis Institute, publishes a wide range of books by and about Jewish women in diverse contexts and time periods. Of interest to scholars and the educated public, the HBI Series on Jewish Women fills major gaps in Jewish Studies and in Women and Gender Studies as well as their intersection.

The HBI Series on Jewish Women is supported by a generous gift from Dr. Laura S. Schor.

For the complete list of books that are available in this series, please see www.upne.com

Ronit Irshai, *Fertility and Jewish Law: Feminist Perspectives on Orthodox Responsa Literature*

Elana Maryles Sztokman, *The Men's Section: Orthodox Jewish Men in an Egalitarian World*

Sharon Faye Koren, *Forsaken: The Menstruant in Medieval Jewish Mysticism*

Sonja M. Hedgepeth and Rochelle G. Saidel, editors, *Sexual Violence against Jewish Women during the Holocaust*

Julia R. Lieberman, editor, *Sephardi Family Life in the Early Modern Diaspora*

Derek Rubin, editor, *Promised Lands: New Jewish American Fiction on Longing and Belonging*

FERTILITY
and Jewish Law

FEMINIST PERSPECTIVES ON
ORTHODOX RESPONSA LITERATURE

Ronit Irshai TRANSLATED BY JOEL A. LINSIDER

Brandeis University Press Waltham, Massachusetts

Brandeis University Press
An imprint of University Press of New England
www.upne.com

Manufactured in the United States of America
Designed by Mindy Basinger Hill
Typeset in 11/14 Garamond Premier Pro by
Keystone Typesetting, Inc.

University Press of New England is a member of the Green Press Initiative. The paper used in this book meets their minimum requirement for recycled paper.

Library of Congress Cataloging-in-Publication Data

Irshai, Ronit.
Fertility and Jewish law: feminist perspectives on Orthodox responsa literature / Ronit Irshai; translated by Joel A. Linsider.—1st. ed.
p. cm.—(HBI series on Jewish women)
Includes bibliographical references and index.
ISBN 978-1-61168-239-7 (cloth: alk. paper)—
ISBN 978-1-61168-240-3 (pbk.: alk. paper)—
ISBN 978-1-61168-241-0 (ebook)
1. Conception—Religious aspects—Judaism.
2. Abortion—Religious aspects—Judaism.
3. Jewish law. I. Linsider, Joel A. II. Title.

BM538. C68178 2012
296.3′662—dc23 2012007839

This book was published with the generous support of the Lucius N. Littauer Foundation.

5 4 3 2 1

To Professor Dafna Izraeli (*z"l*)

Contents

Acknowledgments

Twelve years ago I knew nothing of feminism. At that time I was enrolled as a doctoral student in the field of modern Jewish thought at the Hebrew University of Jerusalem and was engaged in beginning my study of the religious philosophy of Isaac Breuer, a leading figure of early-twentieth-century German neo-Orthodoxy. It was simply by chance that I found myself attending Professor Tamar Ross's course on Feminism and Judaism. This was an earth-shaking experience. I felt as if transported back to my first year as a B.A. student in the philosophy department, studying Socrates and feeling the cogs in my brain turning nonstop.

A month later I informed my advisor at the Hebrew University that, despite my love of modern Jewish thought, I was now captivated by the encounter between Feminism and Judaism and had decided to direct my academic efforts to this field. I approached Professor Ross and asked her to be my new advisor without even precisely knowing the subject of my research or exactly what it was I wished to pursue. Of one thing only was I certain: that I wanted to explore the ways in which feminist theories can influence Jewish halakhic thought. For her trust, and for opening the door to this new and challenging field, I am profoundly in Professor Ross's debt. It is to Professor Ross first and foremost that I must tender thanks for this book. Later on, she was joined by Professor Noam Zohar, who became my second advisor. It was my good fortune to benefit from both Noam and Tamar's knowledge and wisdom.

Bar-Ilan University was the first university in Israel to open a gender studies program at the doctoral level. This program was founded and directed by the late Professor Dafna Izraeli. Dafna's inspiration as a feminist and a scholar illumined my path during this long journey. This book is dedicated to her memory.

Beyond the scope and high level of its offerings, the Bar-Ilan Gender Studies Program became my second home, and its students and lecturers became close friends, and later colleagues. To them I owe many productive discussions and exchanges, but above all the commitment to feminist ideas, their loyalty, and friendship.

After completing my doctoral degree I spent a year at the Women Studies in Religion Program at the Harvard Divinity School. It was during this wonderful year that I had the opportunity to start thinking of revising my dissertation and turning it into a book. I wish to express my sincere thanks and gratitude to director Ann Braude, who even though on sabbatical was available to us, to acting director Joan Branham for doing a great job during this year, and to my colleagues: Sue Houchins, Michelle Molina, Miryam Segal, and Monica Maher with whom I shared many of the ideas found in this book.

The publication of this book received financial support from two institutes at Bar-Ilan University. I thank the Fanya Gottesfeld Heller Center for the Study of Women in Judaism and its chairperson Dr. Elisheva Baumgarten for finding my work in harmony with its objective of advancing feminist research on women in Judaism. I must also thank the Dafna Izraeli chair at the Gender Studies Program and Professor Tova Cohen who succeeded Professor Izraeli as chair of the Gender Studies Program. It was Professor Cohen who not only provided personal support and encouragement for my research but also paved the way for my appointment to the staff of the gender program.

This project would not have been possible without the invaluable contribution of Joel Linsider, the translator of the Hebrew manuscript, whose erudition and linguistic skills are reflected throughout the English translation. I owe him profound thanks. Nor do words suffice to express my heartfelt appreciation to my research assistant, Rachel Furst, an excellent scholar in her own right, who devoted days and nights to helping me complete the difficult task of finishing and editing this manuscript for publication. Her good will, wisdom, and meticulousness made this a better book.

I must also thank the members of the Hadassah-Brandeis Institute, especially Professors Sylvia Barack Fishman and Shulamit Reinharz, and Dr. Lisa Fishbayn Joffe, for supporting my work and affording me the opportunity to publish this book in two distinguished Brandeis series. It is also my pleasant duty to thank the helpful staff at the University Press of New England: Phyllis Deutsch, Amanda Dupuis, and Katy Grabill. Special kudos to editor-in-chief Phyllis Deutsch for her outstanding patience!

And finally my family: I thank my parents, brother, and sisters for their unconditional support; my beloved children, who despite their youth were willing to share their opinions and to discuss some of the ideas, problems, and uncertainties that accompanied my writing; and finally, my husband, who is more than a friend, without whose support and understanding none of this would have happened.

Ronit Irshai

JERUSALEM, SUMMER 2011

FERTILITY AND JEWISH LAW

INTRODUCTION

Epistemology, Jurisprudence, and Halakhah

A FEMINIST CRITIQUE

Jewish law (halakhah) is the product of an exclusively male preserve. Though it governs the lives of men and women alike, it has been formulated and interpreted, for thousands of years, by an all-male scholarly elite. But while that fact cannot be denied, its implications and consequences can be understood in varied, even contradictory, ways.

What significance should be ascribed to the "maleness" of the halakhah? Does the fact that it has been formulated and interpreted exclusively by men necessarily imply that its decision making and its interpretive methods are in some sense "masculine"? If so, in what sense? Does this mean that the halakhah has gender-based leanings, and if so, what are the implications for its objectivity? Do these gender-based leanings differ qualitatively from the subjective qualities that can undeniably be identified in every legal corpus, halakhah included? These questions constitute the infrastructure of the inquiry to which this book is devoted. Most of the book focuses on issues related to reproduction, subjects that illustrate the maleness of halakhic discourse in general. Subjecting the halakhah, as a legal system, to feminist criticism using scientific and jurisprudential methodologies will clarify the way in which gendered assumptions permeate the halakhic system. And while gender criticism is of great value in itself, it can also cast new light on general halakhic processes and thereby make a significant contribution to the philosophy of halakhah, the discipline in which this inquiry is grounded. In that sense, my purpose in subjecting the halakhah to a feminist critique is not only to conduct a "local" analysis looking toward one or another halakhic resolutions to a problem pertaining to women; it is more comprehensive and global, probing much deeper into the halakhic process. In other words, I will not adopt the standard approach of seeking the halakhic tools needed to effectuate change (though I believe this endeavor is important and I do not intend to work against it); rather, I will strive to tell *a different halakhic story*, one that accounts for the female narrative and its missing perspective. Without doubt, some halakhically observant Jews will regard this enterprise as subversive and revolutionary, for it claims that the halakhah fails to properly grasp the world in which we live, and it thereby threatens to change the meaning of halakhah in a drastic way. But what I mean to do is to articulate the sense of a growing number of women and men that the patriarchal picture of the world that lies at the heart of the halakhic system no longer corresponds to the circumstances of their lives. These individuals thereby challenge the halakhic decisors to respond to the self-perception of a target audience both old and new, one that is loyal to the traditional world but lives within a reality that often expresses loyalty to values at odds with those of the traditional world.

Even those of a conservative bent will sometimes recognize subjective proclivities in halakhic decision-making, but it is only natural that they will more often try to depict halakhic decisors as acting in an objective and appropriate manner, heeding the call to rise above their personal inclinations. That perspective, characteristic of the halakhic world itself, rejects as almost abhorrent the idea that halakhic decisors, though male, are unable to rise above the fact of their maleness and resolve halakhic questions in an objective manner, without favoring either men or women. Underlying the conservative viewpoint is the assumption that although the involvement of human decisors entails an amount of subjectivity in decision making, the system itself is able to neutralize that influence, by requiring that its practitioners do what is right and just.[1] In this sense, even "subjectivity" is a product of the halakhah's ethos and the manner in which it shapes the decisor's array of concepts and values.

Those of a more critical bent will call this claim of the system's gender-neutrality into question, however, seeing it as a manifestation of the fact that a halakhic decisor, like a judge (and even a scientist), works within a specific intellectual paradigm and reflects a particular consciousness. The positions taken by a decisor will inevitably be influenced by his particular perspective, based on such factors as his culture and values, his personal characteristics and experiences, as well as his gender. Some will go even further, maintaining that masculine leanings within halakhah are so obvious, inasmuch as the halakhah itself is a clearly masculine corpus, that they don't require explanation or analysis. Consequently, those engaged in academic study of Jewish law have neglected to address these biases in the halakhah, and the issue has been rendered nearly invisible.

The position I will take rejects the naïve view that the halakhah is free of gender biases (in senses to be explained later) but also rejects the claim of triviality, the contention that the masculine leanings of the halakhah are so self-evident that they are not worthy of academic attention. First, if this claim is so trivial and self-evident, why was it not addressed before the advent of feminist criticism?[2] Second, until the problem is clearly defined and its ramifications fully appreciated, it will be nearly impossible to counter these biases and move toward a halakhah that is more inclusive and egalitarian.

My interest here is to examine the claimed objectivity of the halakhah and to question how values that can be characterized as clearly male have made their way into a system that is meant to be devoid of all subjective elements. To do so, I will first have to consider the concept of gender objectivity in a broader context, and particularly the critique that has been developed in feminist scientific and legal theory. The insights provided by this critique of gender objectivity will serve as the background for an examination of the halakhah's masculinity in general and specifically of the gendered considerations that underlie the corpus of halakhic rulings regarding reproduction.

Feminist Critique of Scientific and Legal Methodology

SCIENTIFIC CRITICISM

Feminist criticism of the sciences originated with the growing sense of unease felt by feminist scholars regarding the universal application of studies conducted using almost exclusively male subjects. In addition to highlighting this discrepancy in the interpretation of results, feminist critics maintained that women had been deliberately excluded from power centers by denying the force of their intellects and knowledge. The scientific concept of knowledge was constructed through the use of rational instrumentalities that were defined as masculine, while women were considered to be emotional and incapable of abstract analytical thought. The mythos of "dispassionate investigation" preserved the feminine stereotype and promoted the epistemic authority of the dominant group.[3]

For our purposes, the most significant aspect of feminist criticism of the sciences is the claim that even the realm of knowledge that is perceived as most objective is not immune to subjective biases and predispositions. In general, the sciences are assumed to be a realm of deductive knowledge and inquiry characterized by hard facts and objective conclusions. This positivist-rationalist model used in the natural sciences has shaped the general approach to the social sciences as well, which were understood to be value-free scientific fields in which quantitative studies were focused on identifying the rules of social behavior.[4]

The fundamental premises of traditional science are that "good" investigation takes place in a vacuum; that it has no predispositions; that it is "transparent" with respect to both method and investigator; and that its proofs are objective. Feminist critics reject these claims and argue that there is always a gap between proof and conclusion, a gap in which the subjectivity of the investigator finds expression. Accordingly, all knowledge, including scientific knowledge, is "situated knowledge," conditioned on the knower's situation and grounded in a specific context from which it cannot be severed. Some feminist critics go further, maintaining that these predispositions affect all stages of a study, not only the conclusions. They come into play as early as the point at which the objects of study are identified and determined, and they continue to influence the planning of the study, the definition of key terms, the determination of which proofs are relevant, the collection and analysis of data, and, ultimately, the assessment of conclusions.

For example, feminist critics accuse traditional science of improperly attempting to maintain an unambiguous barrier between the "context of discovery" and the "context of justification." The "context of discovery" deals with the preliminary stages of research—what is worthy of being studied, what are the goals of the study, how the question to be studied is defined, what will be considered relevant proof, and how much proof will be needed to allow for conclusions to be drawn. The "context of justification" pertains to the stage at which proofs are evaluated: what establishes proofs, how to assess them, and what conclusions may be drawn from them. Feminist criticism argues that the sharp distinction between these contexts, and the greater emphasis on the context of justification, conceal, on the one hand, the degree to which the context of discovery fundamentally shapes the research being conducted and, on the other, the extent to which biases make their way into the context of justification as well, making it impossible to assert that that logical rules apply there in any absolute sense.

Ultimately, every investigator perceives reality from his or her own position, and what an investigator considers to be proof is contingent on that positioning. Social, cultural, gender, and class status all affect what individuals regard as proof and how they interpret it. Accordingly, it is impossible to properly assess any knowledge without taking into account the identity of the knower. Paradoxically, the greater the subject's degree of self-reflection, the greater the objectivity of the results, because the disclosure of predispositions allows the public to contextualize the findings.

Among scientists, one of the accepted methods for neutralizing predispositions and attempting to maintain objectivity is to require replicability; that is, a study will be regarded as trustworthy only if other investigators are able to reach the same results. Feminist criticism deems replicability insufficient, for while it may be able to neutralize the predispositions of individuals within the community of investigators, it cannot reveal shared or communal predispositions, such as gender bias. Sandra Harding explains that biases that reflect values or interests that are fundamental to the investigators' worldview, to the point that they themselves are unaware of them, will never be neutralized.[5] Moreover, some biases are incorporated at the earliest stages of inquiry, a part of the scientific process that is generally not subjected to methodological rules, which pertain only to the testing of hypotheses that have already been formulated. Therefore, even self-reflection on the part of the investigator cannot guarantee an unbiased outcome.

Of course, the feminist critique has not gone unanswered, and some critics who accept the principles of its attack on "hard positivism" nevertheless believe that the feminist claims have import only if they are raised within the accepted scientific framework, in an attempt at methodological improvement. According to Sam Rakover, the scientific method is both equipped and obligated to expunge from within itself all traces of prejudice, such as sexist views of women; and he therefore objects strenuously to Harding's claims regarding the need to establish a "feminist science."[6] Feminist scholars respond that since science itself has a history of ignoring these problems, it is nonetheless necessary to address them in a feminist context. They assert that even if Harding's stance is extreme, it is possible to envision scientific studies guided by a "feminist sensitivity"[7] that is based on an empirical understanding of women's experiences within a patriarchal reality. Such studies will be grounded on qualitative methods, including in-depth interviews, observations, and historical texts. This sort of study, to be sure, cannot claim "objectivity" in the accepted sense, nor can it be "public" or "replicable" in the sense empiricism can (or presumes to) be. But neither does this sort of feminist science on that account forfeit its scientific character; it loses only the ability to become more generalized—at the expense of other women or oppressed groups.

LEGAL CRITICISM

Feminist jurists have developed theoretical tools that can be of use in critiquing existing legal doctrines, and the distinctive contribution of their criticism is the argument that in the realm of law, the predominant ideological bias is masculine. According to this critique, the law reflects clearly masculine conceptions of the world, modes of thinking, and values; and its concern is to preserve a social order in which women occupy a position inferior to that of men.

There is, of course, no unanimity among feminist theorists regarding just what it is that makes the law masculine. But while there are substantive disagreements regarding the origin of the law's gender biases, there is somewhat broader agreement regarding the tools and methods advanced for remedying them within the legal system. Despite the vast amount that has been written on the subject,[8] in the following pages I want to consider the work of three prominent feminist theorists, insofar as their writings most clearly represent the split between cultural and radical feminism.[9]

The Origin of Gender Biases in the Law

The first approach, based primarily on the cultural feminism of Carol Gilligan, maintains that the law's male bias derives from *modes of thought* that are patently masculine. Gilligan sees a substantive distinction between the "ethics of justice," which characterizes the way boys think (she draws her example from children's games), and the "ethics of caring," which typifies girls' thinking.[10] An "ethics of justice" applies abstract rules to concrete situations; as such, it resembles the formal character of law. An "ethics of caring," meanwhile, strives to avoid the disputes likely to erupt when rules are applied, and it highlights the value of a connective, personal approach. According to Gilligan, women see questions of morality not in terms of rights and rules but in terms of systems of relationship and responsibility.[11] Applying Gilligan's distinctions to feminist legal criticism allows us to say that the law's male biases result from the law having been produced by men, who are guided by specific thought patterns that do not suit the female personality structure.

In fact, feminist legal scholars who have adapted Gilligan's views to the legal realm have suggested that conflicts should be resolved in a less formal manner, with less emphasis on rules and legal precedents and more on the system of relationships (an idea similar in spirit to mediation).[12] That may be why this approach draws more fire than others and why some believe that suggestions to reform the law in the spirit of cultural feminism are likely to be destructive. In Richard Posner's words: "What is true is that if society goes too far in making the administration of law flexible, particularistic, 'caring,' the consequences will be anarchy, tyranny, or both, which is why 'people's justice' is rightly deprecated."[13]

Catherine MacKinnon also criticizes this approach, arguing that to celebrate feminine distinctiveness is, in effect, to adopt the masculine perspective. In her view, the common differences between the sexes do not involve authentic female characteristics in which one may take pride; rather, they result from male dominance and its systematic oppression and subordination of women. She acknowledges that the recognition of differences has raised the esteem in which feminine moral adjudication is held; but, she asks, when the differences are, in effect, a construct produced by dominant males for their own purposes, how can they be regarded positively?

Still, there are several instances in which the Gilligan-inspired approach has been adopted in American courts, and the growing tendency (at least in Israel) to rely on the tools of Alternative Dispute Resolution (such as mediation) may be attributed to the influence of this approach as well. It is also interesting to note that the few authorities within the Orthodox Jewish world who regard feminism as a positive force promote an approach akin to Gilligan's cultural feminism. But more of that later.

The second theory as to the origin of gender biases within the law is articulated by MacKinnon herself, who represents radical feminism. She suggests that the law's male biases stem from the control exercised by men over women and argues that male interests structure the law in a way that maintains that dominance. Were it not for male dominance, women—and men as well—free of social coercion, would likely develop in other ways, and many would develop inclinations and qualities that now tend to be suppressed within the patriarchal culture.[14] The first wave of feminist criticism, known as liberal feminism, argued that women are not fundamentally different from men in ways that are socially relevant, and therefore there should not be legal distinctions between women and men or barriers to women's full participation in society. Cultural feminism, in contrast, advanced the premise that women *are* different, and therefore require special attention to their voices and their needs, which are no less valuable than those of men. MacKinnon finds both of these approaches distasteful, for both accept the male as the standard, the measuring rod to which women are compared. Why, she asks, "should you have to be the same as a man to get what a man gets simply because he is one?"[15]

MacKinnon believes that the "theory of dominance" raises a whole range of issues not previously considered, pertaining to the centrality of sex in acts of injustice toward women, to sexual violence against women, and to women's right to be protected against such wrongs. Rape, incest, pornography, and sexual harassment are the underpinnings of MacKinnon's critical treatment of law. These phenomena, in her view, affect primarily women; and because they represent the submission of women to male dominance, they can be understood exclusively in terms of male dominion and power.

There are many examples of the law's male biases that bear out MacKinnon's concept of dominance. Noteworthy in the context of this book is her critique of the rationale for allowing women to elect to abort pregnancies during the first trimester.[16] In its 1973 decision in *Roe v. Wade*, the United States Supreme Court used the fundamental right to privacy as the legal basis for overturning state bans on abortion. MacKinnon maintains that the court's rationale is dangerous because it perpetuates discrimination against women by legitimating the continuation of their subjugation to men in the private sphere. If the liberal state does not intervene in the private sphere, in which the greatest wrongs against women are perpetrated, the state itself injures women and strengthens existing social practices.[17] Regarding rape as well, MacKinnon argues, the law reinforces society's prevalent attitude, which fails to determine in absolute terms what "force" is. In its concept of "consent," the law simply confirms male dominance, for it determines at the outset that consent is indicated by the absence of physical resistance, thereby revealing its male biases. In other words, the law accepts the male version of reality, which assumes (or infers) that there is consent to sexual relations in the absence of physical opposition, and that verbal objections, even explicitly saying "no," are not adequate. In the very area where the law should be most sensitive to gender difference, it instead relies on male societal norms and thereby reinforces them. In MacKinnon's view, this is an unavoidable, structural failing of the legal system.[18]

Robin West, representing a third approach, suggests a different origin for the law's masculine leanings.[19] In her view, the differentiation of women is constructed on the basis of their distinct biological experiences, and the maleness of the law is rooted in its failure to reflect—indeed, its disregard for—that distinctive life experience.[20] According to West, liberal and critical theories of law provide two entirely different phenomenological accounts of the human condition, but neither corresponds to women's experience.

Classic legal liberalism asserts the "separation thesis," according to which human beings by definition are distinct from one another, and their distinctiveness encompasses the political right to freedom and autonomy. But because every person is an individual, autonomous entity, every person lives in perpetual fear of danger from the "other," who may be out to destroy him. Accordingly, the "separation thesis" posits the potential for attack by other human beings, for the other always constitutes a source of danger and a threat to one's autonomy. In contrast, the critical approach argues that the fundamental state of human separateness does not generate a celebration of autonomy but, rather, a perpetual aspiration for relationship and association.

The separate individual strives for connection with the other from whom he is separate.

According to West, neither the liberal nor the critical narratives correspond to women's reality. The fact that at some point in their lives women are materially connected, in actuality or at least potentially, to the lives of other human beings has existential implications. Thus, a feminine version of these narratives relies on an inverse assumption regarding the human condition: rather than positing a "separation thesis," it presumes a "connection thesis." But just as liberal and critical theories produce two different masculine narratives, cultural and radical feminism tell two different feminine stories. According to cultural feminism, women's connection to others is a source of gratification, of feelings of intimacy. According to radical feminism, meanwhile, the potential for connection that is experienced concretely through sexual relations and pregnancy is the source of women's degradation, of their disempowerment and misery.

West considers cultural feminism to be the "official story" for women, while radical feminism provides the "unofficial story," much as the liberal approach provides the "official story" and the critical approach the "unofficial story" for men. Each "story" adds to the complexity of the overall human narrative, and therefore no single story can provide a comprehensive picture of reality. Feminine reality, like human reality overall, encompasses genuine contradictions. For example, women's potential for physical connection with others necessarily entails both the capacity for intimacy and the possibility of unwanted "invasion" or "penetration." Correspondingly, the importance for men of physical separation necessarily entails both the yearning for intimacy and the seeds of alienation. Thus, according to West, both cultural and radical feminism tell valid stories, despite the empirical contradiction between them. Women can value intimacy while fearing the incursion and penetration it makes possible, and women can fear separation while yearning for the individualization that it makes possible. Yet even though both men and women live with these internal contradictions, there is a great difference between them: women, in contrast to men, experience these contradictions under the oppressive conditions of patriarchy.

In West's view, all modern legal theories are, in essence, masculine,[21] for the values, dangers, and fundamental contradictions that characterize women's lives are in no way reflected in contracts, constitutional law, or any other area of jurisprudence. The values that derive from women's potential for connection are not legally recognized as values, and the associated dangers are not legally recognized as dangers. For example, neither sexual penetration nor the "penetration" of the woman's body by a fetus is recognized as an actionable tort. Sexual penetration in the case of rape is recognized as tortious only when other harm is involved or when it is accompanied by violence in the form recognized as such by men (that is, actual threat of physical destruction). Similarly, the fetus's "penetration" of its mother's body is not understood as tortious, because the right to self-defense is considered to be the right to protect the body against destruction, not against incursion. The dangers presented by an unwanted fetus, however, are not dangers to bodily security but to bodily integrity; they involve, for the most part, the woman's fear of incursion into her body and the prospect that she will never again be an independent self.[22]

West's complex portrayal of women's conflicted experiences regarding abortion and her assertions regarding the law's inability to account for or respond to these lived realities provides an invaluable tool for analyzing the halakhic discourse on the same topic. As I will demonstrate, the theories of Gilligan, MacKinnon, and West similarly serve as critical lenses for identifying and analyzing gender biases in the halakhic corpus as a whole.

Feminist Legal Methods: Revealing Gender Biases in the Law

The foregoing discussion suggests a range of diverse, sometimes contradictory, theories on the origin of gender inequality in society and in law. On the practical level, however, feminist legal scholars have developed some legal methods about which there seems to be broad consensus. These methods can serve as useful tools for identifying the law's gender biases, dismantling the patriarchal structures concealed within it, and initiating legislation that avoids these pitfalls. When all is said and done, revealing the law's implicit male biases has become a principal goal of feminist legal theorists.

To confront the objectivists' claim that legal discourse is gender-neutral, feminists adopt a "hermeneutic of suspicion." Legal discourse and principles can represent themselves as universal and gender-neutral but still conceal androcentric assumptions insofar as they reflect an exclusively male narrative or perspective. In that context, Katherine Bartlett proposes several essential methods to be used in feminist legal theorizing; the most important for our purposes is that of "asking the woman question."[23] This method aims to identify the *practical* consequences of legal rules and practices that are perceived as gender-neutral and objective but actually result in discrimination against women. "Asking the woman question" means considering: Does the given law consider women as subjects? If not, how can this disregard of women be remedied? Does the law take account of "feminine" values? Do/Can existing legal standards cause harm to women? We will make considerable use of this method in examining halakhic positions on reproductive issues.

Implications for Halakhah

As noted, it is a matter of historical fact that only men have served as accepted authorities within the halakhic system. Women never took part in the halakhic decision-making process; the few exceptional cases are so extraordinary as to have no bearing on the general principle.[24] For the most part, that remains the case today, though some marginal opinions maintain that, in theory, halakhic rulings by women are not problematic.[25] Despite this reality, mainstream halakhic authorities maintain that the ethos of halakhic decision-making is one of objectivity and that halakhic decisions are not affected by considerations outside the halakhah itself, least of all considerations related to the decisors' gender identity.

The question of gender biases in halakhah becomes particularly significant in light of the legal theory that rejects formalism and recognizes the role of judicial discretion in legal decision-making. In the following section I will demonstrate that legal formalism does not accurately describe the halakhic process, which indeed assigns considerable latitude to the decisor in all decisions. This latitude opens the door, at least theoretically, to the influence of biases of various kinds, gender included.

REJECTION OF HALAKHIC FORMALISM

Legal formalism is a school of thought that perceives the law as an autonomous system of rules and norms under which all that is expected of the judge is to engage in deductive reasoning independent of values, goals, or interpretive methods. The claim that halakhah is gender-neutral is conceptually linked to formalistic approaches that portray halakhah as an objective legal system of this nature and halakhic rulings as logically imperative results, arrived at by pure deduction independent of values or other interests.[26]

When speaking of halakhic formalism, however, it is important to distinguish between halakhic language, which may sound deductive although it does not necessarily reflect a process of formalistic thought, and a formalist vision of the halakhic system. A prominent example of such a formalist vision of halakhah appears in the writings of Rabbi Joseph B. Soloveitchik, who describes the "halakhic man" as a scientist who exists in an ideal world of a priori concepts, a world unimpaired by any sort of historical or psychological contingencies.[27] So understood, the halakhah is a complete, closed system with internal rules of inference activated by an interpretive process having no connection to the outside reality; accordingly, the halakhic process is unaffected by any consideration of independent values. In R. Soloveitchik's view, both the act of halakhic conceptualization and the act of halakhic concretization—that is, halakhic decision-making—are untainted by any contingency, subjectivity, or reduction to anything else:

> The halakhah has no need to reflect the character of the halakhist, and neither changes in circumstance nor historical events contribute to shaping it. . . . Psychologization or sociologization of the halakhah are an assault on its soul. . . . If halakhic thought depends on psychological factors, it loses all its objectivity and deteriorates to a level of subjectivity lacking all substance.[28]

The theological benefits of the formalistic approach are clear. Formalism ascribes certainty, stability, and, especially, authenticity to the halakhic system. It affords the community of believers the sense that pursuit of halakhic truth is the decisors' foremost interest and that personal beliefs, transient ideologies, or values that have not passed the test of time cannot distort their assessments and, thereby, the process of interpretation and ruling. This type of certainty, stability, and authenticity bears faithful witness to the divine source and eternal nature of the Torah and the halakhah derived from it. But this concept of halakhah does not merely fail the test of feminist criticism; it also fails to accurately describe the work of halakhic decisors, past or present. Their language, to be sure, is the language of formalism, but closer examination demonstrates that halakhic rulings are guided by values and ideology that even dictate, sometimes from the outset, the rulings' direction and content.

Feminists reject halakhic formalism as a matter of principle, for it is inconsistent with the interests of women. A formalist outlook perceives the halakhic system as a closed corpus with internal decisional rules that are deployed in the interpretive process with no connection whatsoever to the external situation. Accordingly, if women have never been active within the halakhic system and their voices have almost never been assigned any weight, there is no way for formalism, which by definition preserves and reinforces the existing system, to allow for any substantive change.[29]

As noted, I do not believe that an actual examination of the halakhic decision-making process will find a formalistic approach as extreme as that portrayed by Rabbi Soloveitchik. Contemporary academic studies of halakhah have shown that there was never a categorical separation between halakhah and morality.[30] This point is significant in that it allows gender bias to be recognized and contended with as one among many subjective factors that have always existed alongside halakhah and influenced its development.[31]

THE MALENESS OF HALAKHAH

To conclude this discussion, I would like to consider the ways in which gender biases within halakhah are manifested. In the remainder of the book, I will attempt to uncover these biases in specific areas of halakhah in order to provide an alternative to the existing halakhic narrative.[32] Earlier, I presented three principal views regarding the source of the law's male biases. I believe there are three corresponding ways to conceive of the halakhah's male characteristics.

The first claim regarding the "maleness" of halakhah, in the spirit of Gilligan's approach, is that traditional halakhah reflects a distinctly masculine way of thinking and, consequently, that halakhic decision-making by women would look entirely different from halakhic decision-making by men. In other words, the claim is that not only the content of the halakhah but also its form, its analytical tools, its modes of inference, and its modes of interpretation are all affected by a "maleness" that would be altered by "female" ways of thinking. Arguments of this sort are made by those who seek "the female voice" in Torah study—the modes of thought and interpretation characteristic of women, which, it is hoped, will "redeem" the halakhah from its sterile masculine formalism. Rabbi Shimon Gershon Rosenberg (Shagar), for example—a contemporary religious scholar who did not reject the feminist religious revolution out of hand—sought the distinctive feminine voice in Torah study, which would actually redeem Torah study from its lack of relevance and vision:

> Not infrequently, one hears remarks about "the female voice in Torah study." In my view, the problematic aspect of women's Torah study today is that it is merely an imitation of the male voice. The female voice in Torah study is heard all too often as a thickened male voice. But, sad to say, the scholarly and interpretive voices of the yeshiva often turned into standardized voices, a Torah of banalities lacking relevance and vision. And if that is the case with regard to Torah study by men, how much sadder should we be about the effort of women to imitate that voice.[33]

As noted earlier, although these claims seem quite radical and their implications for the integrity of halakhah are far-reaching, it is specifically this approach, which maintains the inherent, essentialist distinction between masculine and feminine "ways of being," that has been adopted by some traditional religious scholars.

The second claim, in the spirit of MacKinnon's radical feminism, is that the halakhah is structured so as to preserve the existing patriarchal order—that is, to maintain the domination of women by men. From that perspective one could argue, for example, that the refusal of religious judges (*dayanim*) to adopt existing halakhic mechanisms for resolving the situation of *'agunot* and women denied bills of divorce[34] stems not from the judges' masculine mode of thought and failure to understand the plight of the women affected but primarily from their desire to maintain and preserve the patriarchal system under which men—be they husbands or the rabbinic establishment—rule over women. Otherwise, it is hard to account for the consistent, sweeping, and systematic refusal to adopt available halakhic solutions to the problem. Similarly, one could argue that the desire to preserve the existing patriarchal order underlies rabbinic interest in preserving the traditional family unit, which would likely be altered fundamentally with the adoption of an egalitarian outlook. Thus, numerous halakhic principles that preserve or reinforce the traditional role of women in the domestic sphere can be seen as part of the same drive for continued dominance.[35]

The third claim, inspired by West's ideas, is that the life experiences of women, their perceptions, feelings, and perspectives, are not and could not be suitably expressed within halakhah because at no stage did women take any active role in shaping the halakhic corpus. Accordingly, the "maleness" of halakhah and the gender biases within the system stem from the fact that halakhah has been interpreted from a perspective informed by the life experiences typical of men. The values and standpoints that derive from a masculine way of life are the building blocks of a halakhic outlook that understandably has difficulty accounting for or integrating the female perspective. The halakhic "story" as told from the male perspective is only a partial story, and that limitation accounts for its gender biases. Even when halakhah presumes to incorporate female experience, it does not regard it as equivalent in value to male experience or as warranting the acceptance of women as equal partners in formulating halakhah. At best, the female perspective will be expressed indirectly, filtered through a male lens.

Numerous examples of the halakhah's male biases accord with this claim, but the paradigmatic examples are related to the laws of modesty. The classic laws of modesty are formulated from a distinctly male perspective and life experience, in the sense that women are assumed to be sexual obstacles that men need to avoid, by means of limiting their visibility rather than limiting the men's activity. The implications of these constraints on the women themselves are simply not considered.[36] Tamar Ross highlights this bias with regard to the prohibition on men hearing women sing (termed *qol be-'ishah 'ervah*, lit. "a woman's voice is nakedness"):

> Women today ask why all the anxiety about the purity of men's thoughts is not accompanied by any concern about women's experiences. Has any halakhist made the effort to weigh the spiritual loss suffered by women through the silencing of their voices against the supposed benefit to men? If modesty is a problem for men, why must women pay the price? Moreover, are women's voices in fact as seductive as they are said to be? A negative answer to that question brings us back to the conclusion that the *halakhah* imposes inappropriate responsibility on women, for the traditional bounds of modesty are always formulated exclusively in terms of women's seductiveness to men.[37]

The halakhic position on the morally difficult and complex question of abortion can likewise be critiqued from this perspective. The prevalent halakhic rulings on the topic focus primarily on the status of the fetus and the morality of terminating its existence. But is that the only relevant issue? Does a determination of the fetus's status provide the exclusive moral basis for such a decision? In other words, does the fetus question tell the entire story, including the female point of view? Does it take into account, as West articulates, the "basic contradiction" in the lives of women, who may want to bear children but also feel threatened by the "invasion" of an unwanted fetus and by the loss of their independence and sense of self?

In light of all these issues, my contention that halakhah is markedly masculine and that gender biases are often a feature of halakhic decisions does not refer exclusively or even necessarily to those areas where there appears to be actual discrimination against women. In most instances, the cases of evident discrimination can be easily identified; indeed, they served as the earliest objects of Jewish feminist criticism.[38] I refer primarily to those areas of halakhah in which women must, in fact, be distinguished from men and cannot be treated similarly to them, as with the reproductive issues that will be addressed in this book. My central argument is that the ideological underpinnings of halakhic decision-making in these areas reflect essentialist concepts of gender that often relate to women as objects rather than subjects and fail to take their interests and perspectives adequately into account. These ideological positions exert a hidden, subconscious influence on interpretive processes—on the reading of sources, on the formulation of questions, and ultimately, of course, on the rulings issued.

Before ending, let me briefly explain some key elements of halakhic methodology, including the significance of precedent, the kinds of precedent and how they are treated, and the differences between private halakhic decisions and those that are publicly issued.

As a general rule, one can say that in Jewish law precedent provides guidance but is not binding in the way it is in Anglo-American law.[39] Several factors may account for Jewish law's rejection of the doctrine of binding precedent:[40]

1. Concern about erroneous application of the precedent
2. The idea that every judge is independent and responsible for his own decisions
3. The judge's obligation to decide the case before him on its own merits

Consequently, the principle of *halakhah ke-batr'ai* (the law is in accord with the view of the later authorities) has become widely accepted. This principle affords substantial, but far from unlimited, decisional latitude. Menaḥem Elon, a leading scholar in the field of Jewish law, puts it this way: "This principle is designed to ensure freedom of decision for later decision-makers while still allowing for deference to earlier decisions, *which are to be consulted and carefully considered*."[41] I emphasize the duty to consult precedent because even though there is no obligation to rule in accordance with it, the Orthodox ethos nonetheless requires its consideration (even if it ultimately is rejected). That point is particularly pertinent to the discussion that follows, as I will attempt to illustrate the ways in which decisors deliberately disregard sources or precedents that they find inconvenient and that, if consulted, might have produced rulings more favorable to women.

It is important as well to recognize the difference between "public" and "private" rulings. The former apply to the community as a whole and are usually published in writing, as with the responsa literature to be considered in this book. In contrast, the latter are issued in camera, typically are not published, and are known, if at all, only through oral accounts. Private rulings may be used to maintain the halakhic ethos and norms of conduct that the decisors regard as appropriate for the community while still recognizing the concrete problems that may arise in specific circumstances and generate extremely difficult situations for individuals observant of halakhah. In the present study, I will consider only the halakhic trends that are manifested in public, written rulings. I am well aware that in the private sphere very different rulings have been rendered, but at this stage scholars lack the data that could shed light on what transpires in that realm.[42]

Overview of the Book

Part 1 of the book deals with "sex without procreation."

Chapter 1 examines the religious mandate to reproduce and presents a diachronic halakhic analysis that offers an alternative to the rhetoric almost universally accepted today. According to contemporary halakhic discourse, the commandment to reproduce is so important that other considerations—economics, family welfare, emotional well-being, and so on—are not significant enough to justify any comprehensive authorization of "family planning." The alternative analysis I propose demonstrates that this outlook is not obligatory or inevitable, for the biblical commandment to reproduce, despite its weightiness, has in the past been qualified and limited to avoid conflicting with other vital interests—or, at least, other vital interests of men.

Chapter 2 focuses on methods of birth control. My goal here is to note reasonable and significant interpretive possibilities that have been excluded, unconsciously or knowingly, from halakhic assessments of birth control techniques. Most often, the disregard for or rejection of these methods stems from hidden, unconscious gender considerations. In some instances, the indirect result of the rulings I consider could actually place women's lives in jeopardy. In others, possibilities that might have significantly improved women's health or quality of life were rejected. I argue that certain interpretive options were preferred for reasons grounded in a gender-based concept of the nature and purpose of women generally. In this chapter I also examine the reasons for the normative halakhic recommendation not to engage in family planning. These reasons are affected by traditional ideas regarding the purpose and essence of women; and only recently, in circles where the status of women has been moving toward equality with men, have we begun to see inklings of change. That change is perceptible in the very formulation of halakhic questions, which have begun to reflect a broader range of women's interests and, of course, in the "discovery" of solutions that were not previously on the table.

In both chapter 1 and chapter 2, the use of feminist theories enables us to sharpen our criticism of concepts of gender that emphasize the reproductive value of a woman at the expense of her value as a person and an independent subject. At the same time, I reject feminist concepts that I regard as inconsistent with the core halakhic ethos, namely, that a person is not "autonomous" in the accepted liberal sense of the term, is not exempt from obligations that limit his or her freedom, and is therefore subject to the command to populate the world.

Chapters 3 and 4 deal with abortion. Their principal thrust is to show, by means of a chronological halakhic analysis, that if contemporary halakhic rulings had adopted a reasonable reading of earlier sources (a reading influenced by a more egalitarian understanding of the role of women), the stringent picture on display today could have been very different. Here I attempt to prove that the more lenient interpretive options have been rejected because the decisors' unarticulated gender assumptions fail to take account of women's fundamental interests and fail to respect them as persons. Even the more lenient decisions are not free of problematic gender considerations, nor are they based on an egalitarian stance toward women, but practically they can eradicate the patriarchal concept of women as being meant almost exclusively for reproduction and child rearing. Here, too, a review of the various philosophical and feminist positions regarding the moral problems raised by abortion enables us to probe the gender concepts implicit in the halakhic decisions. That said, I absolutely reject moral positions (not necessarily feminist) holding that a woman's rights over her body, or the fetus's lack of human characteristics, can justify abortion *on demand* even at the very late stages of a pregnancy. That idea would have to be rejected even if we were to find within the halakhic tradition interpretive possibilities that supported it.

Part 2 of the book considers "procreation without sex."

In this unit, I direct attention to modern technological means for bringing children into the world; these include artificial insemination, in vitro fertilization, and surrogacy. Chapter 5 is a survey of feminist and more general literature on these topics, whereas chapter 6 examines halakhic attitudes toward the use of such technologies.

These issues are treated somewhat differently from those taken up in part 1. Owing to the recent discovery and development of these scientific techniques, the methods themselves were obviously not addressed in earlier halakhic literature (with the exception of a process analogous to artificial insemination). But even on a conceptual plane, halakhic discussion of these reproductive technologies breaks new ground, as it requires an unbundling of processes hitherto considered natural and therefore essential—that is, the separation of genetic from gestational motherhood. Accordingly, the halakhic situation resembles a legal case that addresses a lacuna in the law: in the absence of legal norms, judges are not guided by preexisting rules and standards, and they have broad discretion in their rulings. Similarly, in the absence of clear halakhic rules regarding reproductive technologies, decisors are granted broad discretion. Their tendency to rule leniently, and their evident interest in authorizing the use of advanced technology at almost any cost, attest to the values that they consider fundamental to halakhah. If the value attached to reproduction is so great that it trumps other moral considerations, it is fair to ask what other values are neglected or ignored in the interest of reproduction. The absence of ethical considerations that might well constrain the halakhic rulings and that are intimately linked to gender (as demonstrated by feminist literature that is presented extensively in these chapters) reflects clear gender-related messages, which I consider in this context. Note that, after considering the traditional sources, this book will treat contemporary orthodox halakhah only and not the halakhic verdicts issued in other Jewish movements, which merit separate inquiry.

In summary, the chapters of this book revolve around the axis between sex and reproduction. The first four chapters take a critical look at the link between these spheres and consider the halakhic possibilities available to those seeking to unbundle them. The final two chapters deal with cases of reproduction that do not involve regular sexual relations, which can serve as a litmus test not only for the decisors' thinking about reproduction in general but also for its assumed and assigned significance in the lives of women.

PART ONE

Sex without Procreation

CHAPTER ONE

"Be Fruitful and Multiply"

The hegemonic halakhic discourse of contemporary Orthodoxy speaks of the commandment to procreate in terms that enhance its importance beyond what is implied by the original halakhic sources. In Ultra-Orthodox and even some nationalist Ultra-Orthodox circles, the commandment to "be fertile and increase," and, especially, the attendant directives that will be discussed below, are taken far beyond what would be expected of a halakhic discourse that balances the bearing of children along with an array of other considerations pertinent to a person's life. In many sectors of religious society, the commandment to procreate is understood to require an uninterrupted chain of pregnancies, thereby circumscribing women's lives and opportunities in particular.

I begin my discussion with the feminist positions that attribute women's continued inferior position in society principally to the burdens of child rearing, which they primarily bear. Feminists note that the responsibility of procreation, which gives prominence to a woman's biological qualities, and the responsibility of child rearing, which emphasizes her presence in the private, domestic domain, preserves a twofold gender-based distinction: the distinction between private and public spheres and the distinction between material and spiritual/intellectual spheres. Does the halakhic discourse accept this dichotomy between men and women? Do rabbis understand the worth of women solely in terms of their childbearing and child-rearing function? Is motherhood regarded as an inherent expression of femininity?

My analysis of the halakhic sources will call into question the way in which the commandment to procreate has been construed in recent generations and taken to imply a requirement to engage in ceaseless childbearing, and it will seek out alternative halakhic voices that have been marginalized by contemporary halakhic rhetoric.

Feminist Positions on Procreation and Birth Control

Regulating the birthrate has always been a matter of interest to society because of its implications for sexual behavior, population size, and the role of women. In the professional literature, "family planning" is generally defined as the right of all people to decide, freely and responsibly, on the number of and spacing of their children, including the right to have no children at all.[1] However, "family planning" is recognized as uniquely a right of women, unconnected to questions of responsibility for child care and child rearing. In its deepest sense, the concept reflects a woman's right to protect her body and her health, her right to personal autonomy, pleasure and happiness, her right to develop the full range of her talents and abilities, and the equality of her rights and responsibilities to those of men—not only in the domain of the family but in the economic, cultural, political, and social realms as well.[2] It should be emphasized that the encouragement of "family planning," as here defined, does not necessarily imply less procreation. A reduction in the number of offspring will depend on a wider range of factors, such as socioeconomic conditions or the value ascribed to procreation within a particular society. The point is that because family planning is a basic human right, decisions related to it must be arrived at with full awareness of a birth's actual and potential implications for the couple (especially the woman), the child, the family, and society overall.

In that respect, there is a profound difference between family planning in Malthusian discourse, which calls for its use because of worldwide demographic concerns and is interested primarily in diminishing the number of births, and family planning in a rights-based discourse. The Malthusian League and similar organizations are interested mainly in the danger that an exploding population might outstrip the world's limited natural resources; that is, in the potential imbalance between the demographic situation and the ability of a particular state or the world overall to support it. The discourse they promote treats family planning from the perspective of national and international goals and preferences related to population growth. As such, it does not focus on human rights issues related to family planning—for example, the need to provide information, education, and services that will allow all to determine, freely and responsibly, the size of their families and the intervals between their children. It direct even less attention to the need for family planning in order to enable women to free themselves as individuals, to express fully their rights to social, economic, and political equality.

That multiple pregnancies, births, and children are constraints on a woman's personal and professional prosperity is taken almost for granted, and indeed this assumption has been confirmed by numerous empirical studies conducted in various places throughout the world and on a range of populations.[3] Fullam, accordingly, can argue: "If there is one single factor above all others which is responsible for the low status of women, it is possibly uncontrolled fertility. And there is growing evidence that fertility control is related to educational achievement and employment opportunities."[4]

Studies have shown that in societies in which women are concerned primarily with domestic and child-rearing matters, pregnancy rates are high. Often in these societies, the subordination of women to men and the lack of communication between the members of the couple pose an obstacle to family planning and to a diminished pregnancy rate.[5] The findings suggest that the longer women delay marriage and the start of childbearing, the better able they are to complete their education and professional training and secure interesting, substantive, and high-paying work.[6]

Increasing the participation of women in the workforce and providing higher levels of education are usually suggested as means for diminishing childbearing and increasing women's ability to act autonomously.[7] That suggestion rests in part on the premise that involvement in activities outside the home will provide an alternative source of satisfaction, one that can compete with the satisfaction of child rearing, as well as a higher standard of living—along with greater exposure to information about birth control. The data regarding women show a correlation between larger family size and employment in less professional and lower-paying jobs. Consistent with the United Nations report on the status of women and family planning (1975), many nations are noting correlations between having fewer children and higher educational attainment by women.

The picture conveyed by the data, then, is that procreation is not something freely chosen by individuals in all societies and that it is linked to a lower status for women, to unequal opportunities for education and livelihood, and to conditions of poverty. These facts are both cause and effect of the persistence of a situation in which women occupy a low status and are discriminated against, and this vicious cycle has led many investigators to conclude that family planning programs alone will not be effective and that there must also be an overall improvement, unrelated to questions of procreation, in the status of women.

Pregnancy and motherhood, as capacities unique to women, have been a focus of interest for feminist thinkers who try to explain the inferior position of women in society.[8] Some have considered these female capacities to be the source of women's oppression and have therefore considered abandoning them; others have argued that it is not the capabilities or the experiences that should be given up but the oppressive ideology associated with them. That ideology construes the existence of women as having value only with respect to birthing and raising children; effectively, it restricts women to the private sphere, with no ability to find an appropriate place in the labor market and, therefore, with no real way to improve their social and personal status. Both groups of thinkers believe that motherhood is not necessarily the embodiment of femaleness, and all consider the ability to control procreation to be a basic and legitimate right of every woman. For that reason, they examine birth control solely with respect to safety and effectiveness and not with respect to moral considerations, which, in their view, simply do not exist.

The Commandment to Procreate and Its Religious Significance

The requirement to reproduce first appears in the Bible as a blessing granted to men and women alike in the context of Creation—"God blessed them and God said to them, 'Be fertile and increase, fill the earth and master it; and rule the fish of the sea, the birds of the sky, and all the living things that creep on the earth'" (Gen. 1:28). By the tannaitic period, however, this blessing was understood as a positive commandment applicable to men only.[9] The great importance attached to this commandment is attested to by the profusion of discourses and statements on the topic by the talmudic sages[10] and in their halakhic application in post-talmudic literature. For example, the commandment to procreate is deemed the purpose for which the world was created—"the world was created only for fertility and increase"[11]—and the Talmud asserts that King Hezekiah will be denied a place in the world-to-come because he declined to engage in procreation.[12] However, the words of Ben Azai are perhaps the sharpest articulation of this position:

> Ben Azai says: One who refrains from engaging in procreation is as if he shed blood and nullified the [divine] image, as it is said [Gen. 9:6] "For in His image did God make man" and it continues [Gen. 9:7] "Be fertile, then, and increase, etc." (T Yev. 8:7)

Various parallel texts suggest that the rabbis had reservations about equating one who refrains from procreation with one who sheds blood, but the forceful wording here—"as if he shed blood"; "nullified the [divine] image"—speaks for itself.

As for the post-talmudic literature, the twelfth- and thirteenth-century Tosafists refer to procreation as "a great commandment,"[13] and while the author of *Sefer Mizvot Gadol* and Maimonides do not list it first in their enumerations of the commandments, by the fourteenth century it was listed first by the author of *Sefer Ha-Ḥinukh*, who thereby stressed its special significance.[14] The importance attached to procreation is further demonstrated by the permission granted to sell a Torah scroll if necessary to enable its fulfillment; the only other commandment for which a Torah scroll may be sold is Torah study itself.[15]

In the tannaitic context, Yair Lorberbaum[16] suggests viewing the commandment to procreate as a theurgic duty meant to aggrandize and expand the divine:[17] the fact that man was created in God's image implies that procreation entails the production of more copies of the divine image. To state it differently, God had the same aim in creating humanity and in creating humanity's procreative mechanism: an ongoing augmentation of the divine image. This rationale explains why the sages regarded the commandment as so important and transformed it into so fundamental an aspect of their worldview that they equated its abandonment with the shedding of blood.

Historians take a different tack, placing greater emphasis on the broad social and cultural context. Gafni, Satlow, and Schremer,[18] for example, maintain that the positions taken by Jews in both major centers—Babylonia and the Land of Israel—were significantly influenced by the way marriage was seen in the surrounding societies and cultures. In fact, they argue that the differing concepts of marriage in Roman-Hellenistic society and in the Persian-Zoroastrian world explain some of the differences between attitudes in the two large centers of Jewish life concerning the importance of marriage and procreation, the tension between the intellectual-scholarly world and the institution of marriage, and various solutions proposed for dealing with these problems. In the Land of Israel, men married at a relatively late age, allowing them to study Torah unencumbered by the obligations of married life. In Babylonia, in contrast, men married young but tended to leave their wives for extended periods to study Torah.

Regardless of whether one favors the theological explanation or the historical one, it is clear that for the talmudic sages, the commandment to reproduce was among the most important religious imperatives. Nonetheless, it does not appear to have been regarded as an *absolute* value, trumping all else. I want to direct attention here to the rabbinic voices that challenged the capacity of this commandment, despite its fundamental standing, to overcome all other considerations or interests that might arise during a person's life. Those other considerations and interests include the tension between the commandment to study Torah and the commandment to procreate;[19] the relationship between economic status and fulfillment of the commandment; and the determination of the number of children one must have in order to fulfill one's religious obligation as a matter of biblical (as distinct from rabbinic) law.[20]

WOMEN'S EXEMPTION FROM THE COMMANDMENT

> MISHNAH. A man is commanded to be fertile and increase; not so a woman. Rabbi Yoḥanan ben Beroqa [disagrees and] says: Of both it says "God blessed them and God said to them, 'Be fertile and increase.'"
> GEMARA. How do we know this? Said Rabbi Ilaa in the name of Rabbi Eleazar ben Rabbi Simeon: Scripture said: "Fill the earth and conquer [NJPS: master] it" [Gen. 1:28]; it is a man's way to conquer, but it is not a woman's way to conquer. [But, it might be objected] on the contrary; it says "conquer it" [using a plural verb], implying two [are to do so]! Said Rav

Naḥman ben Isaac: it is written "conquer it" [using a singular verb; that is, the written form, the *ketiv*, uses a singular verb; it is the *qeri*, the vocalized form that is read, that uses a plural verb]. Rav Joseph said: We learn it from this [Gen. 35:11]: "I am El Shaddai. Be fertile and increase [singular verbs]"; it does not say "Be fertile and increase [plural verbs]." (BT Yev. 65b)

This *mishnah* introduces two key innovations: it emphasizes the duty to reproduce, treating procreation as a commandment rather than as the blessing implied by the plain meaning of the biblical verse; and it interprets the verse as addressed exclusively to men, Rabbi Yoḥanan ben Beroqa's dissent notwithstanding.

Women's exemption from the commandment to be fertile and increase is surprising, to say the least. Procreation is not a time-determined positive commandment (from which women, as a rule, are exempt), and the *gemara*'s argument suggests at most that the nature of the commandment ("to conquer") is more suited to the male character. But is that sufficient grounds to exempt women? The Talmud's positive response to that question is difficult for several reasons:

Transforming God's blessing in Genesis into a commandment would seem to necessitate its application to both members of the couple, since it was bestowed upon both man and woman (as per its phrasing in the plural) and it is a requirement that cannot be fulfilled without the participation of both.

The desire to bring children into the world is understood (in a patriarchal worldview) to be a natural and essential characteristic of woman; why, then, exclude her from a religious act that is associated with her more than anything else?

The rationale that it is not a woman's way "to conquer," for all the gender-based distinctions it incorporates, does not really explain why women should therefore be exempt from the commandment to procreate. If the term "to conquer" is understood in its plain, militaristic sense, it is not clear how it relates to the commandment of procreation altogether. If, on the other hand, the term alludes to sexual drive or to assertiveness and initiative in sexual relations, it seems that the Torah means to impose the duty to fulfill the commandment on one who by nature is suited to doing so. But even if we accept the theological claim that the Torah's commandments correspond to human nature, there are, nonetheless, two distinct layers of the commandment to reproduce. There is the sexual act itself, which requires the sexual assertiveness that the rabbis associate with men, but there is also the purpose and result of the sexual act—children who need to be birthed and raised—and the rabbis' worldview regards women as naturally suited to fulfill that role. In that light, woman's exclusion from the commandment is even more surprising; correspondence between character and commandment exists here with respect to the woman no less than with respect to the man.[21]

In order to resolve these peculiarities, we will need to consider the halakhic rule that governs women's obligations and exemptions from commandments in general.

The Mishnah states: "with respect to every positive commandment that is time-determined—men are obligated and women are exempt."[22] In practice, however, that rule is not strictly followed, and there are numerous exceptions both in terms of obligations and exemptions.[23] However, the explanations offered for these exceptions do tend to be rational (at least from the sages' perspective). For example, the explanation for exempting a woman from the commandment of Torah study (which is not time-determined and in theory ought to apply to a woman) is based either on assumptions regarding her cognitive skills, suggesting that she is not intellectually qualified for such study,[24] or on assumptions regarding her character, suggesting that the character traits that develop among Torah scholars are ill suited to women.[25]

Scholars and halakhists have tried to characterize the logic behind women's exemption from some commandments but not from others. Safrai believes that the exemptions reflected the reality of women's lives and were not meant to be a normative determination.[26] In contrast, Zohar claims that "there can be no doubt that a man's more extensive obligations with respect to commandments, in comparison to those of a woman, was seen as an advantage."[27] In other words, according to Zohar, the difference between men's and women's obligations must be understood against the background of their difference in status. Women have less independence (because others have authority over them), and consequently they have fewer duties with respect to fulfilling commandments. In that vein, feminist scholars see the exclusion of women from certain commandments as a clear sign of discrimination against them, evidence of a desire to deny them a foothold within the realm of significant or "prestigious" religious activity.[28] Berman, in contrast, reasons that Judaism in fact does not define a "suitable" or "necessary" role for women but nevertheless encourages women to play the role of wife, mother, and homemaker because Jewish continuity as a nation depends on it.[29] The exemptions from certain commandments ensure that if a woman chooses these assignments, no religious duties will stand in her way and interfere with her discharging them.

Some scholars believe that the exemption from the commandment to procreate reflects a patriarchal worldview that meant to increase a woman's dependence on her husband. David Daube, for example, recognizes that from a certain perspective, exempting women is in line with contemporary liberal tendencies that stress reproductive freedom and a woman's right to decide freely whether to bear children. But he believes that given the historical context, Rabbi Yoḥanan ben Beroqa's position—that women are indeed included in the commandment to procreate—should be read in light of his overall approach, which tends to be more "pro-woman" in other halakhic areas as well.[30] A woman would have been afforded important advantages by being included within the commandment, and her exclusion leads to her subservience to and absolute dependence on her husband.[31] Judith Romney Wegner effectively argues that women's subservience to their husbands within a patriarchal world requires no explanation or justification, and accordingly, when the rabbis of the Mishnah saw a need to establish or even to impose the man's sexual rights, the woman was treated arbitrarily, as chattel.[32] Regarding woman's exclusion from the commandment to procreate, she writes:

> Like Yohanan b. Broqa . . . we wonder at the sages' assertion that the commandment of procreation was directed solely to the *man*. The Mishnah offers no explanation. . . . The only reasonable interpretation is that the sages perceive woman in this context not as a person subject to a duty, but simply as a baby-incubator, a vehicle for the man's implementation of the divine command.[33]

I am not at all sure that these explanations can account for the exemption in our case. As noted, the rationale given by the *gemara* here explains little and primarily raises additional questions. The commandment to procreate is not a time-determined positive commandment, nor is it likely to interfere with a woman's fulfillment of her role as wife and mother; on the contrary, it would only strengthen and confirm that role. It therefore is not clear what purpose is served by the exemption.

I want to suggest that exempting women from the commandment to procreate, even if originally motivated by the factors proposed by Daube and Wegner, had the practical effect of *allowing for flexibility* in carrying out the commandment. It is fair to assume that this flexibility primarily benefited men, facilitating their involvement in Torah study, but it served the needs of women as well.[34] The Babylonian Talmud draws a direct connection between women's exemption from the commandment to procreate and the authorization to avoid pregnancy by drinking a sterility potion. The point is clearly illustrated in the following story:

> Judith, the wife of Rabbi Ḥiyya, had difficulty in giving birth. She donned a disguise, came before Rabbi Ḥiyya, and asked: Is a woman commanded to be fertile and increase? He said to her: No. She went and drank a sterility potion. Eventually, the matter became known [to Rabbi Ḥiyya]. He said to her: If only you had borne me one more pregnancy. (BT Yev. 65b)

There is much of interest in this story, but it is enough to mention here that Judith had to disguise herself in order to gain her husband's attention and, perhaps, even his sympathy for her request to avoid additional pregnancies. What most interests me is the story's halakhic implications. Is a woman permitted to avoid pregnancy only in a case of "difficulty giving birth," or might this be a more fundamental authorization, extended on account of her exemption from the commandment to procreate? The Talmud, to be sure, states that the reason for her wanting to be sterilized was "difficulty giving birth"; theoretically, this suggests that the authorization is conditioned on that difficulty and limited to those cases. But a more careful reading, I believe, suggests that nothing in Rabbi Ḥiyya's ruling implies a direct causal relationship between difficulty giving birth and the authorization to be sterilized. Just the opposite: his halakhic conclusion is formulated as an abstract principle unconnected to the concrete circumstances that provoked his wife's question. From the foregoing, we may infer that one not commanded to be fertile and increase is permitted to use a sterilization potion (referred to as a "cup of roots") in order to prevent unwanted pregnancies. We may not infer that the woman's exemption from the commandment provides unlimited authority to prevent pregnancy—but neither may we infer the converse, that the man's obligation to fulfill the commandment precludes the use of birth control methods that are otherwise halakhically acceptable. My argument here is limited to the following: In the time of the Mishnah and Talmud, there were no known birth control methods for men that did not result in permanent sterility. Since men were obligated to procreate, they could not take actions that would permanently prevent them from fulfilling that duty. On the other hand, women, because they were not bound by the commandment to reproduce, were permitted to become permanently sterilized.[35] In other words, the exemption of women from the commandment to procreate, as a practical matter, served the interests of men who for one reason or another wanted to avoid having additional children. Of course, it could serve the interests of women as well, albeit indirectly.

The Extent of the Commandment

THE MINIMUM NUMBER OF CHILDREN PRESCRIBED BY BIBLICAL LAW

> MISHNAH. One should not refrain from procreation unless he has children. The House of Shammai say: [he must have a minimum of] two males; the House of Hillel say: a male and a female, as it is said (Gen. 5:2): "male and female He created them."
>
> GEMARA. This implies that one who has children may refrain from procreation but may not refrain from having a wife. This supports what Rav Naḥman said in the name of Samuel, for he said: Even if one has several children, he is forbidden to be unmarried, for it is said: (Gen. 2:18): "It is not good for man to be alone." But some say: This implies that one who has children may refrain from procreation and may refrain as well from having a wife. Shall we say that this contradicts what Rav Naḥman said in the name of Samuel? No—[it means that] if he has no children, he should take a wife capable of bearing children; if he has children, he may take a wife incapable of bearing children. What is the practical difference? A Torah scroll may be sold to pay wedding expenses only if the marriage is for the purpose of bearing children.
>
> The House of Shammai say: two males. . . . It was taught in another *baraita*: Rabbi Nathan says, the House of Shammai say: a male and a female;

the House of Hillel say: a male or a female. Rava said: What is the rationale for the House of Hillel's view as reported by Rabbi Nathan? For it is said (Isa. 45:18): "He did not create it a waste, but formed it for habitation," and he has made it [more] inhabited. . . . This *mishnah* is not in accord with the view of Rabbi Joshua, for it was taught in a *baraita*: Rabbi Joshua says: If a man married a woman in his youth, he should marry a woman in old age; if he had children in his youth, he should have children in his old age, as it is said (Eccl. 11:6): "Sow your seed in the morning and don't hold back your hand in the evening, since you don't know which is going to succeed, the one or the other, or if both are equally good." . . . Rav Matna said: The halakhah is in accord with Rabbi Joshua. (BT Yev. 61b–62b)

At the outset, it should be noted that the duty to procreate as delineated in biblical law is minimal, according to both the House of Hillel and the House of Shammai. If the commandment to reproduce is so important, why rest content with only two children? It seems to me that the disagreement between the House of Hillel and the House of Shammai regarding whether it is a son and a daughter or two sons is not terribly important compared to voices of those who want to limit the number even further.

At least according to one of the reported traditions, the House of Hillel requires only one child for fulfillment of the commandment,[36] and the Jerusalem Talmud (*Yerushalmi*) likewise implies that the House of Hillel's position is more lenient than the House of Shammai's, requiring fewer births.[37] According to the *Yerushalmi* on our *mishnah*, the House of Hillel should be understood not as disputing the House of Shammai's view but as agreeing with them that the commandment is fulfilled with two sons or *even* with a son and a daughter. The rationale for that understanding is that otherwise (that is, if the House of Hillel required at least one male and one female and did not regard two males as fulfilling the commandment), this *mishnah* would be one of the relatively rare instances in which the House of Shammai is the more lenient of the two. But this *mishnah* is not included in the listing of those instances set forth in tractate *'Eduyot*;[38] accordingly, the House of Hillel must be read as expanding on the House of Shammai's view rather than as disputing it.

Moreover, the beginning of the passage may suggest that the commandment to reproduce is secondary in importance to the commandment to take a wife (either to relieve the sexual impulse and avoid succumbing to licentiousness or simply because "it is not good for man to be alone"); for if fulfilling the commandment to reproduce were the sole purpose of marriage, why not remain single once the commandment was fulfilled? That possibility is rejected through the distinction between a fertile woman and a woman "incapable of bearing children." Even after a man has fulfilled the commandment to procreate, he must be married; however, at that point he may marry a woman who cannot bear children. As noted, our *mishnah* regards the requirement as fulfilled by two children—a minimalist position. The low number may be driven by the desire to limit the obligation to divorce an infertile or inadequately fertile wife after ten years or take a second wife; if only two children suffice to fulfill the commandment, those circumstances will be less likely to eventuate. Alternatively, the low number may be understood as an effort to limit the scope of the commandment because of its conflict with the commandment to study Torah. In any case, Rabbi Joshua's statement at the end of the passage stands clearly at odds with the *mishnah*'s inclination, as the *gemara* itself states: "This *mishnah* is not in accord with the view of Rabbi Joshua."[39]

"DON'T HOLD BACK YOUR HAND IN THE EVENING": TALMUDIC DISCUSSION

As noted, the Mishnah defines the obligation to procreate to mean the obligation to produce two children. Rabbi Joshua seemingly disagrees with that determination, asserting that one must never stop procreating. The editing of the talmudic passage may reflect polemical opposition to limiting the biblical commandment and support for maximizing procreation. Alternatively, as suggested below, Rabbi Joshua's statement can be seen as an expansion of the mishnaic rule that is not necessarily at odds with it.

Rabbi Joshua's statement appears in the context of a series of homilies on the verse "sow your seed in the morning," whose main purpose seems to be to offer advice on how to lead one's life successfully. Other such recommendations include sowing one's field at various times and studying Torah both in youth and in old age, for one never knows what will endure and what will be lost or forgotten. It can fairly be concluded that the recommendation to continue having children is similar in nature—advice and encouragement to bear more than two children so as to ensure that the biblical commandment will be fulfilled.[40]

In what follows, I will try to ascertain whether that ambivalence regarding Rabbi Joshua's statement made its way into the writings of the medieval and early-modern authorities or whether the statement was taken at face value as a halakhic determination, effectively annulling the limitation on the number of children needed to fulfill, as a matter of biblical law, the commandment to procreate.

VIEWS OF THE MEDIEVAL AUTHORITIES

R. Isaac Alfasi (Rif)[41] determines that Rabbi Joshua does not express disagreement with the *mishnah*. His text of the *gemara* does not include the comment that "this *mishnah* is not in accord with the view of Rabbi Joshua"; moreover, he differentiates between the duty as defined in biblical law and as defined in rabbinic law. According to biblical law, one son and one daughter suffice; Rabbi Joshua's more expansive view is according to rabbinic law.

R. Zeraḥiah Ha-Levi[42] (known as *Ba'al Ha-Ma'or*) disagrees with Rif on the meaning and force of "in the evening." He sees a clear contradiction between the *mishnah*, which limits what needs to be done to satisfy the biblical commandment, and Rabbi Joshua's statement, which rejects any such limit. Consistent with that, he argues against regarding both views as halakhically authoritative; rather, the halakhah accords with Rabbi Joshua, and even if a man has fulfilled the commandment to "be fruitful and multiply," he is not free of his halakhic obligation to procreate. Only in unusual circumstances will it matter, in effect, whether one has already fulfilled the basic commandment: for example, a man is not required to divorce a wife who has been barren for ten years if he himself has already fulfilled the basic requirement to father a son and a daughter. R. Asher b. Jacob (Rosh) takes a similar view.[43]

Naḥmanides's comments on Alfasi explain the difference between the biblical and rabbinic duties in the following terms:

> Said the writer: our rabbi [Alfasi] means to interpret the truth and resolve the statements, for if Rabbi Joshua's view were a matter of biblical law, there would be no point to the dispute between the House of Shammai and the House of Hillel regarding the offspring. . . . Rather, the biblical law is according to the House of Hillel . . . and rabbinic law is that he continues to sow his seed for as long as it is possible for him to do so. . . . For if that were a matter of biblical law, he would be lashed [for failure to comply], but for a rabbinic commandment, not formally enacted but established as a sort of norm for life, we do not treat him so strictly. . . . But because the rabbinic commandment is a sort of custom for proper conduct . . . and there is no prohibition mentioned in connection with it—rather, taking a wife is a commandment from the outset—he is not required to do so and one not wanting to do so is not labeled a transgressor. But he should never cease to have a wife, for that is forbidden. (*Milḥemet Ha-Shem* [Naḥmanides] on Rif, BT Yev. 62b)

Naḥmanides's comments establish a clear hierarchy of values. Marriage has a purpose in its own right, and is not merely a means for fulfilling the commandment to be fertile and increase. As a matter of biblical law, there is an obligation to sire a son and daughter but nothing more, and one who does not want more children than that is not labeled a transgressor.

To summarize, most medieval authorities regarded "in the evening" as a rabbinic commandment having less force than the biblical commandment to be fertile and increase. Nonetheless, some medieval authorities clearly disdained individuals who limited their procreative activity. The Tosafot equate siring only one son and one daughter to decreeing the extinction of the Jewish people: "But the progeny of Abraham will come to an end if people sire only a son and a daughter" (BT BB 60b). Rhetorically, this statement seems critical of the notion that one fulfills the biblical requirement to "be fertile and increase" by having two children. It is unclear, however, whether it was intended as a halakhic determination or merely as practical advice that one should not rest content with only one son and one daughter.

Maimonides, in contrast, does not see the binding purpose of the commandment as maintaining the nation or inhabiting the world, and he avoids citing the verse from Isaiah ("He did not create it a waste, but formed it for habitation") anywhere in his treatment of procreation. To understand his position on the force of "in the evening," let me quote his comments in the order in which they appear in *Hilkhot 'Ishut*:

1. A woman who after marriage gives her husband permission to withhold her conjugal rights from her, this is permitted. When does this apply? When he has children, for in that case he has already fulfilled the commandment [to be fertile and increase]. If, however, he has not yet fulfilled it, he is obligated to have sexual intercourse with her according to his schedule until he has children, because this is a positive commandment of the Torah, as it is said "[Be fertile and increase"] (Gen. 1:28). . . . (Maimonides, *Mishneh Torah, Hilkhot 'Ishut* 15:1; Yale Judaica Series[44] trans., p. 93)

3. He who is so desirous of studying Torah constantly that he is immersed in it like Ben Azai, and cleaves to it all his life, neglecting to take a wife unto himself—there is no sin in his hand, provided that his passion is not wont to overpower him. If, however, his passion repeatedly overcomes him, he is obligated to take a wife, even if he already has children, lest he should fall victim to unchaste thoughts. . . . (15:3; 93–94)

7. One should not marry a sterile woman, an old woman, a barren woman, or a minor female who is incapable of giving birth, unless he has already fulfilled the commandment to be [fertile and increase], or unless he has another wife by whom he can fulfill this commandment. If he marries a woman and she abides with him for ten years without giving birth, he should divorce her and pay her kĕṭubbah, or else take another wife capable of bearing children. If he refuses to divorce her, he should be compelled to do so, by being scourged with a rod until he divorces her. If he says "I will have no sexual intercourse with her, but will abide with her in the constant presence of witnesses, so as never to seclude myself with her"—whether it is she who says so or he, no attention need be paid to it. He must divorce her, or else marry another wife capable of giving birth. . . . (15:7; 94–95)

16. Even if a man has already fulfilled the commandment to be [fertile and increase], he is still obligated by Scribal enactment not to cease being [fertile and increasing] as long as he has the power to do so, because whosoever adds one soul to Israel has as much as built a whole world. It is also a precept of the Sages that no man should live without a wife, in order that he

should not come to unchaste thoughts, nor should a woman live without a husband, in order that she should not become subject to suspicion. . . . (15:16; 97)

Curiously, Maimonides's discussion opens with an exemption to the general rule, phrased in negative terms, rather than establishing at the outset, in positive terms, the duty imposed by the biblical commandment. This surprising editorial choice serves rhetorically to highlight the situation in which a wife might forgo her conjugal rights and thereby exempt her husband from his obligation to engage in procreative activity. Subsequently, in section 3, Maimonides rules that one who craves Torah in the manner of Ben Azai is permitted to refrain from taking a wife, as long as his libido does not overpower him. In other words, Maimonides resolves the tension between the commandment to be fertile and increase and the commandment to study Torah in favor of the latter.[45] When presenting the rabbinic requirement to continue procreating even after fulfilling one's biblical duty, Maimonides adds the qualifier "as long as he has the power to do so." He also suggests that a man who has fulfilled the commandment to be fertile and increase as a matter of biblical law is permitted to marry a woman who is unable to bear children; certainly, it is not forbidden to do so. Moreover, Maimonides takes the view that the commandment of "in the evening" does not preclude a wife waiving her right to conjugal relations.

Maimonides's commentators are perturbed by this position, which effectively permits a man to marry a barren woman if he has already fulfilled his biblical requirement to "be fertile and increase," since it is sharply at odds with Rabbi Joshua's statement in the Talmud. R. Vidal di Tolosa, author of *Maggid Mishneh*, attempts to resolve this contradiction by relying on the distinction between the biblical and rabbinic commandments,[46] but that attempt is unproductive. Maimonides grants permission as matter of principle, and not merely after the fact, contrary to Rabbi Joshua's halakhically accepted statement. Accordingly, R. Abraham di Boton, author of *Leḥem Mishneh*, explains that Maimonides does not believe that Rabbi Joshua differs with the Mishnah. The Mishnah posits that if a man has already fulfilled the commandment to be fertile and increase, he need not sell a Torah scroll in order to wed a fertile woman. However, it is certainly proper, in the

Mishnah's view, that he try to find a fertile woman, and that is what Rabbi Joshua emphasizes. On the other hand, one who has never wed must even sell a Torah scroll if necessary in order to marry a fertile woman.[47]

In practice, Maimonides's formulation implies that one who wants to study Torah is permitted to remain a bachelor, and one who has fulfilled the biblical commandment to reproduce is not *obligated* to bring additional children into the world. His view seems consistent with the line of thought I noted earlier, which aims to limit the scope of the commandment.

In his commentary on the passage from BT *Yevamot*, R. Yom Tov ben Abraham Ishbili (Ritva) supports Maimonides's opinion that, when all is said and done, the commandment of Torah study takes precedence over the commandment to procreate. This approach is also consistent with the analysis presented earlier, in which I argued that in the Talmud itself, the biblical duty to reproduce was defined minimally, so as not to interfere with Torah study. R. Ishbili's contribution to the discussion is that he actually allows a man to take a libido-suppressing drug once he has fulfilled his obligation:

> *What can I do? My soul craves* [*only*] *Torah*. Maimonides of blessed memory ruled that anyone who craves Torah like Ben Azai and is free of any libidinous thoughts is exempt from being fertile and increasing. But Tosafot wrote that no one nowadays can be like Ben Azai in this respect. It is forbidden for a man to drink any sterilizing potion so that he may engage in Torah, but it is permitted [to ingest a drug] to suppress desire and libidinous thoughts. I heard in the name of our great rabbi [Naḥmanides], of blessed memory, that if one has fulfilled the commandment to be fertile and increase and his soul craves only Torah, he is permitted to drink or eat something that will make him sterile so he will not have to neglect his Torah. That is because Rabbi Joshua's commandment is of rabbinic authority, and the rabbis permitted this exception to it. And that explanation is reasonable, and I have heard of great scholars who have done so. (Ritva on Yev. 63b)

Naḥmanides indeed writes that one whose libido has been fully suppressed is not obligated to take a wife if he has already fulfilled the biblical commandment.[48]

R. Jacob b. Asher, author of the *Tur*, cites the two conflicting interpretations of Rabbi Joshua's position that had been presented by his father, Rosh;

and he believes Rosh concluded that according to Alfasi, the obligation to marry a fertile woman is not so great as to warrant selling a Torah scroll. But Rosh's own determination runs counter to Alfasi's; that is, in principle, a man is obligated to marry a fertile woman even if that necessitates selling a Torah scroll, although he would not be obligated to divorce a woman who proves barren. In effect, his ruling is a stringent one.[49]

In any event, it appears that traditions preserved in the responsa of the medieval authorities, both Ashkenazi and Sephardi, show that reality differed substantially from that envisioned by Rabbi Joshua and that decisors refrained from applying the tannaitic rule[50] (of biblical authority!) requiring a husband who is still childless after ten years of marriage to divorce his wife.[51] This restraint attests that other considerations did occasionally prevail over the commandment to procreate, despite its centrality; it may also attest to a decline in that commandment's standing.[52] We turn first to a few prominent examples from Ashkenaz and then to the Sephardi literature.

R. Israel Isserlein, a prominent Ashkenazi authority of the fifteenth century, offers a series of practical explanations for allowing a man to deliberately marry an infertile woman:

> QUESTION: Reuben, having already fulfilled the commandment to be fertile and increase, is widowed and wants to take a wife. He fears that there may be quarrels between his new wife and his children, and he therefore wants to choose a woman widely known not to be at all quarrelsome, but also incapable of bearing children. If he cannot find such a wife, he is thinking of not marrying at all, given his concern about quarrels. Is he acting properly or not?
>
> ANSWER: It appears that he is acting properly in one respect but not in the other. How so[?] If he marries a woman who is not at all quarrelsome, he is acting properly, even though she is totally incapable of bearing children. . . . But in the other respect—that is, his plan, if he fails to find a woman who is not at all quarrelsome, to refrain entirely from taking a wife—we cannot say that he is acting properly, for the sages declared that a man should not remain without a wife. (*Terumat Ha-Deshen* 1:263)

R. Isserlein believes that in no event is the widower permitted to refrain from taking a wife altogether, but he is permitted, even in principle, to marry an infertile woman although he will thereby annul in some sense the commandment of "in the evening." In other words, he believes the commandment of "in the evening" can be superseded by considerations of "household peace" in the broad sense, referring not only to relationships between husband and wife but to relationships between parents and children as well. Overall, the author of *Terumat Ha-Deshen* conveys the sense that, in the hierarchy of values, the obligation to take a wife is paramount and bringing additional children into the world is not a goal to be pursued at all costs.

R. Moses Minẓ (Maharam Minẓ), another fifteenth-century Ashkenazi authority, goes even further than R. Israel Isserlein. The obligation to (re)marry after fulfilling the basic commandment to procreate is incumbent only on those who cannot overcome their sexual drives; those who can devote themselves to Torah and forgo conjugal relations are not obligated to remarry once they have fulfilled the commandment to "be fertile and increase." He even adds that "if that is so, it follows that one who would be kept from study by domestic obligations is better off not marrying."[53] In other words, R. Minẓ seems to resolve the tension between Torah study and procreation in favor of Torah study (as long as the man is able to overcome his libido), as did Maimonides.

In the Sephardi tradition, in addition to the previously noted comments of Maimonides and R. Ishbili, there is a responsum by R. Isaac b. Sheshet (Rivash) that is consistent with both his Sephardi predecessors and the Ashkenazi tradition: Rivash attests to a social reality in which the authorities compelled compliance neither with Rabbi Joshua's rule nor even with fulfillment of "be fertile and increase" as a matter of biblical law.[54]

THE LATER AUTHORITIES

The multivocality that emerges from the writings of the medieval authorities, in which procreation is weighed against other values, continues to resonate in the halakhic determinations of the *Shulḥan 'Arukh*. Although the normative requirement is to have many children, this rule is immediately qualified by reference to the individual's economic capacity. Extreme measures (such as selling a Torah scroll) need not be taken in order to enable a man to take a (second) wife who is fertile. It follows that the obligation to remarry overrides the requirement of "in the evening," once the commandment as prescribed by biblical law has been fulfilled. R. Moses Isserles (Rama) cites a number of circumstances in which a man may marry a woman who is infertile:

> ANNOTATION: But if he knows that he is no longer capable of siring children, he should take a wife incapable of bearing children. . . . Similarly, if he has many children and fears that if he takes a wife capable of bearing children, quarrels will ensue between his children and his wife, he may take a wife incapable of bearing children. But it is forbidden to remain unmarried, on account of that concern [about potential sinful conduct]. (*Shulḥan ʿArukh*, *ʾEven Ha-ʿEzer* 1:8)

We find that the positions of the medieval authorities are renewed and reinforced here.[55] Some of the commentators on the *Shulḥan ʿArukh* effectively disagree with Rama (and thereby with Maimonides as well),[56] but that simply strengthens the contention that for them (Maimonides and Rama), "in the evening" was not a commandment with significant halakhic weight. With that in mind, we will consider more recent positions.

R. Moses Sofer (*Ḥatam Sofer*) understands "in the evening" as a rabbinic commandment (and emphasizes its importance by referring to it as "a positive commandment"). He therefore regards it as preferable for a woman who would find additional pregnancies difficult to accept a divorce from her husband, thereby enabling him to take another wife and continue fulfilling the commandment. Yet, the *Ḥatam Sofer* also writes that because a woman is not obligated to suffer on account of her husband's obligation to procreate, it is possible that countervailing considerations may supersede his requirement "in the evening":

> In my humble opinion, a woman who has not yet borne a child and not fulfilled "habitation" may not drink a "cup of roots" except to save her from jaundice or difficult childbirth or similar matters. But if "habitation" has already been fulfilled, then it is permitted even if childbirth is not at all difficult. . . . now that we are subject to the ban enacted by Rabbeinu Gershom *Meʾor Ha-Golah* [which forbids polygamy and nonconsensual divorce], she is not permitted to drink [the "cup of roots"] without her husband's consent . . . or else she should be willing to accept a divorce from him. But if he wants neither to divorce her nor to grant permission, it seems

> to me that she is not required to make herself suffer on account of her subordination to her husband, and this appears to be great suffering. And it is impossible to go into all aspects of this. (*Ḥatam Sofer* on *'Even Ha-'Ezer* 1:20)

Depending on the reader's own interpretation, R. Sofer can be understood to be ruling either stringently or leniently. On the one hand, the rhetoric attests that he not only accepts the strict position of the *Ba'al Ha-Ma'or* and of Rosh; he even emphasizes their position by determining that the commandment of "in the evening" requires a woman to obtain her husband's consent before drinking a sterilizing potion or, in the absence of that consent, to "be willing to accept a divorce from him." Only where no alternative is possible is the commandment of "in the evening" superseded by countervailing consideration of the woman's suffering. On the other hand, one who wants to take account of a woman's interests will emphasize that she is not bound to suffer on account of her subservience to her husband for purposes of fulfilling the commandment to procreate and that the definition of "great suffering," on account of which a woman is permitted to keep her husband from fulfilling the commandment of "in the evening," is subject to interpretation in light of the cultural reality of the decisor and the affected public alike.

The comments of the *'Arukh Ha-Shulḥan* next cited suggest that the force of "in the evening" does not outweigh all economic considerations; on the contrary, economic considerations related to the ability to support more children are certainly pertinent to deciding whether to expand the family. We have seen economic factors taken into account before, but they have pertained only to the man himself and the economic resources he must expend in order to father additional children: is he obligated, for example, to sell a Torah scroll to be able to take a fertile wife? Here, for the first time, we see consideration given as well to the good and welfare of the children who are destined to be born:

> And so the sages commanded that if he sees himself as still fit to father children, he should take a wife capable of bearing children *if his situation is adequate to support them*. . . . Regarding the general matter of taking a wife capable of bearing children, Naḥmanides of blessed memory wrote that according to no opinion is he compelled to do so, for there is no such

enactment; rather, it is a rule of sound conduct, and it is not treated so stringently. And Maimonides' words suggest a similar result. (*'Arukh Ha-Shulḥan, 'Even Ha-'Ezer* 1:8; emphasis mine)

The *'Arukh Ha-Shulḥan* here formally places "in the evening" within the category of "enhancement of a commandment and sound conduct." That categorization is attributed to Maimonides as well and is likely to bolster the distinction suggested earlier between insisting on fulfilling the commandment unless there is a significant countervailing consideration and not so insisting. In any case, even more than the *'Arukh Ha-Shulḥan*'s author emphasizes the legitimacy of considering economic factors, he stresses that deciding whether to bring more children into the world is a personal decision. The decision must be reached in light of a person's concrete situation; even more, there is no "objective" test for examining that situation. The standard is worded as "if he sees himself as still fit to father children," meaning that the decision is up to the individual looking at himself and his personal situation.

The opinions of the later authorities regarding "in the evening" reflect an effort on their part to balance the duty to procreate against a range of other considerations and interests that may arise in the course of a person's life. An additional illustration of that attitude is provided by the next topic we will examine, halakhic discussions concerning conjugal relations in a time of famine.

The Prohibition on Sexual Intercourse in a Time of Famine

The Babylonian Talmud forbids conjugal relations during a time of famine. Let us consider the reason for the prohibition and its scope:

> Resh Laqish said: A man is forbidden to engage in sexual intercourse during years of famine, as it is said (Gen. 41:50): "Before the years of famine came, Joseph became the father of two sons." A sage taught: Those who are childless engage in sexual intercourse during years of famine. Our rabbis taught: When Israel is sunk in sorrow, and one person withdrew from involvement in it, the two ministering angels that accompany a person come and place their hand on his head and say, "this person who withdrew from the community will not see the consolation of the community." It was taught in another *baraita*: When the community is sunk in sorrow, a man

should not say "I will go to my home and eat and drink, and it will be well with my soul" . . . rather, one should be sorrowful with the community. (BT Ta'an. 11a)

Resh Laqish's statement can be understood in two ways. He may believe it is wrong to bring additional children into the world in a time of famine for economic reasons, so that there are not extra mouths to feed. From the ensuing discussion, however, it appears that the prohibition is based on a concern for social solidarity rather than economics. A person is part of a community, and he may not act for the sake of his own household without paying attention to and identifying with the troubles faced by the community as a whole. Times of trouble require setting aside personal interests, even on a symbolic level.

The Jerusalem Talmud words it this way:

Rabbi Avun said: It is written [Job 30:3], "Wasted [*galmud*, which also means 'lonely' or 'abandoned'] from want and starvation"—When you see want come into the world, let your wife be lonely. Rabbi Levi said: It is written [Gen. 41:50]: "Joseph became the father of two sons." When? "Before the years of famine came." It was taught in the name of Rabbi Judah: Those who crave children engage in sexual intercourse. Rabbi Yosi said: Only on the day of her [postmenstrual] immersion. (JT Ta'an. 1:6)[57]

The *Yerushalmi* may help clarify whether the prohibition is intended to promote solidarity in suffering or conservation of scarce resources. The reference to "want," a term parallel to "starvation" in the verse from Job, suggests that the prohibition is designed to avoid exacerbating a tenuous economic situation. What follows, however, allows for an alternative explanation. The *baraita* cited in Rabbi Judah's name allows "those who crave children" to engage in intercourse as long as they do so in accordance with Rabbi Yosi's qualification, that is, only on the wife's day of immersion (when her potential to conceive is greatest). This *baraita* seems to suggest that the prohibition on conjugal relations in a time of famine is not motivated by economic concerns; if it were, why permit the act to those who want children? Rabbi Yosi's qualification emphasizes this further, for it seems intended to limit pleasure as much as possible—to one day a month—while still allowing individuals to take advantage of the potential for fertility. Once again, the emphasis is shifted to social solidarity, and the beginning of the passage may be read in that light as well. The passage first establishes the principle of refraining from conjugal relations in time of famine and then explains the reason.

Rashi's interpretation likewise suggests that the principal reason for the prohibition pertains not to practical concerns about increasing the number of mouths to feed but to the ethical standard that should guide a person's conduct when the society in which he lives finds itself in difficult straits: "*A man is forbidden to engage in sexual intercourse during years of famine*—For a man must conduct himself in a sorrowful manner" (Rashi on BT Ta'an. 11a).

The Tosafists, however, understand Resh Laqish's statement not as a sweeping prohibition but merely as identifying a characteristic of pious behavior:

> *A man is forbidden to engage in sexual intercourse during years of famine*—You might ask: Was not Yokheved [Moses' mother] born between the walls [of the Egyptian border, as the Israelites were descending to Egypt] during a time of famine, in which case they engaged in sexual relations during years of famine? One may answer: All agree that there is no prohibition except for a person who wants to conduct himself piously. Joseph did not engage in sexual relations, but others did. (Tosafot on BT Ta'an. 11a)

The author of *Qorban Netan'el* disagrees with this understanding:

> *A man is forbidden to engage in sexual intercourse during years of famine*—This [interpretation offered by Tosafot] is surprising, for Resh Laqish said: "A man is forbidden." It may be resolved by saying that all certainly agree it is forbidden, but for Levi [Yokheved's father] and Joseph, who had not yet fulfilled "be fertile and increase," it remained permitted as a matter of law, but Joseph acted piously. (*Qorban Netan'el* on Rosh on BT Ta'an. 11a)

The Tosafist's interpretation suggests that adherence to the ban on sexual relations is considered an act of piety only for an individual who has not yet fulfilled his biblical obligation to procreate. But if he has already fulfilled the commandment, sexual relations are forbidden.

R. Nissim b. Reuben (Ran) limits the scope of the prohibition to situations in which Israel is suffering but not the other nations.[58] Maimonides and the *Shulḥan 'Arukh* rule that one who has already fulfilled "be fertile and increase" is indeed forbidden to engage in sexual intercourse during years of famine.[59] Rama significantly expands the scope of the prohibition, maintaining that "years of famine" is merely an example and that the prohibition applies in other troubling and sorrowful circumstances as well.[60]

R. Judah Ayyash provides insight as to which circumstances are regarded by the halakhah as "years of famine":

> Whenever normal market prices are doubled, it is a famine; and even if a person subject to the prohibition himself has produce, it is still forbidden on account of the sorrow of others, as in the case of Joseph. (*Beit Yehudah, 'Oraḥ Ḥayyim* 40)

In other words, according to R. Judah Ayyash, famine is defined as price inflation of 100 percent, and the reason for the prohibition is to identify and express solidarity with the suffering of others, even if one is not himself suffering on account of that famine.

The overall impression conveyed by both Talmuds, by the medieval authorities, and by the later authorities is that the prohibition on conjugal relations in time of famine is motivated by social solidarity rather than economic scarcity and is directed toward avoiding the pleasure of sexuality and the joy of bringing children into the world at a time of sorrow and distress. As R. David b. Naftali Hirsch Frenkel, author of the *Qorban Ha-'Edah* on the *Yerushalmi*, puts it, "The Holy One blessed be He is engaged in destruction of the world and he should build?"[61] The focus is on the Jewish people or perhaps the entire world, with no direct connection to the familial or economic situation of any individual. At the same time, it is clear that a sharp distinction is drawn between one who has already fulfilled the biblical commandment to procreate and one who has not fulfilled it. Most opinions hold that one who has already fulfilled the commandment is forbidden to engage in sexual relations during these hard times, providing additional proof that the commandment of "in the evening" is superseded even for reasons of symbolic identification with one's community.

Summary

The principal course of interpretation we have considered to this point pertains to the proper understanding of how the commandment to be fertile and increase, defined as biblical law, relates to Rabbi Joshua's invocation of "don't hold back your hand in the evening." We have seen how the Talmud itself perceives procreation to inherently conflict with the commandment to study Torah. On the one hand, the rabbis of the Talmud strive to affix procreation in religious consciousness as a weighty commandment. On the other hand, they limit the requirement to procreate so as to avoid conflict with the duty to study. To state it differently, establishing procreation as a commandment while simultaneously limiting its biblical scope to one son and one daughter reflects two sides of the same coin: the belief that one is obligated to engage in procreation coupled with the understanding that this existential duty has the potential to delay or even impair realization of the commandment to study Torah. Attempts to balance these two commandments have been fraught with dialectical tension through the generations.

The commandment of "in the evening" could have been interpreted as upsetting that delicate balance, on the premise that it represented a rejection of any limitation on the scope of the biblical commandment. But a survey of the sources reveals that the attitude toward "in the evening" has undergone many changes from talmudic times to the present. A survey that encompasses so many historical periods can direct attention only to the major trends that are evident in the decisional literature; accordingly, the foregoing discussion does not cover the range of connections and contradictions between the duty to procreate and all the other obligations of the observant Jew. Still, it seems to me that a clear line of thought can be identified that assigns relatively little weight to Rabbi Joshua's position and regards the duty of "don't hold back your hand in the evening" as subject to other considerations—among them the desire to study Torah, the need to respond to various economic or familial factors, and even the expression of social solidarity. There are many, of course, who do not engage in Torah study, and for them the tension between the two commandments is not relevant. But that does not affect the *principle* that I want to stress here: the willingness to narrow the scope of the commandment when it comes into conflict with other values.

This balanced picture, which situates the value of procreation within an array of other values, has clear gender-related implications for how the purpose of women is understood. The interests that are brought into balance, to be sure, have their weights assigned from a male perspective, and the entire discourse is conducted from a male point of view. Still, the balancing can lead, indirectly, to women being seen as having functions other than bearing children. As we have seen, at least some decisors have regarded marriage as something having independent value, and the husband's duty to engage in conjugal relations with his wife is independent of the commandment to procreate. That conclusion is important in the ensuing discussion, for when we reach contemporary decisors, we will need to see whether this balancing, with its gender implications, is preserved or abandoned.

CHAPTER TWO

Birth Control and Family Planning

In the previous chapter, we considered the religious obligation to be fertile and increase—its moral significance; its definition as a matter of biblical and rabbinic law; and its implications for the weighing of various obligations and interests that arise over the course of one's life. Our analysis clearly demonstrated that the requirement to procreate is not absolute, and thus in principle there are circumstances under which family planning and contraception may be permitted. In this chapter, we will focus on the use of specific birth control mechanisms from a halakhic point of view.

Birth Control

NEUTERING AND STERILIZATION

Treatment of the Issue in the Talmud and by Medieval Authorities

Neutering (*sirus*)[1] and sterilization (*'iqqur*) connote intentional impairment of the reproductive organs or of the capacity to bear children; usually, the reference is to a total and permanent impairment. In the course of our discussion, we will try to clarify the difference between these terms, for they appear in the talmudic and halakhic literature in an imprecise and sometimes confusing fashion.[2]

For men, castration is biblically prohibited, as derived from the verse "You shall not offer to the Lord anything [with its testes] bruised or crushed or torn or cut. You shall have no such practices in your own land" (Lev. 22:24). The sages differed, however, about whether the prohibition applied to women as well:

> How is it known that women are included in [the prohibition on] neutering? It is learned from "for they are mutilated, they have a defect" [Lev. 22:25]. Rabbi Judah says [the pronoun in the verse is masculine in form]; women are not included in [the prohibition on] neutering. (*Sifra, 'Emor* 7:7, par. 12)[3]

The anonymous *tanna* takes the view that the prohibition on neutering applies to women and men alike; Rabbi Judah disagrees. The Tosefta records various traditions on the matter. The version in the Vienna manuscript follows the anonymous *tanna* in the *Sifra* and forbids neutering a woman:

> A person should not forgo procreation unless he has children. . . . A man is not permitted to drink a "cup of roots"[4] so as to become incapable of fathering a child, and a woman is not permitted to drink a "cup of roots" so as to become incapable of bearing a child. . . . Rabbi Judah says one who neuters a man is liable; one who neuters a woman is not liable. (T Yev. 8:4)

Saul Lieberman notes that, in contrast to the version quoted, the Erfurt manuscript reads, "a woman is permitted to drink . . . ," and he believes that to be the correct reading.[5]

The discussion in the Babylonian Talmud (Shabbat 111a) likewise reaches the conclusion that the use of a drug that causes sterilization is permissible only for a woman, for she is not bound by the commandment to be fertile and increase. A man, however—even if he has already been neutered—is not permitted to take a drug of that sort.[6] In other words, there is a sweeping prohibition on causing the sterilization of a man, but no such prohibition applies to a woman (except according to the view of Rabbi Yoḥanan ben Beroqa regarding women and procreation, as discussed in the previous chapter). That conclusion is bolstered by the story about Judith, the wife of Rabbi Ḥiyya.[7] Judith did not ask Rabbi Ḥiyya directly whether a woman was permitted to drink a sterilizing drug; rather, she asked whether a woman was bound by the commandment to be fertile and increase. In so doing, she confirmed the straightforward conclusion that exemption from the commandment allows for drinking a sterilizing drug.

The Tosafists seem to believe that *sirus* of a woman is impossible; it follows that *sirus* connotes physical injury to the reproductive organs (with which its translation here as "neutering" is consistent), while *'iqqur* means indirect impairment of the reproductive capacity.[8] The Tosafists seem to be saying that because a woman's reproductive organs are internal, there is no way to injure them so as to preclude childbearing, something that can be done to a man. But it could be argued that they do not mean neutering a woman is impossible but that the prohibition of neutering does not apply to a woman. That interpretation may be, in fact, the more reasonable one, as many of the later authorities claim.[9]

As a practical matter, Maimonides rules that "one who neuters a female—whether a human or some other species—is not liable"[10] (meaning that he has not violated a biblical law); however, the act is forbidden as a matter of rabbinic law. Yet in the following passage, Maimonides continues:

> One who gives a "cup of roots" to a man or to any other species to neuter him [to accomplish *sirus*] has committed a prohibited act but is not subject to the penalty of lashes. But a woman is permitted to drink a "cup of roots" potion in order to be neutered [to accomplish *sirus*] so that she cannot bear children. (*Mishneh Torah, Hilkhot 'Issurei Bi'ah* 16:12)

As the author of *Maggid Mishneh* notes,[11] to avoid a contradiction between the two halakhot, one must assume that Maimonides distinguishes between *sirus* and *'iqqur*. Maimonides seems to take the view that *sirus* of a woman is possible, just as is *sirus* of a man; accordingly, the distinction between his rulings in the two passages relates to the distinction between the two actions. *Sirus* of a woman is forbidden by rabbinic law, but *'iqqur* is entirely permissible. This interpretation is supported by the wording of the second passage: "to drink a 'cup of roots' in order to be neutered [to accomplish *sirus*]." This suggests that Maimonides distinguishes between direct *sirus*—physical neutering, which he refers to in the first passage—and drinking a potion for *'iqqur*, which achieves the same result, but indirectly.

The authors of *Sefer Mizvot Gadol* and the *Tur* follow Maimonides and confirm the determination that one who performs *sirus* on a woman is exempt (though the action is rabbinically forbidden) but that *'iqqur* by means of a potion is entirely permitted.[12]

Review of the *rishonim* thus establishes that there is a distinction between *sirus* (physical neutering) and *'iqqur* (drug-induced sterilization). A woman is entirely permitted to prevent herself from bearing children by drinking a sterilizing drug, but she is forbidden as a matter of rabbinic law to subject herself to physical neutering.

Treatment of the Issue by Later Authorities

The *Shulḥan 'Arukh* rules in accord with Maimonides,[13] but some later commentators to this work distinguish between a determination in principle that a woman may drink a "cup of roots" and a determination that she may do so only if she has difficulty in childbirth. It seems to me that distinction is new and is not found in the writings of the medieval authorities (notwithstanding the reference in the talmudic story about Judith to her difficulties in childbirth, on account of which she wanted to bear no more children). R. Solomon Luria, author of *Yam Shel Shelomoh*, is the first of the later authorities to adopt it:

> A man is commanded to be fertile and increase but not so a woman; Rabbi Yoḥanan said the commandment applies to both. . . . The halakhah is according to the rabbis, and a woman is not required to be fertile and increase . . . and she is permitted even to drink a sterilizing potion; thus wrote the [author of] *Sefer Mizvot Gadol.* And his proof is from the passage at the end of that chapter, regarding Rabbi Ḥiyya's wife. . . . But I say that this cannot be cited as proof except for a woman, like Rabbi Ḥiyya's wife, who has difficulty in childbirth. And it is all the more forbidden if her sons do not walk the straight and narrow, and she is afraid she cannot raise them, as if the right [not to bear more children] were hers. (*Yam Shel Shelomoh, Yevamot*, chap. 6, sec. 44)

R. Luria's comments here are surprising, for the conclusion of *Sefer Mizvot Gadol* does not rely specifically on the story about Judith; it is also based on the passage from tractate *Shabbat*, presented earlier, as its author expressly states: "In the chapter *'Shemonah Sheraẓim,'* it is proven that it is forbidden to give a 'cup of roots' to a man so as to cause *sirus*, but it is permitted to give it to a woman."[14]

Moreover, it is not only *Sefer Mizvot Gadol* that rules this way. The author of *Bayit Ḥadash* (*Baḥ*) on the *Tur* reaches the same conclusion. He rejects the view of the *Maggid Mishneh* (offered to explain the seeming contradiction between two adjacent passages in Maimonides) on the basis of his understanding that the Tosafists believe it is impossible to neuter a woman by direct injury to her reproductive organs. In order to resolve the seeming contradiction between Maimonides's statements, he rejects any distinction between self-inflicted sterilization (*'iqqur*) and sterilization inflicted by another, and the only distinction he is left with, for purposes of resolving the contradiction, is one between sterilization for a woman who has difficulty in childbirth, which is permissible, and sterilization for a woman who does not have such difficulty, which is forbidden as a matter of rabbinic law. But that interpretation is nowhere alluded to in Maimonides's words nor is it a necessary implication, as I understand it, of the story about Judith.

In contrast to the authors of *Yam Shel Shelomoh* and *Baḥ*, other interpreters of the *Shulḥan 'Arukh* do not draw a distinction based on difficulty in childbirth:

> *A woman is permitted, etc.*—This implies that it is permitted even in the absence of any difficulty in childbirth. (*Beit Shemu'el* on *Shulḥan 'Arukh, 'Even Ha-'Ezer* 5:11–12, sec. 14)
>
> *A woman is permitted to drink*— . . . It likewise is far-fetched to say that a woman, too, is not permitted to drink except where there is difficulty in childbirth—the distinction drawn by the *Baḥ*—because the *Tur* makes no mention whatsoever of difficulty in childbearing. (*Be'er Heiteiv* on ibid., 12, sec. 11)

The author of *Turei Zahav* (*Taz*) expressly rejects the *Baḥ*'s conclusion, and his comments are the most definitive:

> A woman is permitted to drink a "cup of roots"— . . . And the distinction regarding difficulty in childbirth *is not at all implied by the decisors.* (*Taz* on ibid., 12, sec. 7; emphasis mine)

The conclusion suggested by all this is that women are permitted to sterilize themselves (with no distinction regarding who administers the drug) by drinking a "cup of roots" or by any other means that does not cause direct physical injury to the reproductive organs themselves and that no specific condition, such as difficulty in childbirth, must be satisfied to invoke that authorization. The position that permits drinking a "cup of roots" only on account of difficulty in childbirth seems to be a radical and innovative interpretation with clear gender implications, for it limits a woman's control over her fertility and heightens her dependency on the halakhic-interpretive establishment, which is authorized to determine what constitutes sufficient "difficulty in childbirth" to warrant preventing pregnancy.

As for physical neutering—destruction of the reproductive organs—most authorities regard it as forbidden for women only by rabbinic law. The exception is R. Elijah of Vilna (Gra), according to whom the biblical prohibition on neutering applies to women as well.[15] According to R. Elijah, the dispute between the anonymous *tanna* and Rabbi Judah pertains not to the inclusion of women in the prohibition on neutering—both agree that she is included—but only to whether she is subject to the penalty of lashes if she violates it. It follows that R. Elijah believes the prohibition on neutering applies to women as a matter of biblical law, just as it applies to men—a position contrary to the plain meaning of Maimonides's ruling, to the *Tur*, to the *Shulḥan 'Arukh*, and to all their commentaries. In contrast to the picture that emerges from the rulings of all the other decisors—namely, that the issue is resolved in accord with Rabbi Judah—R. Elijah takes the view that the halakhah is in accord with the sages.

In this context, we should note as well the position of R. Noah Ḥayyim Zvi Berlin, author of *'Aẓei 'Arazim*. In his view, the story about Rabbi Ḥiyya's wife implies no authorization to drink a "cup of roots," which is no different from engaging in sexual intercourse using a *mokh* (a cloth that prevents conception by absorbing seed, next discussed), and it should be permitted only in cases where pregnancy would be dangerous:

> The story of Rabbi Ḥiyya's wife . . . [concludes] and she did so herself; but it seems to me, on the contrary, that Rabbi Ḥiyya was angry with her, and it appears that if she wants to avoid difficult childbirth, she should separate from her husband rather than actively transgress a prohibition. (*'Aẓei 'Arazim, 'Even Ha-'Ezer* 5:52)

The interpretation of the author of *'Aẓei 'Arazim* implies that the concern about "wasting seed" that is raised in connection with a *mokh* pertains as well to drinking a "cup of roots." Other decisors, however, find that view hard to understand and reject it.[16]

"THREE WOMEN USE A *MOKH*"

Notwithstanding the conclusion that indirect means of sterilization that do not directly injure the reproductive organs are permissible for women, the "cup of roots" did not become the primary halakhic rubric for discussion of birth control. That initially seems odd, for the legitimacy of this mechanism —certainly in cases of danger—is unquestioned. It is possible that the potential harm to a woman's body associated with ingesting the drug and the permanence of the sterilization made many women reluctant to use it and decisors hesitant to recommend it.[17] It is also possible that, over time, the precise recipe was lost or ingredients became unavailable. These factors may be able to explain why, despite the simpler remedy of the sterilizing potion, it was the model of "three women who use a *mokh*" that became the central locus for all discussions related to birth control and has been extensively considered in the responsa literature of the last several centuries.[18]

Discussion of the *mokh*, at least since the medieval authorities, has not dealt with the legitimacy of preventing pregnancy, for, as we have seen, women are permitted to make themselves sterile. The central issue that has been considered is the legitimacy of using a *mokh* given the concern it raises about wasting seed.[19] That is a fundamental concern with respect to all "mechanical" methods of birth control, which do not work indirectly in the manner of the "cup of roots," including contemporary mechanisms of this sort. As I will show in the analysis that follows, the concern about wasting seed goes entirely unmentioned in the tannaitic and amoraic sources. Beginning with the medieval authorities, however, it becomes the focus of all discussions pertaining to use of the *mokh*.

Talmudic (Tannaitic and Amoraic) Sources

> Three women use a *mokh* in sexual intercourse: a minor, a pregnant woman, and a nursing woman. A minor, lest she become pregnant and die. Who is a minor? One whose age is from eleven years and one day to twelve years and

> one day; one younger or older than that engages in intercourse normally and has no such concern. A pregnant woman, lest her fetus become a *sandal* [flattened or otherwise damaged]. A nursing woman, lest she kill her child [by becoming pregnant and ending lactation]; for Rabbi Meir said, all twenty-four months [of nursing] he [her husband] treads inside and sows outside [that is, uses coitus interruptus so she does not become pregnant], but the sages say he engages in intercourse in the usual way and God protects him, as it is said, "the LORD protects fools." (T [Zuckermandel] Nid. 2:6)[20]

This *baraita* first appears in the Tosefta, and its rendition there differs slightly from the version that appears in the Talmud. The variance may have a significant bearing on its meaning, and the interpretive differences it engenders will be considered below.

Understood in accord with its plain meaning, the *baraita* recommends that three categories of women use a mechanism for preventing pregnancy in order to avoid risk to the woman, a fetus,[21] or a nursing child. Rabbi Meir's words may be understood in two ways. He may be agreeing with the statement in the first part of the *baraita* according to which three women may use a *mokh*, adding that they may also use other means of preventing pregnancy, such as coitus interruptus; alternatively, his recommendation may apply only to a nursing mother.

The talmudic sources whose wording differs from that of the Tosefta give a different impression:

> Rav Bibi taught before Rav Naḥman: Three women use a *mokh* in sexual intercourse—a minor, a pregnant woman, and a nursing woman. A minor, lest she become pregnant and lest she die. A pregnant woman, lest her fetus become a *sandal*. A nursing woman, lest she wean her child [prematurely] and he die. Who is a minor? One whose age is from eleven years and one day to twelve years and one day; one younger or older than that engages in intercourse in the usual way; that is the view of Rabbi Meir. The sages say: It is the same for every woman; she engages in intercourse in the usual way and Heaven will have mercy, as it is said (Ps. 116), "the LORD protects fools." (BT Yev. 12b)

According to this version, which appears in identical form whenever the *baraita* appears is cited in the Talmud,[22] Rabbi Meir's statement comprises the entire first portion of the *baraita*, in which the only mechanism under discussion is the *mokh*. A significant addition appears in the words of the sages: "It is the same for every woman." The dispute, then, is no longer a localized one regarding a nursing woman or the birth control mechanism proposed by Rabbi Meir in the Tosefta; rather, it has become a difference in principle regarding the acceptability of using a *mokh* under any circumstances.

On the one hand, the dispute may be understood as a simple one: all agree that women who are not at risk are forbidden to engage in intercourse using a mechanism to prevent pregnancy. The dispute pertains only to the three categories of women mentioned. Rabbi Meir believes they must use a *mokh* when engaging in intercourse; the sages, however, believe they are forbidden to do so; rather they should engage in intercourse in the usual way, and "Heaven will have mercy." The expression "she engages in intercourse in the usual way"[23] reinforces this strict reading, for in the Tosefta the wording is "he engages in intercourse in the usual way" (the Hebrew differs only by one letter, indicating the gender of the verb), and the expression is meant to reject the option of coitus interruptus. It is reasonable to assume, therefore, that the version appearing in the Talmud, where the verb is feminine, pertains to maintaining natural conjugal relations without the use of any artificial mechanisms and with no change from usual practice.

But if we have reservations about what is implied by the sages—that women may subject themselves to danger[24]—it is also possible to understand the *baraita* in an alternative way, in which the fundamental premise is reversed. According to the second reading, in the absence of dangerous circumstances, women are permitted to use a *mokh*. The question is whether women whose pregnancy entails special dangers are required to use a *mokh*, or whether it is simply recommended, but if they want to incur the risk (albeit not a serious one), they are permitted to do so. According to this reading, when Rabbi Meir says "they engage in intercourse using a *mokh*," he means they are obligated to use it; the sages, however, say its use is permitted but not required. I believe this interpretation is consistent with the *baraita* appearing in *Niddah* and elsewhere that mentions specific women who use a *mokh*.[25] One might claim, therefore, that the Talmud was aware that many women use a *mokh* in intercourse[26] and did not disparage the practice or warn against it. As we shall see, however, the medieval authorities understood the subject in a manner inconsistent with what I believe to be the more reasonable reading of the talmudic sources; and in so doing, they gave the matter an almost entirely unprecedented meaning.

But before turning to these authorities, we should note the position of R. Hai Ga'on:

> *As for the matter of the three women*: The rabbis said she uses a *mokh* in intercourse and said all of them engage in intercourse in their usual way. It does not mean they forbade use of a *mokh*; rather, they are permitted to engage in intercourse in their usual way, and Heaven will have mercy. But it always is permitted to engage in intercourse using a *mokh*, and where women do not rely on "Heaven will have mercy," they and their husbands should use a *mokh* in intercourse, and there is no concern whatever about doing so.[27]

R. Hai's interpretation lends support to the second reading of the *baraita* suggested above. In his opinion, women are generally permitted to use a *mokh*, and the three specific categories of women may also use a *mokh*, though they are not required to in spite of the medical danger not using it would entail. R. Hai does not mention whether he is referring to precoital or postcoital use of a *mokh*, which suggests that until the medieval authorities took up the issue, as we shall see below, the premise was simply that a *mokh* was used during intercourse (as implied by the present-tense phrasing: "use a *mokh* in intercourse").

Treatment by the Medieval Authorities

The primary disputants regarding the use of a *mokh* are R. Solomon b. Isaac (Rashi) and R. Jacob b. Meir (Rabbeinu Tam). To a great extent, their differing views of the matter shaped the interpretations and rulings of the later medieval and modern authorities.

RASHI'S POSITION Rashi comments on the issue at several different points,[28] and it is pretty clear that he understood Rabbi Meir to permit the use of a *mokh* only for the three specific categories of women and, accordingly, to forbid its use by all others. The sages, in Rashi's view, say that despite the danger to these women (or their fetuses or infants), they may not use a *mokh*, and "Heaven will have mercy."[29]

Rashi's comments, however, introduce an additional variable: whether the *mokh* is inserted before or after intercourse. All his statements except the one on *Ketubbot* 37a suggest that the *mokh* is placed before intercourse. At issue there is the wayward woman; but it is not clear how, if at all, that bears on the question of when the *mokh* is placed. How should Rashi's references to placing a *mokh* before or after intercourse be understood? Does his statement on *Ketubbot* 37a contradict the others? I see no necessary contradiction. It is fair to assume that Rashi's references to precoital and postcoital *mokh*s are meant to demonstrate that he saw no difference between them; with regard to both, he asserts that Rabbi Meir believes the danger supersedes the prohibition on a *mokh*, while the sages believe it does not. And it seems reasonably likely that he assumes a postcoital *mokh* is not a sufficiently effective contraceptive; accordingly, in interpreting Rabbi Meir's opinion, he assumes precoital placement because that is the only way the *mokh* can ensure that pregnancy will not ensue.[30]

THE POSITION OF TOSAFOT Before considering the position taken by Tosafot as set forth in the printed texts, we should clarify the position of Rabbeinu Tam. In *Sefer Ha-Yashar*, he writes:

> *Three women use a mokh in intercourse.* This means they must use a *mokh* because of the risk [of not doing so], as it goes on to explain. And it should not be interpreted to mean [only] that they are permitted to use a *mokh*, for that [applies] even to all women, who are not commanded to be fertile and increase. . . . And it is not a case of wasting seed that would lead us to say it is forbidden for other women, as said at the beginning of the chapter. (Editor's note—the reference is to [BT *Niddah*] 3a above, the implication of which is that all women may engage in intercourse using a *mokh*.) (*Sefer Ha-Yashar*, sec. 166, p. 120)

Rabbeinu Tam does not believe that women are subject to the prohibition against wasting seed; in any event, in his view, the use of a *mokh* does not invoke that question. Reading the statement at BT *Niddah* 3a in accord with its plain sense, Rabbeinu Tam acknowledges that the use of a *mokh* is treated there as something routine and is therefore permissible for all women. But he notes no difference between precoital and postcoital placement of a *mokh*, and the plain meaning of the passage seems to deal with the former. At the same time, he emphasizes that one should not follow Rashi in understanding that three women are permitted to use a *mokh*; rather, they are required to use it, and other women are permitted to do so.

The version of Rabbeinu Tam's ruling that appears in *Sefer Ha-Yashar* is consistent with the comments of R. Samson of Sens on the passage in *Ketubbot,* which formed the basis for the standard Tosafist commentary on that tractate:[31]

> *Three women use a mokh in intercourse.* Rashi interpreted that they are permitted to use a *mokh*; even though other women are forbidden [to do so] because of wasting seed, these are permitted. And this is not evident to Rabbeinu Tam, for it is permitted to engage in intercourse with a minor or a barren woman even though they are incapable of bearing children, and doing so is not considered a waste of seed because [the seed is emitted] through intercourse. Here, too, with the use of *mokh*, it is through intercourse and it is not forbidden. He therefore interprets "use a *mokh* in intercourse" to mean they must use a *mokh*, and it is good advice. (R. Samson of Sens on *Ketubbot* 39a)

A reconstruction of Rabbeinu Tam's original position on the basis of the foregoing two sources seems to me to suggest that he believed all women are permitted to insert a *mokh* before engaging in sexual intercourse. His position as it appears in the printed versions of Tosafot, however, is entirely different:

> *Three women use a mokh in intercourse. . . .* And Rabbeinu Tam interprets "use . . . in intercourse" to mean they must use a *mokh after* intercourse, and it is good advice. . . . (Tosafot on BT Ket. 39a; emphasis mine)
>
> *Three women use a mokh in intercourse. . . .* And Rabbeinu Tam says that it certainly is forbidden to place a *mokh* there before intercourse. . . . But if she places the *mokh* following intercourse, it appears it should not be forbidden, for the man is engaging in intercourse in his usual way. . . . And "use a *mokh* in intercourse," as taught here means they are required to use a *mokh*.[32] (Tosafot on BT Yev. 12b)

According to Tosafot's interpretation, Rashi opposes use of a *mokh* regardless of whether it is inserted before intercourse or after, because he believes women, too, are subject to the prohibition on wasting seed. Placement of a *mokh* before intercourse entails forbidden action on the husband's part; placement after intercourse entails forbidden action on the wife's part. Rabbeinu Tam's position is presented as disagreeing with Rashi regarding postcoital placement. According to this reading, Rabbeinu Tam agrees that precoital placement is forbidden, but he permits it after intercourse because the woman is not forbidden to waste her husband's seed inasmuch as she is not commanded to be fertile and increase.

The reconstruction of Rabbeinu Tam's position presented earlier suggests, however, that the positions attributed to him in the printed versions of Tosafot fail to reflect his original stance and were no doubt edited to suit a stricter mind-set, influenced by those who recoiled from blanket authorization to use a *mokh*. The position of R. Isaac reported in Tosafot on *Ketubbot*, which maintains Rashi's view, illustrates the editing process, and Urbach's argument supports the explanation I have proposed. Urbach maintains that in Tosafot on *Yevamot*, Rabbeinu Tam was represented by many of his French and German students, whose statements provide a first layer of commentary, on top of which a second layer of material contributed by the students of R. Isaac was superimposed.[33] That fact may explain the difference between Rabbeinu Tam's original position—which did not refer specifically to postcoital use of a *mokh*—and the altered version that appears in Tosafot on *Yevamot*. The position attributed to him there renders his opinion on use of a *mokh* by all women closer to the opinion of Rashi, according to whom precoital placement of a *mokh* is forbidden because of wasting seed.

Additional support for my surmise regarding the reworking of Rabbeinu Tam's original position can be gleaned from a version reported in Tosafot on *Ketubbot*, where he refutes Rashi's opinion: "and it is not waste of seed because it is [emitted] through intercourse." Even if a woman is incapable of bearing children (because she is a minor or because she is barren), the emission of her husband's seed during regular intercourse is not considered wasteful. Rabbeinu Tam suggests that this model guides the halakhah's attitude toward the use of a *mokh* as well: so long as regular intercourse occurred, the seed is not considered wasted. But if Rabbeinu Tam is referring only to postcoital placement, it is self-evident that the emission was "through intercourse," since the *mokh* had not yet been put in place, so there is no need to say so.[34] This interpretation strengthens the inference that the words "after intercourse" are a later addition and do not reflect Rabbeinu Tam's original position. The writings of other medieval authorities suggest that they, too, had the version of Rabbeinu Tam that appears in *Sefer Ha-Yashar*, with no reference to any prohibition on precoital placement of a *mokh*.

It appears from this brief survey that the better understanding of Rabbeinu Tam's view is the one that appears in *Sefer Ha-Yashar* and in Tosafot on *Ketubbot*, a view that is also supported by the earlier statement of R. Hai Ga'on. If that is so, and if I am right that Rashi did not forbid postcoital placement of a *mokh*, then the essential dispute between Rashi and Rabbeinu Tam boils down to whether women are bound by the commandment that forbids wasting seed. Rashi believes they are; and therefore, in his opinion, women are generally forbidden to use a *mokh*. Rabbi Meir *permits* its use by three categories of women and allows both precoital and postcoital placement, and the sages forbid it even for those women. Rabbeinu Tam, in contrast, believes women are not bound by the prohibition on wasting seed. In his view, therefore, all women are permitted to use a *mokh*, without distinction between precoital and postcoital placement. Rabbi Meir *requires* three categories of women to use it because of the of risk of becoming pregnant; but the sages, who permit the use of a *mokh* by those women, do not require it.[35]

Despite the foregoing, later generations likely knew Rabbeinu Tam's position only through the version printed in Tosafot. But I believe the reconstruction of Rabbeinu Tam's original position has halakhic significance, especially since R. Solomon Luria, as I will show, understands Rabbeinu Tam in the way I have described and therefore permits all women to use a *mokh*. The later decisors' complete disregard of R. Luria's position becomes even more troublesome given what appears to me to be the consistency of Luria's position with the correct understanding of what Rabbeinu Tam actually said.

RASHI AND RABBEINU TAM AS UNDERSTOOD BY LATER RISHONIM

An examination of how the medieval authorities understood Rashi and Rabbeinu Tam[36] shows, first, that all reject Rashi's position regarding the three women and understand the matter as did Rabbeinu Tam: women in a situation of danger are permitted (per the sages) or required (per Rabbi Meir) to use a *mokh* (though it may be that they are permitted or required to use it only after intercourse). Regarding women in general, there appears to be no clear trend; some permit use of a *mokh* and others forbid it. Those who permit it believe that women are not bound by the prohibition on wasting seed or that use of a *mokh* may not constitute wasting seed because the seed is emitted "through intercourse." It is fair to assume that those who regard women, too, as bound by the prohibition on wasting seed reject only precoital, but not postcoital, use of a *mokh*;[37] but whether that in fact is so depends on their understanding of the nature and scope of the prohibition, and there is ample room for interpretation on the part of the later authorities.

This analysis would not be complete without taking account of the positions of Maimonides and the other decisors. Maimonides stands out among the medieval authorities in that he pays no attention at all to the question of the three women who use a *mokh*. Many later authorities have attempted to account for his omission, some taking it to imply permission to use a *mokh* and others to imply a prohibition on its use.[38]

From a halakhic perspective, Maimonides is not unusual in failing to apply some halakhic rule to use of a *mokh* (that is, whether it involves waste of seed and whether its use by women in general is permitted). Alfasi before him and Rosh after him did the same. But while their perspective on the matter is evident from their commentaries on the Talmud, in Maimonides's case, we lack even that. And the matter similarly goes untreated by the authors of *Sefer Mizvot Gadol*, *Tur*, and *Shulḥan 'Arukh* and by Rama.

It may be that the systematic rejection of Rashi's view by all medieval authorities effectively eliminated the prohibition on use of a *mokh* by women in general. Rabbeinu Tam's words, accordingly, were interpreted more as sound advice against entering a dangerous situation. That would explain Maimonides's disregard of the *baraita* dealing with use of a *mokh*.

To sum up the positions of the medieval authorities, we may say that Rabbeinu Tam's authentic position is that precoital placement of a *mokh* is permitted for women in general and required for the three categories of women at risk. Nevertheless, the redacted version, according to which he permits only postcoital placement of a *mokh*, gained currency in Ashkenaz and appears in the printed versions of Tosafot and in the writings of Rosh. And while Ashkenazi authorities disagreed about use of a *mokh* by women in general, Naḥmanides and his students seem to forbid it.[39] The principal halakhic compendiums omit the issue, which may be taken to mean they permit it (though proof from silence can never be certain).

Treatment by the Later Authorities

Use of a *mokh* is treated extensively in the responsa literature. In what follows, I present a chronological account of the principal approaches. I first consider pre-twentieth-century authorities and then turn to modern and contemporary decisors who are familiar with novel and more advanced means of birth control.

SIXTEENTH CENTURY: R. DAVID B. SOLOMON IBN ZIMRA (RADBAZ) First, it should be noted that Radbaz refers to a *mokh* during intercourse and says nothing about the possibility of postcoital placement (Radbaz 3:596). In his view, intercourse using a *mokh* entails waste of seed (the prohibition applies to men but also to women, who are forbidden to waste their husbands' seed), and he therefore accepts the view that the statement in the *baraita* means that three categories of women are permitted to use a *mokh* and other women are forbidden to use it. Inasmuch as the halakhah follows the view of the sages, it would appear that even the three women whose pregnancy would be dangerous are nonetheless forbidden to use a *mokh*. In fact, however, Radbaz believes the sages meant not to forbid use of a *mokh* by the three women but only to say that in these particular circumstances, they are permitted to endanger themselves by not using a *mokh*, but they are not required to do so (that is, they are free to use a *mokh* to avoid the danger). According to this interpretation, the dispute between Rabbi Meir and the sages (at least according to Rashi) becomes very narrow: Rabbi Meir believes that three categories of women are permitted to use a *mokh*; the sages do not disagree but merely emphasize that their use of the *mokh* is permitted but not required and they are free to incur the risks at issue if they wish.

This characterization of the dispute draws Radbaz's interpretation closer to that of Rabbeinu Tam, according to whom Rabbi Meir maintains that the three categories of women are required to use a *mokh*, while the sages permit it but do not require it. In other words, Radbaz adopts Rashi's view with respect to precoital but not postcoital placement of a *mokh* but believes, like Rabbeinu Tam, that according to the sages, the three women are permitted to use a *mokh*. The significant difference pertains to women in general. While Rabbeinu Tam permits women in general to use a *mokh*, Radbaz forbids it because it entails wasting seed. The interpretive option adopted by Radbaz is especially interesting because it brings us one step closer to the twofold leniency adopted by his Ashkenazi contemporary R. Solomon Luria, despite their opposing positions with respect to women using a *mokh* in general.

R. SOLOMON LURIA R. Solomon Luria, a sixteenth-century Polish authority, discusses use of a *mokh* in his work *Yam Shel Shelomoh* (*Yashash*).

Although that work was written to clarify and rule on halakhic issues, his views on this subject are presented through an interpretation of the passage about the three women rather than as a response to a concrete question; accordingly, they can be taken as a statement of principle that does not depend on specific circumstances. As already noted, his interpretive stance is very permissive, for he believes that use of a *mokh* does not entail waste of seed and is therefore allowable for women in general:

> It nevertheless appears to me that Rashi's interpretation is correct and that it is speaking of precoital placement of a *mokh*, which does not resemble emission of seed onto wood; for when all is said and done, it is through intercourse, as one body takes pleasure in the other, and it resembles intercourse with a minor [unable to conceive]. . . . But it nevertheless appears that Rabbeinu Tam's opinion also is correct in that even other women [than the three] are permitted [to use a *mokh*], for there is no prohibition on women doing so inasmuch as they are not commanded to be fertile and increase; and the three women are singled out to say they must [use a *mokh*]. . . . And it follows that all women are permitted [to use it]. (*Yam Shel Shelomoh*, *Yevamot* 1:8)

R. Solomon Luria thus permits all women to use a *mokh* and to do so both before and after intercourse because it raises no concern at all about wasting seed. His conclusion rests on several arguments, but I think his unique and possibly most important contribution is the claim that the issue of waste of seed simply does not arise in the context of intercourse using a *mokh*, for sexual intercourse proceeds in its natural way; as he puts it, "one body takes pleasure in the other."[40]

To sum up the position of *Yam Shel Shelomoh*, we can say that if we accept (1) my conclusion that Rabbeinu Tam never referred to postcoital placement of a *mokh* and (2) the surmise that Maimonides's omission of the subject follows from his belief that it poses no halakhic issue inasmuch as the sages believe use of a *mokh* is permitted but not required, then R. Luria's authorization to use a *mokh*, regardless of whether it is placed before or after intercourse, makes excellent sense.

Nevertheless, as we shall see, a preponderance of later authorities do not accept R. Luria's position.[41]

The Eighteenth and Early Nineteenth Centuries

The eighteenth century and early nineteenth century witnessed the emergence of a strict tendency that forbids use of a *mokh* even in situations where pregnancy would pose a danger to the mother or the fetus. As a matter of legal interpretation, this constitutes an entirely novel and unprecedented stance, found neither among the medieval authorities (except for Tosafot *Ha-Rosh* on *Yevamot*, who maintains that in dangerous conditions it is better simply not to engage in intercourse) nor among the early modern authorities. I will discuss in detail only the view of the *Ḥatam Sofer*, but the strict position can be found also in the *Beit Mei'ir*, the *Rosh Mashbir*, the writings of R. Akiva Eger, and the *Binyan Ẓiyyon*.

ḤATAM SOFER The question posed to R. Moses Sofer (the *Ḥatam Sofer*) was whether a woman who faced "great danger" while pregnant and nursing would be permitted to use a *mokh* during intercourse to avoid becoming pregnant.[42] He responded that it could not be permitted even for women in dangerous circumstances because "I have not found anyone who permitted it at all," and he therefore saw no room for "elaborate argumentation." Accordingly, in situations of danger it might be permissible to place a *mokh* after intercourse, but then, too, only with the husband's express consent:

> The rule is, in my humble opinion, that [use of a *mokh*] during intercourse should not be permitted, but after intercourse there may be a basis for leniency, but it is subject to the will and authority of the husband. (*Ḥatam Sofer*, *Yoreh De'ah*, 172)

The *Ḥatam Sofer* explains "three women use a *mokh*" as follows: Rashi did not believe a postcoital *mokh* was sufficiently effective, so he based the entire analysis on a *mokh* placed before intercourse. Rabbi Meir, according to that view, permitted a precoital *mokh* in cases of danger, but the rabbis forbade it, and the halakhah follows their view. Rabbeinu Tam, meanwhile, was even stricter than Rashi, seeing no possibility of permitting a precoital *mokh* even in cases of danger. In his view, Rabbi Meir required a postcoital *mokh* in cases of danger, while the sages permitted but did not require it. It follows, according to the *Ḥatam Sofer*, that in Rashi's view, in cases of danger, it might be required to use a postcoital *mokh*, but in Rabbeinu Tam's view, it would only be permitted but not required, consistent with the opinion of the sages.

The *Ḥatam Sofer* goes on to consider the responsum in which Rosh, as we have seen, appears to refer explicitly to a precoital *mokh*. The *Ḥatam Sofer* comments that Rosh certainly could not have meant to rule in accordance with Rabbi Meir and against the opinion of the sages: "Even if we say that the case involves use of a *mokh* during intercourse, as Rashi understood it, it need not mean that he ruled in accord with Rabbi Meir and against the sages, for how could he have so ruled? Rather, he meant that this [see immediately below] is worse than use of a *mokh*, which Rabbi Meir permits, but in our view, both are forbidden."[43] In other words, a blockage of the womb is even worse than intercourse using a *mokh*, which Rabbi Meir permits, but in our view (that is, the view of Rosh), both are forbidden—intercourse with a woman whose uterus is blocked, and use of a *mokh* during intercourse. This interpretation of Rosh seems rather far-fetched to me, but it must be recalled that Rosh's comments appear to be contradictory at several points, though the *Ḥatam Sofer* does not specifically consider that.

In a responsum written in 1820,[44] the *Ḥatam Sofer* bolsters his halakhic positions with respect to using a *mokh* and to drinking a "cup of roots." Regarding the former, he reiterates his view that it may be permitted only after intercourse, but with respect to the latter, his position takes an interesting turn. In a slightly later responsum, written in 1821,[45] he permits a woman to drink a "cup of roots" even without her husband's consent. In the 1820 responsum, however, his view is somewhat different. First, he emphasizes the importance of the husband's consent as a precedent condition:

> With regard to a cup of roots, which we find R. Ḥiyya's wife to have drunk, I have already written . . . that nowadays, when the ban of Rabbeinu Gershom *Me'or Ha-Golah* forbids one to divorce his wife against her will or to take an additional wife, she is not permitted to drink a cup of roots or to use a *mokh* to preclude pregnancy against her husband's will and without his consent. (*'Even Ha-'Ezer* 20)

Second, in the earlier responsum he suggests he is not happy about allowing use of the "cup of roots" because it may entail mortal risk.

From all the foregoing, it appears that even if the "cup of roots" is easier to deal with from a halakhic perspective and is something the wife may do without her husband's consent (if we assume that the *Ḥatam Sofer*'s more fully developed position is the one expressed in the later responsum), the potentially mortal danger in using it seems to rule it out. If follows that the only remaining, halakhically acceptable methods for preventing pregnancy, whether or not danger is present, are postcoital use of a *mokh* or sexual abstinence. But the *Ḥatam Sofer* himself (in the responsum at issue, *Yoreh De'ah* 172), suggests that a postcoital *mokh* may not be sufficiently effective—as Rashi, in his opinion, similarly believed—leaving abstinence as the only option.

The *Ḥatam Sofer*, R. Akiva Eger, and R. Ettlinger were among the leading decisors in their communities, and their rulings and novellae became part of the universal Jewish heritage. Much has been written about their struggle against reformist trends and their efforts to fortify Orthodoxy. If we take account of the historical and cultural milieus in which they worked, we may be able to see their inclination to rule stringently on the issues at hand as part of a broader halakhic worldview. But this is not primarily a historical study, and what I want to do instead—thereby neither detracting from nor adding to the importance of local-historical context to an understanding of trends in halakhic rulings—is to examine the gender implications of these decisors' interpretive moves and of the ways in which they read the earlier halakhic literature.

Assessing the material from this perspective, it is striking, to say the least, that not one of the three great decisors makes any attempt to grapple with the sweepingly permissive ruling by the author of *Yam Shel Shelomoh* (R. Solomon Luria); indeed, none of them so much as mentions him.[46] Moreover, at least R. Akiva Eger and the *Ḥatam Sofer* wrote that they found no previous authority who had permitted a *mokh*, even though, as I shall show later, they were familiar with *Yam Shel Shelomoh* on *Yevamot*.

Feldman believes that because R. Luria's position was unknown or was voided as an individual's opinion, the more stringent rulings emerged as dominant and shaped the halakhic stance toward birth control. He believes that the *Ḥatam Sofer* and R. Akiva Eger were unaware of R. Luria's position:

> What direction, however, would the course of subsequent Responsa legislation have taken if the position of Luria had been known to these fountainheads of the non-permissive school? That it was in fact not known to them is evidenced in many ways. First, they make no reference at all to him. Second, with regard to pre-coital *mokh* even in cases of danger, they state explicitly at the outset, "I have not seen any authority who permits it."[47]

But Feldman seems to have erred here, for there is proof that both R. Akiva Eger and the *Ḥatam Sofer* well knew *Yam Shel Shelomoh* on *Yevamot*. The evidence is quite straightforward: they themselves cite the work at other points.[48]

We cannot date the pertinent responsa with precision, and it might be argued that the responsa on use of a *mokh* were written before their authors came to know of *Yam Shel Shelomoh* on *Yevamot*. But that argument strikes me as strained at best with respect to all three decisors, and at least in the case of the *Ḥatam Sofer* it lacks all support, for it can be shown beyond doubt that he knew of *Yam Shel Shelomoh* on *Yevamot* when he wrote his responsum on birth control.

The *Ḥatam Sofer*'s principal responsum on the subject (*Yoreh De'ah* 172) is undated, but other, dated, responsa show him referring to *Yam Shel Shelomoh* on *Yevamot* as early as 1800[49]—a mere four years after his initial venture into the writing of responsa.[50] Responsum *Yoreh De'ah* 172 was directed to R. Naftali when he was rabbi of Miklash, a post in which he appears to have been serving by 1814;[51] accordingly, that is the earliest date for the responsum at issue. In other words, even though we have evidence that *Ḥatam Sofer* knew of *Yam Shel Shelomoh* on *Yevamot* by 1800, he wrote later he had found no one who permits a precoital *mokh*, something explicitly permitted in *Yam Shel Shelomoh*.

The foregoing evidence demonstrates, in my judgment, the clear tendentiousness of the strictly nonpermissive halakhic rulings and the deliberate disregard of R. Luria's contrary view. I am not accusing the writers of conscious misogyny, nor do I believe they meant to place the lives of women in danger; that is certainly not the case. The *Ḥatam Sofer* himself expressly stated, as we have seen, that a wife has no obligation to afflict herself for the sake of her husband's performance of a commandment, much less to place herself in mortal danger.[52] For that reason, he does not even recommend drinking a "cup of roots."[53]

The question we must ask, then, is not whether these rulings were consciously misogynistic—they were not—but how they affected people, directly and indirectly, and what those effects tell us of the subconscious gender concepts that shaped them. On the most straightforward plane, what troubled the writers was the prospect of seed being wasted—a concern so serious in their eyes that it warranted, at least indirectly, marginalizing a woman's needs. According to the least permissive authorities, who forbid both precoital and postcoital *mokh* (R. Ettlinger), and even according to the *Ḥatam Sofer*, who forbids precoital *mokh* and recognizes the ineffectiveness of postcoital *mokh*,[54] the only remaining options are the sterilizing potion and sexual abstinence. The potion turned out to be dangerous, and even if decisors were not aware of that (something I doubt with respect to R. Ettlinger, who certainly was familiar with the *Ḥatam Sofer*'s comments on the issue), it is fair to assume that women knew it and avoided using it. As a practical matter, then, abstinence becomes the only option. But that option, though halakhically valid and equally difficult for both sexes, is potentially dangerous *only for women*, for it is fair to assume that husbands and wives alike would fail in their efforts to avoid all sexual contact for extended periods. It seems likely, then, that women would have "paid the price" and become pregnant at the risk of their lives, or, at least, at the risk of considerable pain and suffering (of the sort that the *Ḥatam Sofer* said they were permitted to avoid once the commandment to be fertile and increase had been fulfilled). In other words, the interpretations adopted by the nonpermissive decisors, together with their blatant disregard of R. Luria's ruling, which could have been adopted at least in the presence of danger, had the likely effect of endangering women's health and subjecting them to permanent sterilization if they drank a "cup of roots," or of subjecting them to dangerous and unwanted pregnancies if they could not remain entirely abstinent and used an ineffective postcoital *mokh*. To put it differently, "asking the woman question," as suggested by the feminist legal scholar Bartlett, produces different scholarly conclusions, conclusions having clear gender implications, especially with respect to the positions of the *Ḥatam Sofer*, which are usually accepted as being permissive with respect to women.

The tendentious nonpermissiveness of the halakhic decisions may also be explained against the background of a lowered birthrate in European countries, especially France, and the strict position taken by the Roman Catholic Church in response to that trend.[55] It may be that the halakhic decisors did not want to adopt a more lenient stance than the Church, lest they be portrayed as permissive or as encouraging sexual permissiveness—something that, in their view, would desecrate God's name.

The Late Nineteenth Century

If the eighteenth and early nineteenth centuries witnessed a clear tendency to rule nonpermissively and forbid use of a *mokh* even in the presence of danger, the remainder of the nineteenth century saw a degree of change in that posture. Decisors adopted a critical stance toward those extremely stringent tendencies and found a way to rule permissively at least in the presence of danger. Many, of course, felt bound by the rulings of the *Ḥatam Sofer* and R. Akiva Eger, and one can hardly say that the changes were revolutionary.[56] Still, it appears that interpretive options closer to those we suggested at the outset were being more widely adopted. The *Ḥatam Sofer*'s own son, the author of *Ketav Sofer*, disagreed with his father. In a responsum written in 1859, he is troubled by enforcing the prohibition on wasting seed even when there is danger, and he notes the problematic nature of relying on abstinence:

> Danger is treated as more weighty than a prohibition, and where life is at stake, we do not rely on the premise that, in most instances, the danger will not eventuate. Therefore . . . the prohibition is nevertheless set aside because of the possible danger. But, it may be asked, why not say that husband and wife should not engage in intercourse at all? We must say that because he has the duty to engage in conjugal relations with his wife at specified intervals, it is permitted for him to do so using a *mokh*. (*Ketav Sofer*, *'Even Ha-'Ezer* 26)

It should be noted that he permits intercourse with the use of a *mokh* even in a case of potential but nonconfirmed danger. Later in his responsum, he mentions R. Luria's permissive ruling, and he concludes by permitting the husband to engage in sexual relations with his wife even by means of "treading inside and sowing outside" if that is the only way to fulfill the commandment to engage in conjugal relations until she is cured and able to sustain a pregnancy. The *Ḥatam Sofer*'s grandson, R. Simeon Sofer, likewise follows R. Luria rather than his grandfather.[57]

The approach that permits use of a precoital *mokh* in the presence of danger attains its clearest and most comprehensive expression in a responsum by R. Shneur Zalman of Lublin, author of *Torat Ḥesed*. The responsum is one of the longest, most basic, and most exhaustive treatments of the issue.[58] The question presented to R. Shneur Zalman involved a woman who, according to her physicians, would be exposed to great danger if she were to give birth; the question was whether she could use a precoital *mokh*. R. Shneur Zalman begins by noting that since the two great scholars of the generation, R. Akiva Eger and the *Ḥatam Sofer*, had ruled nonpermissively, it might not be proper for him to consider the issue at all, "for who could follow them and be permissive?" Nevertheless, he believed both of them "had overlooked the words of the *Yam Shel Shelomoh*," and he thought it right, therefore, to take up the matter. He begins his analysis with the approaches of Rashi and Rabbeinu Tam and determines, on the basis of several sources, that Rabbeinu Tam wrote precoital, not a postcoital, *mokh*. In his opinion, when the medieval authorities reject Rashi's view in favor of Rabbeinu Tam's, they are taking the position that the sages permit the three women to place a *mokh* before intercourse. Moreover, R. Shneur Zalman believes that when the sages say that a woman should engage in intercourse in the usual manner and "Heaven will watch over fools," they are referring to a situation in which the danger is uncommon and heavenly mercy can therefore be relied on; but where the danger is clear and present, even the sages would no doubt acknowledge that a woman is obligated to use a *mokh*.[59] In other words, the majority of medieval authorities, who adopt Rabbeinu Tam's approach, would require a woman facing danger to use a precoital *mokh*. On the other hand, he does not recommend drinking a "cup of roots," for in his opinion (formed, he says, after discussions with physicians), it can damage the womb and bring about permanent sterility.

Given the analysis presented by R. Shneur Zalman, who construed Rabbeinu Tam's position consistently with our reconstruction of it and similarly understood the *Yam Shel Shelomoh*, it is unclear why, when all is said and done, he permits use of a *mokh* only by women faced with danger. I believe his interpretation is but one step away from a stance that permits all women to use a *mokh*, as does the *Yam Shel Shelomoh*, and it seems to me that R. Shneur Zalman tacitly acknowledges the legitimacy of that position.

In sum, even the decisors who take a more permissive approach, allowing use of a precoital *mokh* where danger is present, do not permit women in general to use this device. As a practical matter, we should recall that the analysis of "three women use a *mokh* in intercourse" turned primarily on the question of wasting seed and not on the legitimacy in principle of preventing pregnancy. In the absence of other effective birth control mechanisms, and after it became clear that the "cup of roots" could harm one's health or produce permanent sterility, women to a great degree were left exposed to unwanted, or even mortally dangerous, pregnancies (although, as I have said, that was a likely, indirect effect of the rulings and certainly not the intended purpose).

Had the decisors thought of women as having essential value independent of their procreative function, the strict rulings that forbid use of a *mokh* in the presence of danger—and even the more permissive rulings that forbid it only in the absence of danger—might have been rendered quite differently. On the premise that prevention of pregnancy is permitted as a matter of principle (except when the biblical commandment to be fertile and increase has not yet been fulfilled, a subject to which I shall return), and recognizing that until the twentieth century, the *mokh* was the primary mechanism available for doing so, halakhic rulings on the subject cannot be considered without taking account of these factors.

An Ideology of Procreation in Contemporary Halakhic Discourse

To this point, we have considered the halakhic genealogy of two central subjects: in chapter 1, the commandment to be fertile and increase, and in this chapter, the prevention of pregnancy. We have discovered a highly complex "halakhic narrative" related to these two aspects of procreation, a narrative that assigns great significance to the commandment to reproduce but, at the same time, accords substantial weight to other considerations that can balance what seems at first blush to be the unyielding duty to procreate. We have seen how, through the ages, recognition was given to the need for reasoned implementation of "in the evening," not only to avoid unduly compromising the husband's duty to study Torah but also to maintain domestic peace, to ensure one's ability to educate and support one's children, and to promote social solidarity.

How do contemporary halakhic rulings deal with these questions? Does the hegemonic halakhic discourse maintain the tendencies described above, or does it embark on a different course?

My central contention is that the weight now given to the commandment to procreate deviates from the balance struck in earlier halakhic discourse and that the overwhelming importance recently assigned to procreation—to the point of investing it with an aura of sanctity—is closely tied to an ideology of fertility and fostered by a gender perspective that allows for that ideology's forceful deployment.

The inquiry that follows will be focused primarily on the *rhetoric* of contemporary halakhic analyses, on the way in which they construe the sources, and on what I see as the hegemonic halakhic discourse they reflect. The specific question I want to pose is *how these analyses understand—and whether they even consider—the proper balance between the duty to procreate and the other needs and interests of men and women*. Of particular interest is whether any weight is given in halakhic discourse to a woman's needs beyond those related to her physical and mental health, for to consider those factors but no others is to maintain and bolster, even if unconsciously, the notion of woman as procreative vessel. Exclusive attention to health concerns suggests that the halakhah's underlying concern is to maintain a woman's ability to continue functioning in her procreative role.

Let me begin with the position of Rabbi Prof. Abraham Steinberg, which reflects much contemporary writing about procreation.[60] His understanding of halakhah and his construction of the sources are manifestations of an ideology with clear gender-based elements that bear examination. R. Steinberg's basic position on the importance of procreation is expressed quite clearly:

> Such an approach [world population control] is *contrary to Jewish thinking and Torah Law*, which requires each couple to enlarge their family and have many children as part of the precepts of procreation and populating the world. From a *Jewish demographic* standpoint, there is no justifiable fear of a population explosion. On the contrary, the survival of the Jewish people depends on procreation because they are among the smallest nations. Jews have suffered from *pogroms* and *forced conversions* and . . . Nazi holocaust. Jews suffer from *constant wars* with their Arab neighbors, as well as from *traffic*-related deaths. . . . However, procreation in Judaism may be limited according to the physical and mental health of the mother.[61]

Elsewhere he writes:

> There are some who have tried to show, on the basis of the law in the *gemara*, and even more so from the *Yerushalmi*, that a man is forbidden to engage in intercourse in a time of famine. . . . and Rama inferred from that a prohibition on engaging in intercourse in times of other troubles that are like famine. On that basis, they tried to show that when there is concern about adequate sustenance, the birthrate should be reduced; and since there is talk today of economic troubles resulting from the population explosion, Jews should take that into account and diminish their birthrate. But it is clear for several reasons that such a view has no merit.[62]

In addition, R. Steinberg sees a need to clarify that:

> Earning a livelihood is, in general, not sufficient justification for allowing contraception. Even if the husband is ill and unable to raise children, some Rabbis do not allow the wife to use contraceptives. However, if a man already has a large family and cannot afford more children, contraception may be allowed, particularly if the birth of additional children might lead to marital strife.[63]

The clear tendency here is to promote families that are as large as possible—for national, demographic, and religious reasons.

It seems to me that Steinberg reads the halakhic sources in a startlingly one-sided manner. For example, he offers several reasons not to rely on the prohibition of conjugal relations during a time of famine as a model for limiting procreation, even under difficult circumstances. First, he asserts that conditions in the world today differ substantially from those considered in the halakhic literature, and insists that there is no merit to the claim that the population explosion today requires reducing the birthrate. He seems to suggest that even in the face of actual famine, the halakhah limited the degree to which births should be avoided for economic reasons.

As a second reason for rejecting any diminution in the birthrate on the basis of a "time of famine" argument, Steinberg cites the statements in both Talmuds that people who have no children or who crave more children may engage in conjugal relations during times of famine, despite the general prohibition. On that basis, he infers that the commandment to be fertile and increase trumps the prohibition. But he fails to note that while the biblical commandment indeed trumps the prohibition, the prohibition continues to apply to one who has already fulfilled the biblical commandment. In other words, one might get the impression that a person who eagerly wants to have more children is permitted to engage in conjugal relations during a famine, but the actual picture is quite different: the permission extends only to one who has not yet fulfilled the commandment. Moreover, he cites the Tosafists' view that the prohibition is not normative law but only a recommendation for those motivated by personal piety; as I have already shown, however, that understanding is rejected by several leading interpreters. Maharsha and *Qorban Netan'el* explain that observance of the prohibition is a mere act of piety only on the part of one who has not yet fulfilled the commandment to be fertile and increase; but for one who has already fulfilled it, the prohibition is absolute. Steinberg mentions those who disagree with the Tosafists, but he does so only in a footnote.

In addition, and without any reference to the "years of famine" issue, Steinberg writes that personal economic considerations, or considerations of the family's welfare, do not as a rule justify the use of birth control. As I have shown, however, taking account of these factors is entirely legitimate, as proven by the comments of the author of *Terumat Ha-Deshen*, of Maharam Minẓ, and of the author of *'Arukh Ha-Shulḥan*, reviewed earlier.

In his article, Steinberg criticizes the lowered birthrate of Jewish women worldwide as compared to the populations among which they reside. He presents two tables that are meant to demonstrate the decreasing Jewish fertility rates in Israel between the years 1949 and 1963. Steinberg does not explicitly take note of the fact that these same tables relate the women's average birthrates to their levels of education and countries of origin.[64] The data in fact show a high degree of inverse correlation between education and birthrate; the higher a woman's educational attainments, the fewer children she bears.

The feminist critique presented at the beginning of the previous chapter has pointed out the connection between women's procreative potential or the "myth of motherhood" and their continued oppression. On the premise that education serves as the key to social mobility and to the attainment of higher social status and economic power, it appears that the data showing an inverse relation between years of education and number of children bear out the feminist critique. As egalitarian models of family life become more firmly established, of course, it becomes less necessary to posit a direct link between a woman's education and status and the number of children she bears. Nevertheless, as long as patriarchal cultural models remain deeply instilled in society, exceptions should not be seen as undercutting the rule.

Returning to Steinberg, for whom raising the Jewish birthrate is of paramount importance, the implication of his silence regarding the correlation between education and birthrate is that he is willing to allow women to bear the cost of this national goal. Immediately after presenting the tables, he offers the following comments:

> It should be noted that the general decline in the natural growth of the Jewish population is even more pronounced and serious against the background of the increased natural growth of the Arab population in Israel. In view of this worrisome trend, the government has found it proper to establish, within the Prime Minister's office, a special center to deal with demographic problems. . . . But that is not enough, and the disturbing fact is that the trend in the birthrate remains downward.[65]

Is it not startling to find weight being given, in a halakhic discussion, to a government policy with which the writer identifies? Does he regard women as a means for doing battle against demographic trends at the expense of their education, social status, and personal welfare?

To sum up the impression conveyed by Steinberg, we may say that his moral orientation is clear and unambiguous. Explicit demographic and national considerations, encompassing implicit gender-based considerations (that is, the assignment of higher value to procreative women than to educated women), generate a tendentious halakhic analysis that not only construes the sources so that they correspond to the writer's position but even disregards sources that are not conducive to that sort of construction.

A similar line of reasoning can be seen in an essay by Rabbi Shlomo Aviner addressed exclusively to a married or soon-to-be-married readership.[66] In a straightforward response to the question of how many children one is commanded to bear, he says that the requirement imposed by biblical law is one son and one daughter but that one is also bound by the rabbinic commandment of "in the evening." As for the question of whether, after bearing some number of children, one may cease having further pregnancies (that is, use birth control), he offers the following:

> One can never decide that he has begotten enough sons and daughters, for there is the commandment of "don't hold back your hand in the evening." Our rabbis, to be sure, disagreed over the severity of this law. . . . In any event, whether one takes it strictly or somewhat less so, this is a rabbinic commandment. And Maimonides wrote as follows: "as long as one has the strength, one is commanded to reproduce the image of God." And Tosafot wrote that if every Jewish family were satisfied with but one son and one daughter, "the progeny of Abraham [would long since have] come to an end."[67]

R. Aviner selectively cites those statements by Maimonides that are compatible with his own values, but he avoids presenting the full complexity of Maimonides's position. As we have seen, Maimonides writes that one does not violate "in the evening" by marrying a barren woman or refraining from regular conjugal relations at his wife's request or with her consent. To say that one can never decide that he has begotten enough children is to assert that even substantial difficulties must somehow be overcome in the name of conforming to the religious standard. R. Aviner concedes that when there is a specific difficulty related to mental or physical health, the halakhah will certainly take those factors into account; but the unambiguous message to young couples (and especially to the women) is that the higher their level of religious commitment, the higher they must set the bar with respect to enduring the hardships inherent in raising a large family. Even if the halakhah leaves room for the use of birth control in various circumstances, responsa formulated in this way construe such leniencies as an occasionally necessary evil, meant for "weaklings" of lower religious stature.

A comprehensive treatment of issues related to birth control can also be found in the rulings of Rabbi Elijah Judah Waldenberg, author of the *Ẓiẓ 'Eli'ezer*. He summarizes his perspective in the following principles, which suggest that birth control should not be permitted in the absence of concern about the wife's health:

> When there is no concern about a dangerous pregnancy, no illness, and no difficulty in childbirth but [a couple] wishes to prevent pregnancy for other reasons, the rules are as follows:

1. One should not permit the use of birth control in cases of concern about an adequate livelihood caused by lack of faith in God, who feeds and sustains all and prepares food for all His creatures.
2. One should not permit the use of birth control in order to avoid the difficulties of raising children.
3. Where illness or weak health makes it difficult for the wife to raise more children and a physician so determines, there may be a basis for temporarily permitting her, as the halakhic authority sees fit, to take an oral medication that indirectly brings about temporary sterility or to use postcoital birth control mechanisms.
4. Some are permissive . . . in cases where all of her children have strayed from the proper path and she is afraid of having additional children. Likewise, there are some who permit even direct action [as a means of birth control].
5. The halakhic authority must be extremely cautious and deliberate when approached with questions such as these, giving abundant consideration to when a permissive ruling may be issued. One must be very cautious in view of the liberties taken by the current generation in these areas and of frivolous women who lead one another astray. Accordingly, it is necessary to examine each situation in detail and to know when to draw near and when to be distant. (*Ẓiẓ 'Eli'ezer* 9:51; *sha'ar* 2, chap. 4; summary, 6)

These remarks, I believe, support my claim regarding the normative assumption of large families and the link between large families and faith in God. The final paragraph attests to the ideological and gender-based concept that guides him: from a gender perspective, it is clear that he believes women's primary, if not exclusive, role to be bringing children into the world and raising and caring for them. He evidently sees the accessibility of the birth control pill, and the absence of any formal halakhic reason to forbid its use, as something that threatens to undermine the foundations of the family and the desired augmentation of the commandment to be fertile and increase; otherwise, why the need to speak in terms of "the liberties taken by the current generation" or "frivolous women who lead one another astray"? Do the liberties take the form of smaller families, and does the disparaging label connote women who use the pill in order to bring fewer children into the world so they can develop in other ways and realize their talents in areas other than motherhood?

It should be noted here that decisors occasionally prefer to issue unwritten responses on these matters, which allow them to take account of pertinent factors in individual situations; and it is fair to assume that these responsa, delivered face to face, tend to be more permissive. But I believe that the refusal of these authorities to commit their more lenient responsa to writing, and the emphasis in their writings on the use of birth control only when pregnancy would be medically dangerous, are themselves indications of a certain gender bias. They are meant to impress on the reader's consciousness that birth control is a modern, alien import and that, as a normative matter, pregnancy should never be avoided except for health-related reasons. Moreover, this "modern, alien import" is associated primarily with the rise in legal and social status of the women who carry most of the burden of bearing and raising children. It follows that to treat birth control solely from the perspective of physical or mental health is to view the totality of a woman's essence in terms of her procreative capacity. In turn, women's feelings of obligation to raise large families can lead, in some sectors of the religious world, to extreme measures. For example, a woman having difficulty conceiving an additional child (after having already borne five!) may feel obligated to use artificial fertilization techniques to bring about the desired result.[68]

Birth Control Methods in Contemporary Halakhic Discourse

The contemporary analogue to the "cup of roots" is the birth control pill; accordingly, the theoretical conclusions reached with regard to the "cup of roots" become very relevant, given the pill's wide and easy availability. The pill, of course, is superior to the "cup of roots" in that its effects are only temporary, it does not damage the reproductive organs, and it has a relatively high degree of reliability.[69]

In view of the halakhic analysis I presented above, it is fair to assume that halakhic decisors would have no basis for restricting use of the pill in principle[70] (except when it had only recently been invented and it was not yet clear how well it worked, whether it was safe, and whether it might promote bleeding—and consequent menstrual impurity—between a woman's periods). As we have seen, a decisive majority of commentators and decisors believe that the "cup of roots" is the least halakhically problematic way to prevent a woman from becoming pregnant (even in the absence of difficult births).[71] But despite the clear implications of the sources we have considered, we find a pronounced tendency in contemporary halakhic rulings to reject these very simple and straightforward conclusions.

Rabbi Isaac Weiss, among the leading decisors in the Ultra-Orthodox community in Jerusalem, was asked whether a woman is permitted to take birth control pills for a limited time on account of weakness and fatigue. The interpretive moves he adopts in responding to the question leave no doubt, in my judgment, as to the ideological predisposition that drives his ruling. A reading of his analysis reveals a conscious interpretive course that patently contradicts the positions of all the earlier interpreters. At the very beginning of his responsum, as he sets out to summarize the interpretations of the issue that have been offered, one can already see his construction of the sources in a way that conflicts with reality:

> To briefly summarize the opinions regarding a woman drinking a cup of roots, there are three approaches. The first permits it even in the absence of any difficulty [in childbirth], and it is the approach taken by *Ḥelqat Meḥoqqeq* and *Beit Shemu'el*. . . . The second considers it to be the same as a precoital *mokh*, which is permitted only in the presence of danger, and that is the approach of the *'Aẓei 'Arazim*. . . . The third, which is determinative, is that it is permitted only where there is difficultly in childbirth or similar problems, and it is the approach of the *Baḥ* and Maharshal, cited in the decisors, and it appears to be the approach accepted by the great halakhic authorities. . . . If so, then in the case before us as well, with respect to the woman [who wants to use it] to be able to recuperate, since [her fertility] will be annulled only temporarily, there is no prohibition here. (*Minḥat Yiẓḥaq* 5:113)

Weiss identifies three approaches to drinking a "cup of roots." His summary gives the impression that the first and second approaches are of equal weight measured by the number of opinions supporting them, but that is not, in fact, the case. The first approach is in the mainstream, adopted by all the medieval authorities and most of the later decisors, while the second, that of the *'Aẓei 'Arazim*, is an individual's opinion that is refuted in several rulings.[72] Beyond that, his claim that the third approach—the one permitting use of the "cup of roots" only in cases of difficult childbirth—is the determinative one, *has absolutely no basis in the sources*. It is at most the opinion of a minority, adopted by the *Baḥ* and Maharshal in opposition to all the others. But even if he is speaking here only of the *Shulḥan 'Arukh* and its commentators, how can he ignore the *Taz*? True, Weiss concludes that the pill is permitted (subject to the limitations noted); but for our purposes, his construction of the sources is no less important than the conclusion he arrives at. If his view is that pregnancy may be prevented only after the commandment to be fertile and increase has been fulfilled, and, even then, only on account of difficult childbirth or infirmity, then there is no room left for consideration of a woman's emotional or intellectual needs beyond simple physical health. The gap between the views of the earlier decisors and R. Weiss's summary of those views is so great that it displays, in my judgment, a gender-based assessment, latent or blatant, of a woman's place and role with respect to bearing children. If a woman is not permitted to avoid pregnancy even in the absence of difficult childbirth, then she cannot escape being construed exclusively as a "mother machine."

A line of interpretation with similar gender assumptions appears in Rabbi Moses Feinstein's responsum on *sirus* of a woman. As I showed earlier, a decisive majority of authorities consider physical neutering of a woman to be forbidden only rabbinically (as distinct from neutering of a man, which is forbidden by biblical law), and a permissive ruling should be possible in cases of danger. Rabbi Feinstein, however, chooses to adopt R. Elijah of Vilna's view that the prohibition is biblical and rules accordingly—without mentioning that it is a lone opinion that the contemplated act is forbidden.[73] He concludes the responsum by permitting the specific woman in question to use a *mokh* in intercourse, because pregnancy would endanger her medically; that is consistent with his view that a *mokh* is forbidden except in the presence of danger. But, as in Weiss's responsum, the obvious gap between the decisional tradition and the minority position that is adopted can attest to a set of values that dictates a nonpermissive halakhic decision.[74]

Feinstein's decisions on birth control were issued over the course of many years,[75] but it appears that we can extract from them a consistent, fundamental position that permits use of a *mokh* solely in the presence of danger. The principles that underlie Feinstein's rulings on use of a *mokh* (which he identifies with the modern diaphragm[76]) can be summed up as follows:

1. Use of a *mokh* is forbidden in principle because it is entails wasting seed.
2. Use of a *mokh* is permitted where an additional pregnancy and birth would be dangerous for the woman or for an existing child. The basis for consent is the novel idea that in the presence of danger, the prohibition on wasting seed is not applicable.
3. The definition of danger is flexible and fluid; it depends on the situation and on the extent to which the questioners are God-fearing.

I would like to focus on Feinstein's first and central responsum on the subject, issued as early as 1935. As noted, this responsum is especially interesting because of its innovative contention that danger can annul the prohibition on the wasting of seed that is entailed in use of a *mokh*. Also of interest are his interpretive moves with respect to the positions of the medieval authorities.[77]

R. Feinstein infers from Rashi's comments that it would make no sense to read the sages as forbidding use of a *mokh* in cases where the danger clearly exceeds the natural risk of pregnancy. That interpretation opens the door to the claim that Rashi's approach allows a precoital *mokh* in circumstances of danger. But still, one may ask: regardless of the danger, how can a precoital *mokh* be permitted if it entails violation of the severe prohibition on wasting seed? Would it not be preferable to abstain entirely from conjugal relations and avoid violating the prohibition? Feinstein's innovative response is that the prohibition on wasting seed applies only where the potential for pregnancy exists and is deliberately avoided. But a woman for whom pregnancy would be dangerous is forbidden to become pregnant, and it follows that there is no potential pregnancy in such a situation. Meanwhile, the husband remains subject to the commandment of providing his wife periodic conjugal relations; therefore, it is permissible to use even a precoital *mokh*, so that both the prohibition and the obligation may be observed. In other words, R. Feinstein does not reason that the danger trumps the prohibition on wasting seed (though it would appear as a practical matter that seed is wasted); rather, his interpretation is that where pregnancy would be dangerous, the act of intercourse using a *mokh* does not constitute waste of seed at all. The emphasis on that point is important in clarifying the remainder of his approach and in understanding why he is careful to stress the danger itself and the danger to the wife in particular; without that danger, the use of a *mokh* would entail commission of a prohibited act. Feinstein completely disregards R. Solomon Luria's opinion that intercourse using a *mokh* does not entail waste of seed.

In his other responsa, Feinstein consistently reiterates the prohibition on using a *mokh* except in cases of danger. In a later responsum, from 1958, he writes:

> And what his exalted Torah highness [an honorific applied to the addressee of the responsum] heard from some rabbi, to the effect that in Lithuania, all women were permitted [to use a *mokh*] for two years after giving birth, is a lie; for I know of many rabbis who were extremely strict, and I never heard of anyone who permitted [use of a *mokh*] by women in general, for the entire discussion involves only cases where danger is present. (*'Iggerot Mosheh, 'Even Ha-'Ezer* 1:64)[78]

He stresses that use of a *mokh* is forbidden even if the husband has already fulfilled the commandment to be fertile and increase and even where there is difficulty in earning a living or where an additional pregnancy *would impair the woman's health*.[79] It is permitted solely in circumstances of actual and present danger, for only then can the prohibition on wasting seed be overcome.

How is "danger" to be defined? It evidently depends on the situation. In one instance, R. Feinstein writes that he has heard that kidney disease does not pose a danger as long as the woman remains confined to bed throughout the pregnancy; accordingly, use of a *mokh* is not to be permitted in that case.[80] On the other hand, with regard to a case in which a couple reports beating their children "because of their being too weak to raise children," R. Feinstein deems the woman clinically depressed and regards the situation as dangerous enough to warrant use of a *mokh*.[81] And in another case when he knew that the woman posing the question was truly God-fearing, he permits use of a *mokh* even where the danger is only potential, but he admonishes her not to publicize the ruling.[82]

In a still later responsum (1981), R. Feinstein rules that use of a *mokh* during intercourse is permitted in a case of danger to an existing child (consistent with the *baraita* itself) but emphasizes that here, too, the danger must be real. Thus, he forbade the use of birth control by a woman who was caring for a three-year-old daughter who was ill with cancer; he reasoned that it was possible to find an alternative caregiver and that the mother's pregnancy would not necessarily jeopardize the care of her child. (In this particular case, the husband had not yet fulfilled the biblical commandment to be fertile and increase.)[83]

With the invention of the pill, the concern about wasting seed—the principal problem associated with use of a *mokh*—would appear to have been obviated. During the early years of the pill, however, it frequently caused bleeding between menstrual periods, and R. Feinstein therefore continued to regard the *mokh* as preferable to the pill:

> As for the recent invention of a pill to be swallowed as a medicine that prevents pregnancy, it appears that most women taking the pill see a drop of blood that makes them *niddah* [menstrually impure]. . . . My son-in-law . . . Rabbi Moshe David Tendler . . . inquired of the doctor who invented this pill and [the latter] acknowledged to him that sixty percent of women taking the pill see some blood, but non-Jews are not concerned about it. And so it is necessary to allow her to use the rubber [diaphragm] that she places in her body. (*'Iggerot Mosheh, 'Even Ha-'Ezer* 1:65)

This concern about bleeding, and the broader concern that the pill itself might harm a woman's health, led to the reservations about its use that pervade Feinstein's rulings on the issue. Still, the availability of the pill brought about a certain easing of his approach, and after resolving the bleeding issue—by directing the woman to examine herself over the course of a month to be sure the pill was not inducing bleeding[84]—he permitted its use in the following circumstances:

> With regard to the pill that prevents a woman from becoming pregnant, it certainly does not invoke the prohibition on wasting seed. And if pregnancy would be difficult for the woman because of illness, or even because of weakness making the pregnancy more difficult than for most women, it may be permitted even if "be fertile and increase" has not yet been fulfilled. If she is weak, she may wait a short interval [before becoming pregnant] until she becomes stronger. And that is even more the case if "be fertile and increase" has already been fulfilled, in which case a delay of up to three years may be permitted so she may regain her strength. But if she is ill, even if [pregnancy] would not endanger her but only make her illness worse, it is reasonable to

> say that if "be fertile and increase" has already been fulfilled, she may entirely avoid [pregnancy] in this manner, for a woman is not subservient to her husband to the point of becoming more ill than women in general for the sake of [fulfilling] the commandment of "for habitation." (*'Iggerot Mosheh, 'Even Ha-'Ezer* 3:24)

Elsewhere, R. Feinstein even permits use of the pill to avoid pregnancy for "an economic reason or some other pressing reason,"[85] as long as the commandment to be fertile and increase has already been fulfilled.

In light of the foregoing, it would be interesting to examine R. Feinstein's stance regarding a woman who wanted to avoid pregnancy for the sake of her own intellectual or professional development; in such a case, would he find a basis for ruling permissively? R. Elyakim G. Ellinson posed that very question to R. Feinstein, but it is unclear from the formulation of his response whether the question pertained to a woman delaying marriage because she wanted to study or to the more general question of whether it was preferable to defer marriage or to marry but defer pregnancy. But even if the question was formulated generally, it is clear that R. Feinstein believed marriage should not be deferred, and that use of effective birth control measures should not be permitted; the couple should rely, at most, on the method of "safe days."[86] However, we have to ask here: if the pill entails no violation of the prohibition on wasting seed, why permit only the use of a birth control mechanism known to be unreliable? In other words, if the commandment to procreate is already being deferred, why not permit the pill if its use contravenes no prohibition? It may be that this responsum bolsters the claim that R. Feinstein's reservations about use of the pill (expressed in responsa issued over the course of many years) do not derive solely, or even primarily, from formal halakhic concerns about interperiod bleeding or about the health risks of taking the pill. The greater concern, perhaps, is that the pill's relative availability, ease of use, and reliability may lead to "licentiousness" or facilitate "family planning," which he regards as a way to evade God's will.[87]

R. Feinstein's explicit comments about a woman's principal roles in life clarify why these discussions take her into account only in cases of certain danger, possible danger, or physical or psychological weakness:

> For ordinary women in the world are not wealthy, and they are assigned the task of raising boys and girls, which is the labor that is most important to

> God, may He be blessed, and to the Torah. And so God, may He be blessed, made it in the nature of every animal species that females raise the young, and He did not exclude the human species from that rule; for women by their nature are better equipped to raise children. And for that reason He eased their burden, exempting them from Torah study and from time-determined positive commandments. And so even if the ways of the world change for all women, and [are different] for wealthy women at all times, and even if it is possible to assign child rearing to certain men and women, as [is done] in our lands, there is no change in the law of the Torah or even rabbinical law. And no battle [for change] will be effective, for there is no power that can change anything even by universal consensus; and women who stubbornly want to battle for change are considered *deniers of Torah*. (*'Iggerot Mosheh*, *'Orah Ḥayyim* 4:49; emphasis mine)

The gender significance of this type of understanding is that a woman is viewed primarily through the prism of procreation. Considerations foreign to that purpose, such as her desire to prevent pregnancy for significant reasons other than physical weakness or more serious health problems, are treated as simply irrelevant to the discussion.

Family Planning (Deferring Births; Intervals Between Children)

Contemporary halakhic studies treat the use of specific birth control mechanisms and the manner in which they operate (does it waste seed?) separately from the more general question of family planning (is it permitted to circumscribe one's fulfillment of the commandment to be fertile and increase?).[88] For methodological reasons, I will adopt the distinction as well, though I am not convinced that the dichotomy is all that sharp. It seems to me that deliberations over the permissibility of the *mokh*—which became the dominant, if not the exclusive, question addressed in the responsa literature on premodern birth control mechanisms—involved more than the formal halakhic question of whether it entailed waste of seed. In the absence of other effective methods of birth control, the argument that the *mokh* indeed entailed wasting seed was transformed into a political issue in the full sense of the word. The emergence, worldwide, of concerns regarding population control and modern attitudes toward childbearing that tend to diminish its value elicited a restrictive halakhic reaction that sought to counter those trends through halakhic control or force. Consequently, the nonpermissive approach, which forbade use of the *mokh*, came to dominate—even though alternative interpretations might have led in a different direction. Limiting the permissibility of using a *mokh* was an effective way to ensure maintenance of the birthrate in the face of undesirable trends.

This may explain the strict rulings of Hungarian and German rabbis in the late eighteenth and early nineteenth centuries and of many who followed them. Since the invention of the pill, it is harder to dismiss birth control as wasting seed, because the predominant method does not violate this prohibition. Accordingly, most halakhic analyses now focus directly on the question of family planning. Questions include deferral by a married couple of the commandment to be fertile and increase, intervals between births, and overall size of the family. Here too, as we shall see, halakhic force has been deployed, sometimes only implicitly or allusively, to maintain the ethos of large families.

Thus far, we have considered the legitimacy in principle of a woman making herself sterile or using a *mokh* to prevent pregnancy, but that is not the complete picture. In a monogamous environment, a woman is also obligated to enable her husband to fulfill the commandment to be fertile and increase. Accordingly, one must ask not only which birth control mechanisms are permissible but also at what stage and under what circumstances she is permitted to use them.

A central halakhic text regarding family planning is the statement by Maimonides in *Hilkhot 'Ishut*:

> A woman who after marriage gives her husband permission to withhold her conjugal rights from her, is permitted to do so. When does this apply? When he has children, for in that case he has already fulfilled the commandment [to be fertile and increase]. If, however, he has not yet fulfilled it, he is obligated to have sexual intercourse with her according to his schedule until he has children, because this is a positive commandment of the Torah, as it is said ["Be fertile and increase"] (Gen. 1:28). (Maimonides, *Mishneh Torah, Hilkhot 'Ishut* 15:1; Yale Judaica Series trans., p. 93)

This approach seems to suggest that one may not defer fulfillment of the commandment to be fertile and increase; on the contrary, one must begin striving to fulfill it as soon as one is married and not stop until the biblical commandment has been fulfilled. Accordingly, once the halakhic principles regarding permissibility of particular birth control methods have been settled, the question to be answered is whether a man is permitted to temporarily defer his fulfillment of the biblical commandment to be fertile and increase. It seems to me that our inquiry into the commandments of "for habitation" and "in the evening" as well as R. Feinstein's treatment of the issue have shown that no particular difficulties are posed by using birth control to ensure intervals between births once the biblical commandment has been fulfilled.

In today's environment, the question can be worded as follows: is it permissible for a couple to defer bearing children if the only alternative to using birth control is to delay marriage? One may further ask whether the decisors would rule differently if the requested deferral were for the husband's benefit (for example, to allow him to continue studying Torah or to complete his professional training) than if it were for the wife's benefit, for similar reasons. (The husband is bound by the commandment to be fertile and increase; the wife herself is not bound by the commandment but, in the *Ḥatam Sofer*'s words, "is subservient to her husband" for the sake of fulfilling the commandment to procreate.) I will first examine the Ultra-Orthodox approach to this issue and then consider Nationalist Orthodox and Modern Orthodox perspectives.

THE ULTRA-ORTHODOX OUTLOOK

Virtually no Ḥaredi decisor treats the question of family planning as we have just formulated it. In their view, the sole halakhic category that justifies use of any form of birth control is "danger" or possible danger, a category whose limits are defined by a given woman's strength or frailty, insofar as it pertains to pregnancies and child rearing. I have found no halakhic formulation of the issue that raises, even theoretically, the question of deferring pregnancies for reasons other than mental or physical health, and certainly not to enable the woman to pursue studies or professional development. This is hardly surprising, given the clear division of roles within the Ḥaredi world; but I think the situation is likely to change in the future, thanks to the growing number of Ḥaredi women who are working outside the home to support their families and allow their husbands to devote themselves exclusively to Torah study.

A few examples will illustrate the point. Rabbi Samuel Ha-Levi Wosner, one of the leading contemporary Ḥaredi decisors, has frequently written on the subject of birth control. It is evident from his writings that he considers the use of contraceptives only by women for whom pregnancy is or might be dangerous. He permits such women to use a *taba'at* (lit. a "ring," probably referring to a diaphragm; see below) but only for a limited period (up to half a year), following which their situation must be reexamined, "lest permissive rulings become excessive."[89] Of birth control in cases where danger is not a factor, he writes:

> In any case, I reiterate that what we have said applies, in my humble opinion, only in a case of possible danger. It is not like those among the people who transgress, regarding their actions as permitted even though they lack any basis in halakhah; and [what they do] entails annulment of "be fertile and increase" and waste of seed, and it impedes the indwelling of God's presence among the Jews.[90]

To similar effect are the comments of Rabbi Yekutiel Judah Halberstam (of Sanz),[91] though his concern about wasting seed leads him to forbid even a *taba'at* (most likely a diaphragm, for he depicts the *taba'at* as covering the opening of the uterus) and allows only spermicidal jelly. Neither rabbi, as far as I could tell, refers to women interested in spacing pregnancies or deferring births.

Rabbi Moses Judah Landau writes more explicitly of "family planning," which he equates with treachery against the Jewish people and considers an impediment to the redemption:

> Various agents have recently undertaken a course of treachery against our people, a campaign of propaganda and incitement in favor of "family planning" and a diminished birthrate. . . . This apostate notion of [reliance on] "my strength and the might of my hand" is the origin of "family planning" that takes account of the parents' economic circumstances or their "comfort." But we know that truth is the complete opposite of this, "and I was created only to serve my Creator." . . . It is certainly proper to gather one's strength to stand forcefully against such actions . . . and to the women of

> Israel, I issue this urgent call: protect your souls! Do not heed the advice of those who would incite you to abandon your [share in the] world [to come] and to be among those who impede the redemption.[92]

Rabbi Joshua Isaiah Neubart refers expressly to the prevention of pregnancy not for the purpose of avoiding danger but to allow an opportunity to complete one's studies or become economically established:

> Lately I have been hearing questions regarding family planning, which is to say, imposing on ourselves decrees of annihilation, Heaven forbid. Of course, I do not expect a "baby factory," Heaven forbid. But why should we intervene for "medical" reasons in the growth of the Jewish people? Where has the subject of family planning been heard of among us? Moreover, I have read, young couples are getting married with the intent from the outset to live as animals until the wife completes her studies, until they have finished paying off the mortgage on their magnificent apartment, and certainly one cannot make do without a splendid car, all of this at the cost of the birthrate.[93]

It is worth noting that R. Neubart does not speak disparagingly of the fact that childbearing might be deferred to allow the man to complete his professional training; he rejects only a deferral of pregnancy to allow the woman to complete her studies. He characterizes the couple as living *like animals*—no less—if the woman, as a subject in her own right, weighs her interests and desires against the duty to procreate, even though childbearing is merely being deferred, not permanently avoided. His ideological posture, to say nothing of his gender-based understanding, requires no further discussion.

NATIONALIST ORTHODOX AND MODERN ORTHODOX PERSPECTIVES

In contrast to the Ultra-Orthodox rulings, in Nationalist Orthodox[94] and Modern Orthodox halakhic writings, we do find explicit consideration of deferred childbearing and of allowing intervals between children for the purpose of allowing the wife to work outside the home.

R. Aviner is among the prominent decisors who forbid deferring conception of a first child. He relies on the opinion of his teacher, Rabbi Dov

Auerbach, who forbade use of birth control immediately after the wedding for any reason other than danger to the wife:

> It is certain that in this circumstance, there is no way to permit it, for the reason they marry is to be fertile and increase. And so there is no possibility of becoming exempt from it, except in cases of danger. And even if he wants to do so in order to study Torah, there is no basis for permitting it.[95]

He does permits some spacing of children, however, even before the biblical commandment to procreate has been fulfilled, when there is great need for it, as when caring for a number of children in quick succession becomes very difficult for the woman or when spacing is necessary to ensure that all children receive adequate attention.[96] Nonetheless, as I have already shown, R. Aviner leaves no room to doubt that the number of children a couple produces is linked to their degree of religious faith. As a result, even his seemingly permissive position regarding intervals between births must be ideologically contextualized as the position of one who encourages large families and the gender-based notion that a woman's primary role is in the home, raising children. In the voice of an imaginary woman, R. Aviner writes as follows with respect to the role of motherhood, birthrate, and women's education:

> Yes, I will be a professor. My husband is completing a doctorate in physics; I am not jealous of him, but I will be a professor. I sense that I have the capacity to do it. I want degrees and a career; I will be a professor, I will succeed, and my students will hold me in esteem. I want equality. This isn't my suggestion; it was the master of the universe who created man and woman as equals, equally in the image of God. I have a pure soul, and I believe in myself. I certainly differ from my husband but I am not inferior to him. I will be a professor. This is a dream I have nurtured since my school days. I am committed to it, and I even know in what field: a professor of education, of childhood education, with lots of degrees—a degree in femininity, a degree in marriage, a degree in motherhood.
>
> Why are you smiling? This is no joke. My husband creates electronic components for some important instrument, and I will create children. I will create souls. So why are you laughing? Is that less important? No, it is much more important; I will be a professor of the education of my children . . .

> motherhood is a profession and also sacred work. It is a huge task. . . . And my kingdom is the home. I will be a professor of the home.[97]

Rabbi Yehuda Henkin takes an interesting view of the rationale for permitting or prohibiting the planned spacing of children. In a responsum written in 1978,[98] he recounts that his grandfather permitted women to prevent pregnancy for as long as four or five years following a child's birth when that was necessary to enable the mother to care for her child, regardless of whether her husband had already fulfilled the commandment to be fertile and increase. R. Henkin himself rules that way as well. The permissive ruling is based on the welfare of the child, the promotion of which R. Henkin considers to be an element of fulfilling the commandment to procreate. Still, one must note his following comments:

> If a question arises, I ascertain whether the woman wants to avoid pregnancy to promote the benefit of the child or to be able to go out to work. In that regard, it is necessary to distinguish one country from another. In the United States, children remain home until the age of five, when they go to kindergarten. That is not the case in the Holy Land, where they go to preschool at the age of three or less and the woman then goes out to work. In such cases, *one should not rule permissively* [emphasis mine].[99]

R. Henkin's responsum seems premised on the idea that all child-rearing problems are obviated by the existence of well-run preschools and kindergartens; when such arrangements are available, the professional or financial interests of the woman must yield to the interest of bringing another child into the world. When the good of a child is at stake, birth control may be permitted, but when what is at issue is the good of the woman—as when she wants to work outside the home—birth control will not be allowed.

As we have already seen in the responsa of other decisors, no consideration whatsoever is given to the woman as a subject, having her own desires, needs, and interests, *except in cases of danger*. Where danger is not an issue, posing the halakhic question from the woman's point of view results in a nonpermissive ruling. A woman therefore must choose between waiving her standing as an independent subject, thereby gaining a more sympathetic ear with respect to family planning, and asserting her standing at the risk of receiving a ruling at odds with her interests. To put it differently, as long as women fulfill their destiny as determined in the patriarchal view of the world, they may find, paradoxically, that the practical effects of the resulting halakhic rulings tend to compromise that worldview. Conversely, a woman who tries to avoid playing by the rules of the patriarchal game almost certainly will be denied a hearing. Both alternatives show the continued dominance of the gender-based notion that sees the primary, central role of a woman to be the bearing and raising of children (in order to facilitate her husband's fulfillment of the commandment) even where women are no longer satisfied with that role alone—and perhaps because of that dissatisfaction.

Nationalist Orthodox and Modern Orthodox thinking about family planning—primarily, the desired intervals between pregnancies—has been further illuminated by recent discussions of the issue in the pages of the journal *Ẓohar*.[100] Those discussions manifest a veiled conflict between conservatives and liberals and between positive and negative perspectives on women's desire to find fulfillment beyond the reproductive sphere.

The discussion opened with an article by Uri Levy, a gynecologist,[101] whose central argument is that the latest scientific studies show the ideal interval between a birth and the next pregnancy to be from eighteen to twenty-three months. He sees this conclusion as consistent with the talmudic view,[102] which he understands to be that a woman needs a recovery period of two years after giving birth and that becoming pregnant sooner can harm her physically and psychologically. Levy points as well to what he perceives as the widespread understanding within the contemporary observant community that birth control is permissible only for a woman for whom pregnancy or childbirth is particularly difficult, and he asks why the rabbinic view that a woman requires a two-year recovery period is not applied. Halakhic authorities claim that women who bear many children with only a year or less between birth and pregnancy "seem 'well' and their children seem 'well.'"[103] But Levy does not accept that argument, for a person's state of health cannot be reliably assessed simply by looking at her. He believes the studies showed impairment of a woman's health and the health of her children when births and pregnancies are very close. He concludes that because there is no prohibition on a woman preventing a pregnancy or even making herself sterile, she is required (not merely permitted) to prevent pregnancy for eighteen to twenty-four months following a birth, and he urges physicians and halakhic decisors to recommend that they do so.[104]

In response, Rabbi Joel and Dr. Hannah Katan (a gynecologist) strongly dispute Dr. Levy's conclusions. Challenging both his understanding of the talmudic passage and the conclusions he draws from the medical studies, they argue that he meets neither the halakhic nor the medical burden of proof. It seems to me that the dispute does not really turn on how one talmudic passage or another is to be understood. Joel and Hannah Kattan systematically promote their position in numerous articles making plain their underlying preference for families that are as large as possible. Regarding a woman who has been married four years and, by her own choice, has not yet borne a child, Hannah Kattan writes: "She has given voice to the hedonist, selfish, spoiled way of life that is spreading even within the modern religious camp in many areas."[105]

Rabbi Yigal Ariel's reaction, more than any other, attests to the cultural construct implicit in the treatment of family planning.[106] He points out that a leading decisor, Rabbi Kalman Kahana, included the following statement in his popular, contemporary manual *Tahorat Bat Yisra'el*:

> Preventing pregnancy in any way at all is among the most severe prohibitions. A husband and his wife therefore must be extremely careful not to stumble into committing this serious sin. Even if the physicians find reason for concern that pregnancy would pose a mortal risk, they should not rule on the matter for themselves but should pose the question to a sage.[107]

R. Ariel himself finds it hard to imagine that so prominent an authority could have formulated the prohibition on birth control in such harshly absolute terms:

> Many families no doubt took these words simplistically, as an absolute obligation, which tended to encourage a high birthrate within the religious community. But the decisor must also envision the women who paid for that with shortened lives marked by suffering and illness; and who will be called to account for that?[108]

Consequently, R. Ariel believes that R. Kahana's statement is the product of "historical accident." He suggests that the book was written at a time when birth control necessarily entailed either unrealistic abstinence or forbidden wasting of seed, and though the treatise was widely disseminated during the 1960s, when the pill had already been developed, the wording for some reason remained unchanged in later editions. But it seems to me that the failure to modify the wording grew out of the ideological strain that sees an abundance of children as a religious obligation of the first order. This was no "historical accident"; rather, the absence of any change in the later editions reflects the deliberate and well-thought-out realization of an ideological agenda.

R. Ariel objects to depicting large families as the model mandated by the halakhah. The family, to be sure, is highly esteemed and bears the mantle of "the sanctity of a commandment," as he puts it; but there is no clear guide as to its proper size. Large families were not the norm in every generation; at times, the opposite may have been true. Economic, medical, and cultural circumstances clearly have a bearing on the issue, and R. Ariel notes that "most of my teachers and rabbis had small families, which seems to have been typical of the entire previous generation."[109] Although he does not explicitly consider the question of family planning for purposes of allowing a woman to pursue her career, R. Ariel's sharp critique of strictly nonpermissive trends with regard to birth control amounts to an almost subversive voice. But while we can rejoice in his view of the revolutionary expansion of families in our generation, it remains true that:

> There exist families larger than can be physically, emotionally, economically, and educationally sustained, and their circumstances border on the tragic. The mother does not have the strength to maintain herself, they cannot care for the children. . . . and it is a great desecration of God's name to commit the error of thinking that the situation is imposed by the halakhic norm and that doing anything to change it is forbidden.[110]

Of all the opinions voiced in the *Ẓohar* debate, only Naomi Wolfson's refers sympathetically to the *intellectual* needs of women.[111] Wolfson identifies two principal sets of circumstances in which young, religious couples consider deferring childbearing. Either the wife finds herself torn between her yearning to have children and her yearning to realize her talents and develop her distinctiveness as a person, or both husband and wife want to solidify their marriage before having children. Wolfson considers these interests to be "genuine, deserving of serious consideration."[112] Not one of the male participants in this debate has written so explicitly of the considerations raised by women in support of deferring pregnancy before the biblical commandment to procreate has been fulfilled. Moreover, Wolfson calls on decisors to heed women's voices with respect to the intervals between births: "In my humble opinion, when the practical question is brought before a halakhic decisor, it is fair to rely on the woman; and just as she is believed in all matters related to her [menstrual] purity, it seems she should be relied on in this matter as well."[113]

AN ALTERNATIVE PERSPECTIVE ON GENDER

Despite all the foregoing, a different sort of halakhic thinking has recently begun to emerge.

Already in 1977, noting that the question of family planning had been raised by a significant number of young couples, R. Getsel Ellinson expressed surprise that no halakhic authorities had adequately addressed the issue in their written response.[114] R. Ellinson's own analysis suggests that two ways of deferring the commandment to be fertile and increase must be considered, namely, delaying marriage and marrying but practicing birth control. Finding no practical difference between them, he concludes it is preferable to marry and use birth control, for marriage itself is greatly valued. R. Ellinson also asks whether fulfillment of the commandment can be deferred to enable the *wife* to complete her professional training.[115] As far as I can tell, he is the first to pose this question from the woman's perspective and is among the few authorities to suggest that there may be more permissive halakhic options. He reasons that it is the man who is bound by the commandment to be fertile and increase, and that a woman certainly is permitted to defer marriage until she has completed her training. As long as she remains single, she is under no obligation with respect to the commandment. Accordingly, if she asks her husband-to-be, before they are married, to waive temporarily his right to have her bear his children, it is permissible to delay childbearing so she can pursue her professional training. I believe that underlying R. Ellinson's permissive ruling is the treatment of a woman's education as something of value, something religiously legitimate. Without that threshold determination, there would be no basis for adopting a permissive interpretation on the formal-halakhic plane.

R. 'Aharon Lichtenstein offers a similar analysis and also finds that childbearing may be deferred in certain circumstances:

It should be noted that, as a practical matter, it is not uncommon for quarrels to arise between a husband and wife over such matters, though it is difficult to define precisely what constitutes a "quarrel." To the extent there are more children, the burden, as a rule, falls primarily upon the wife: the physical burden of pregnancy and, thereafter, the burden of child care. The burden acquires added bite when the woman wants to advance her personal career, and her bearing the principal burden is likely to generate tensions.[116]

R. Lichtenstein applies the halakhic rubric of "quarrel," used by earlier decisors in other contexts,[117] as the vehicle for legitimating the woman's interests. His position seems to stem from his moral outlook, which accords legitimacy to the question of family planning, a conflict that arises from a clash between values—and, perhaps, commandments—that should not necessarily be seen as contradictory: personal development and fulfillment of the commandment to be fertile and increase. In contrast to the position of the Ultra-Orthodox decisors cited above, R. Lichtenstein writes as follows:

Some see family planning solely as an expression of debased modernism. Were that the case, it would be relatively easy to rule in this area. . . . [But] I would say that, in most instances, we find a clash of values or even of commandments. From a communal perspective, we face the inclination to grow the nation and to increase its human resources. . . . From an individual perspective, [however] . . . the commandment to establish and expand a family may come into conflict with the realization of inclinations that can certainly be regarded as personally and religiously legitimate: continued Torah study, acquiring a trade, professional advancement, maintaining personal tranquility, providing a proper education to one's children, etc.[118]

Rabbi Jacob Ariel renders women's concerns even more central to his analysis. He finds a basis to permit the deferral of continued childbearing for economic or educational reasons, including to allow the wife to complete her studies. However, he does not permit a couple to forgo childbearing entirely or to delay conception of a first child.[119] He infers from his analysis of Maimonides that the commandment to be fertile and increase may be fulfilled throughout one's life; it is desirable that one seize the opportunity to fulfill it as soon as possible, but there is no obligation to do so immediately when there is good reason to defer it. Like R. Lichtenstein before him, R. Ariel is among the few halakhic authorities who empathize with a woman's need for education and professional training and recognize the possibility of conflict between those considerations and continued childbearing. His responsum assumes that women nowadays acquire an education as do men, that "the professional degree gained through one's studies today is tantamount to wealth,"[120] and that a woman is not obligated to sacrifice her wealth to facilitate her husband's fulfillment of the commandment to procreate.

R. Yigal Ariel, as another example of this line of reasoning, bases his position in part on Maimonides's statement in *Hilkhot 'Ishut*[121] that links the commandment to be fertile and increase with a man's variable obligation regarding conjugal relations. Sailors, for example, are expected to engage in conjugal relations only infrequently, yet they are not obligated to change their way of earning a living until after they have fulfilled the commandment to be fertile and increase. In other words, considerations of livelihood are relevant even before the biblical commandment has been fulfilled.

We can see further development in this area in the writings of the younger generation of rabbis, especially within the Modern Orthodox community. Their rhetoric, which formulates the problem from the woman's perspective, including her need to study and develop as a person, shows that the changing status of women within that society, and the legitimization of that change, are bringing about new ways of looking at the question and producing new answers not previously offered. That fact in itself can bear out retroactively my claim that birth control, through the ages, has been a question not only of halakhah but also, and inseparably, of policy and gender.

Rabbi Benjamin Lau considers deferral of the command to be fertile and increase from a broader theological-conceptual perspective regarding the purpose of marriage as a social institution.[122] Through an analysis that is both conceptual and halakhic, he identifies three positions regarding the purpose of marriage:[123]

1. Functional—to facilitate the commandment to reproduce
2. Moral—to overcome human isolation
3. Spiritual—to attain human perfection through unity of man and woman

R. Lau formulates the halakhic question regarding deferral of a first child as follows:

> It is one of the questions most often posed by young couples, at least in religious Zionist circles, *where the woman's social status is equal to the man's*. . . . The reasons for this desire on the part of young couples [to defer having their first child] are numerous: completion of the woman's higher education, a sense of insecurity (whether personal or economic) during the initial stages of married life, or various personal plans.[124]

He later emphasizes the importance of the question and offers halakhic decisors several possible lines of reasoning by which a couple might be permitted to defer childbearing. Analyzing the writings of contemporary decisors, such as R. Aviner, who do not permit deferring the first birth, he traces that position to Maimonides and his implicit determination that the purpose of marriage is exclusively functional, that is, to facilitate procreation.

R. Lau, however, believes the situation to be more complex. His halakhic analysis proceeds on the premise that a woman is not obligated to marry at all; from her perspective, accordingly, putting off the commandment poses no difficulty whatsoever. The question then reverts to the man and whether he, having decided he wants to marry a particular woman, is permitted to defer the marriage. His positive answer to that question is based on the comments of R. Joseph Trani (Maharit),[125] which suggest that deferring a commandment is not tantamount to nullifying it.[126] That leads, of course, to the further question of whether it is preferable to delay the marriage or to marry and defer fulfillment of the commandment to be fertile and increase. R. Lau believes that if decisors see the purpose of marriage as something of independent value, beyond the facilitation of procreation, they must help young couples build their homes and permit them to defer, for a limited time, fulfillment of the commandment. He shies away from any sweepingly permissive ruling that might treat the institution of marriage as resting entirely on intimacy and companionship; but that does not diminish the value of what he does say.

R. Elyashiv Knohl likewise offers a sympathetic ear to requests of this sort from young couples. In his book on the subject, he treats their questions as legitimate, though he does not undertake an ordered halakhic assessment of the matter.[127]

It is not only the substantive halakhic positions taken by R. Lau and R. Knohl that herald a turning point; there is significance as well to the very fact that they are willing to publicize them. Until now, the rhetoric of halakhic decisors in this area has tended to keep permissive rulings under wraps or treat them as personal rulings issued to individual couples in accord with their own circumstances. These decisors, too, call on couples to participate in a private and personal examination of their situation, but they do not hesitate to declare publicly the principles they are applying and the directions in which they are moving.

Halakhic Discourse and Feminist Discourse

The principal halakhic reservations about the use of birth control may be summed up as follows:

1. A man is bound by the commandment to procreate, and until that commandment has been fulfilled, at least on a biblical level, neither member of the couple is permitted, a priori, to use birth control.
2. When a couple is permitted to use birth control, they may use only those methods that do not result in wasting the man's seed. Accordingly, the pill is the preferred method (and a condom, if allowed at all, is least preferred).
3. As a rule, it is preferable for birth control to be practiced by the woman, who is not bound by the commandment to be fertile and increase. But physically neutering her reproductive organs may be permitted only in certain circumstances, since it is forbidden as a matter of rabbinic law.
4. Birth control by the man is likely to be permitted, a priori, only by indirect means that result neither in wasting seed nor in physical neutering of the reproductive organs, both of which are biblically forbidden for men.

The principles that emerge from feminist literature are almost diametrically opposite:

1. There is no reason to impose any limitation whatsoever on birth control. On the contrary, it should be encouraged inasmuch as it enhances reproductive freedom and women's sexual freedom, paralleling the continued development of equality in society as a whole.
2. Birth control methods should be selected with an eye toward

minimizing side effects, health risks, and potential injury to women; it follows that methods having long-term effects or causing permanent sterilization should be avoided. Accordingly, use of a condom, spermicide, diaphragm, or "female condom" is preferred; the pill and the intrauterine device are least preferred. Any factor that might limit a woman's options on account of male interests, of course, is considered irrelevant.

3. According to some feminist thinking, it is preferable as a rule for birth control to be practiced by the man. Most feminists, however, favor an egalitarian model in which responsibility for birth control is borne by both members of the couple; they oppose casting full responsibility on the woman, even though that might appear to grant her additional control over procreation. Sterilization, if recommended at all, is preferably applied to the man rather than the woman, for women regard injury to their sexual organs as harmful to their femininity or their sexuality.[128]

Those differences notwithstanding, I do not believe a halakhic-feminist conversation is impossible. Neither the feminist positions nor the contrary interpretations adopted by most halakhic decisors in this area should be accepted in their entirety. If a feminist position minimizes to the point of denial either a woman's procreative function or the overall institution of motherhood (freed of its patriarchal baggage), that position deserves to be rejected. Such a position cannot be consistent with the halakhic notion that inhabiting the world is a commandment of the highest order. In that sense, the individual, whether man or woman, defers or even subordinates his desires, needs, and interests to promote a value to which he ascribes important religious significance. But to the extent feminist thinkers assign importance (as most do) to procreating, establishing a family, and raising children, they ask whether and to what extent these roles are constructed in a manner that conflicts with the values of equality and partnership and to what extent they reflect male control over women and an attitude that treats women as means to an end rather than as an end in themselves. Accordingly, they raise important issues of principle regarding the gender significance of these roles.

At the same time, one must inquire into whether the hegemonic halakhic position described above is, in fact, necessarily implied by the sources or whether there exist interpretive options that might shift the balance more in the direction of women's equality in these matters. I am convinced that such options exist, and I have already shown that respected legal interpretations permit both delaying childbearing and maintaining longer intervals between births. The problem, however, is not the absence of those options but their having been suppressed and kept out of the public view. In that context, let me cite a young rabbi's call, Harel Gordin, for halakhic decisors to disclose the halakhic possibilities that go hand in hand with the establishment of egalitarian values that promote a more nearly equal division of labor between men and women:

> The "pure" model promotes marriage at the earliest possible age as a way to channel sexual impulses, as fulfillment of a commandment, and as a manifestation of the belief in "growth." It espouses the bringing of children into the world without delay and maximal fulfillment of the commandment to be fertile and increase. . . . But we should disregard neither the cost imposed by that model nor the problems it has difficulty dealing with. These include child-marriage, or, sometimes even worse, "impulse marriage," entered into and encouraged out of a desire to avoid sinning, arrested development; fatigue associated with the burdens of frequent births. . . . There appears to be room to consider, seriously and openly, the possibility of strengthening the family unit through halakhic rulings that permit temporary deferral of childbearing under the rubric of "It is a time to act for the LORD." *Concealing the halakhic possibility* and relegating it to "closed" rabbinic consideration and personal rulings allows, to be sure, for close supervision of the cases that are considered, but it makes it more difficult for many couples tormented by religious and halakhic struggles to find their way to halakhic decisors and literature. . . . Concealing and silencing these possibilities may serve as a defense against doubts and other concerns, but it does not permit properly treating and effectively responding to the weighty questions that are brought before us.[129]

What might account for the concealment of halakhic possibilities in this area? Why do most contemporary halakhic decisors continue to adopt a rhetoric that maximizes the commandment to be fertile and increase beyond the point required by the halakhic sources? How can we explain the halakhic ideology that encourages childbearing at almost any cost?

Some believe that this ideology is motivated by national-demographic considerations,[130] particularly in the wake of the Holocaust and the Israeli-Arab conflict. But I do not believe it could have been so forcefully deployed were it not based on a concept of gender in which a woman's primary role lies in procreation and motherhood and those activities are taken to define femininity. This concept regards a woman not as "an end in herself" but as "marked for birth and child-rearing," as R. Isaac Aramah puts it. Implicit in this concept is a significant (though not necessary) potential to maintain decidedly patriarchal notions that take no account of women's existential interests and tend to define women primarily in terms of "substance" rather than of "form" or that maintain women's inferior status by emphasizing their role exclusively in the private sphere.

Moreover, recognizing women as subjects having desires, aspirations, and needs transcending the procreative function may contribute to a growing exodus of women from the domestic sphere and thereby, it is feared, undermine the way of the world. For example, it may cause young women, and young men as well, to establish smaller families so that both members of the couple—but primarily the wife—can realize talents beyond their parental roles. It may undermine the social standing of men and their place in the labor market. If men are called upon to take an equal part in running the household and become more involved in family life, they will no longer be able to devote all their time and ability to personal, intellectual, or professional development.[131]

It may be argued, to be sure, that men as well as women are burdened by the tendency of contemporary halakhic rulings to encourage large families—it is the men, after all, who are required to support those families and divert their energies from Torah study—and that it is mistaken, therefore, to view the matter solely from the woman's perspective. But it seems reasonably clear that nature and social convention alike make the trend more burdensome to women than to men. It is women, for the most part, who suffer the weariness that results from endless pregnancies, child rearing, and the inability to develop spiritually, intellectually, or professionally. Moreover, the dichotomies between the public and private spheres and between the physical and the spiritual are greatly intensified. The woman's roles are fixed within the private sphere, and she is thought of in material and biological terms, for her procreative and motherly roles prevent her from developing her other abilities.

The question of birth control is thus central to women's progress in recent times, and halakhah appears to be maintaining a last stand in a losing battle. With the development of birth control techniques that entail no halakhic violation and the existence of an interpretive approach that does not consider "in the evening" to embody an unending obligation to bear more children, it appears that the question of birth control poses no particularly difficult halakhic problems. But because the issue necessarily involves a challenge to the traditional role of women and undermines the existing social order, it has become a matter of control and of power relationships. As such, it leaves the domain of pure halakhah and becomes a political issue in the full sense of the word. When I say a "political issue," I mean, in Foucault's terms, to insert the question of power into the halakhic discourse, that is, to ask just whom that discourse is meant to serve.[132] Foucault believed the foundational discourse to be more basic than scientific truths. In his opinion, no discourse may be analyzed in epistemic philosophical terms; rather, one must look to the circles of power within every form of discourse or human practice.[133] Paraphrasing his words, one may say that in the case of halakhic rulings regarding birth control and family planning, the foundational discourse, which promotes childbearing, is more fundamental that the halakhic "truths," for the latter in most cases are contingent (that is, subject to interpretation), as I have tried to show throughout this chapter. To state it differently, if we look beyond formal terms in thinking about the subject, and uncover the moral and gender concepts that shape the pertinent halakhic rulings, we are unable to escape the conclusion that the halakhic power structure has an interest in creating a halakhic foundation for the maintenance of traditional gender notions that consider a woman's primary functions to be the bearing and raising of children. At the same time, this infrastructure means to fortify the halakhah against the penetration of "debased modernism" that could undermine its way of ordering the world. The tendency to encourage childbearing at any cost constitutes, in effect, a defense against what is perceived as an attack on halakhah from within the halakhic discourse itself.

I see no necessary contradiction between maintaining a nonpatriarchal perception that treats women honorably, as subjects, and affirming and fulfilling the commandment to be fertile and increase, even in a more extensive manner than biblically required. It depends, of course, on the willingness of men to give up their power positions and dichotomous concepts with respect to the differences between the sexes—or, alternatively, on the power of women to forge an alternative halakhic discourse that will reflect the contingency of halakhic "dicta" so as to allow for change.

CHAPTER THREE

Halakhic Rulings on Abortion

A HISTORICAL SURVEY FROM THE RABBINIC TO THE MODERN PERIOD

Introduction: Liberal and Feminist Views of Abortion

The mantle of feminist consensus with regard to abortion conceals an array of conflicts over the nature of women, the value of children, the role of the family, and the social significance of sexual relations between men and women. At times, a radical feminist position regarding power relationships between men and women engenders a conservative position on abortion. We thus find "pro-life" feminists who oppose abortion on the grounds that the freedom to abort only increases women's sexual availability to men, for it frees men from the need take responsibility for the consequences of their actions.[1]

The various liberal positions on abortion may be summed up as follows:

1. *The fetus is not a "person" until it is born.* Those who take this view distinguish between a "person" and a "human entity." Positing a discontinuity between biological-physiological qualities and those that are clearly

human, they maintain it is only the latter that transform a purely biological entity into a full person, possessing defined characteristics and endowed with moral rights. The fetus, according to this view, is a "human entity" in the biological sense alone; it belongs to the human species (*Homo sapiens*), but it bears no moral rights.[2]

2. *The fetus acquires human characteristics during pregnancy*. Adherents of this position believe that once a specified point in the pregnancy has been reached, abortion will be permitted in some cases but forbidden in others; however, they debate the crucial point in the pregnancy at which the fetus begins to acquire human characteristics and abortion becomes morally problematic.[3]

Within this group, Ronald Dworkin is a bit of an outlier, for he does not analyze the issue of abortion from the perspective of whether the fetus enjoys the rights of personhood.[4] Nevertheless, he does not justify abortion at any price and is therefore consistent with other intermediate positions. In Dworkin's view, the debate over abortion is actually a debate over how to protect the sanctity of life.[5]

Indeed, Dworkin portrays the dispute between liberals and conservatives as stemming from the different weights the two sides assign to the "natural" and "human" components of a person's life. Conservatives believe that the natural component of human life, that is, the gift of life itself, is more important than anything a human being may do with his life, however significant his accomplishments. As a result, conservatives tend to think that killing a fetus strikes a mortal blow at the principle of life's sanctity, unrelated to the nature and quality of that fetus's future life. Liberals, on the other hand, assign more weight to the human component. They regard life as the outcome of human choice, decisions, and undertakings, and therefore are more likely to permit abortion:

> It may be more frustrating of life's miracle when an adult's ambitions, talents, training and expectations are wasted because of an unforeseen and unwanted pregnancy than when a fetus dies before any significant investment of that kind has been made.[6]

Dworkin's analysis bears on a crucial question: does abortion entail some sort of desecration of human life? His response, in principle, is negative. Abortion, in cases where it is warranted, does not detract from the substantive value of human life; on the contrary, it constitutes an act of respect for human, especially female, freedom and autonomy. That is so because reverence for human life means honoring the human qualities and values that make life so unique and sanctified. This is not to say that adherents of the liberal position will permit abortion in every case; but in cases of conflict, the woman's rights should prevail over those of the fetus, which has not yet been the recipient of much human investment.

3. *Even if the fetus is a "person," aborting it is permitted.* The philosopher most identified with this position is Judith Thomson.[7] I cannot treat her arguments in detail, but they may be summed up as asserting that the right to life does not encompass the right to use another person's body. The extent of the fetus's "personhood" is not the sole factor that is pertinent to the question of abortion, for even if the fetus is a person, its right to life does not include the right to use its mother's body in order to realize that right. Thomson argues that the right to life does not imply the right not to be killed; it implies only the right not to be killed unjustly. When a woman aborts a pregnancy, she does not violate the fetus's right to life, for she is not acting unjustly in denying the fetus the use of her body. It would be more generous of her to allow the fetus to reside within her, and her refusal to do so may be considered distasteful, but it certainly is not unjust. This does not mean that abortion will be justified at any cost. If the woman accepted responsibility for the pregnancy, used no birth control, and failed to abort early in the pregnancy, she could not reasonably argue later that she was "forced" in one way or another to accept the fact of the pregnancy. If she consented to "host" the fetus within her body, she cannot arbitrarily send it away. In such a case, the abortion would be considered an unjustified killing, not a legitimate act of self-defense.

4. *The feminist view—the personhood of the fetus is not the principal question.* Feminists treat the question of abortion from the broadest possible perspective. They are interested in the gender-based power relationships that provide the context for the sexual relations that are likely to bring about unwanted pregnancy, but they also consider the effects of unwanted pregnancy on the lives of women. In what follows, I will consider primarily the latter.[8]

Robin West suggests seeing rights and responsibilities as intertwined and therefore emphasizes that the fetus is a being with moral implications, primarily for the life of the pregnant woman.[9] Respect for rights is more than a necessary condition for personal liberty; it is also a condition for the personal responsibility without which freedom would lack importance and be morally problematic. If that respect is not extended to the responsibilities implied by freedom within a liberal society, those liberties will not be ensured. A woman must make reproductive decisions with absolute freedom in order to strengthen her ties to others, to plan a family that can meet her needs, and to raise children appropriately. The decision with respect to abortion is almost always caught up in a net of responsibilities that sometimes conflict. Accordingly, in every debate over abortion, one must emphasize not only reproductive freedom and the right to privacy and bodily integrity, but also—perhaps primarily—the responsibility that follows from these liberties.

Indeed, in Susan Sherwin's view, the principal difference between feminist approaches and others lies in the relative degree of attention afforded to the interests and experiences of women.[10] Feminists consider the *effects* of unwanted pregnancies on the lives of women, individually and collectively, to be the central component of any moral inquiry into the subject of abortion. In their view, it is self-evident that the woman is the primary factor in the discussion of abortion. Nonfeminist discussions, in contrast, not only fail to treat the woman as central; they generally treat her as "invisible," for their analyses are centered primarily on the question of the fetus's personhood. And, in fact, most ethicists take the latter position. Even those who maintain the legitimacy of abortion accept the logic of focusing on the fetus and direct their efforts to proving that it lacks significant human value. It is the nature of the fetus as an independent being that determines the abortion's morality. The woman, on whom the life of the fetus depends, is regarded as secondary (if even that) to these discussions. The actual experience and responsibilities of women are not treated as morally relevant to the discussion unless the woman is considered an innocent victim of rape or incest.

Because the public debate is presented as a rivalry between the woman's rights and those of the fetus, feminists feel a need to reject claims about the value of a fetus's life even if they do not believe it to lack all value. To put it more precisely, from a feminist perspective, a fetus has moral significance, but the value of its life is more relative than absolute. Its existence is defined by its interrelationship with the woman carrying it. No person, and certainly not a fetus, can exist without a framework of relationships. Accordingly, the attempts to speak of the fetus in and of itself, as if it were separate from the body of the woman in which it is developing, are inappropriate and misguided. The value assigned by a woman to an individual fetus will vary from case to case. The fact that the fetus's life can be neither preserved nor terminated without affecting the woman implies that whatever value is assigned to the fetus by others cannot outweigh that assigned to it by the pregnant woman herself.

Sherwin and others emphasize that there is more involved in the battle over abortion than protecting the potential lives of fetuses. What is at stake is the sexual freedom of women and their reproductive liberty, to which the religious establishment is systematically opposed. When the subject of abortion is placed in the broader political context, it becomes evident that most groups who oppose abortion likewise oppose various forms of birth control and object as well to placing women in positions of political, ecclesiastical, or domestic authority—that is, they support additional conservative measures to maintain patriarchal forms of control. Their actions, in typical form, thus serve to protect the interests of the favored social classes while disregarding the needs of the weaker underclass.

This position highlights a critical point with respect to abortion, namely, the equivalence or lack thereof between the right of the fetus to remain alive and the right of a woman to maintain the *quality* of her life.[11]

It seems to me that every liberal position on abortion, whether or not it is rooted in a feminist worldview, is required to address the question of the fetus's personhood. At the same time, I would argue that one's assessment of that status will be influenced by the weight one gives to women's interests and by regarding women as a subject in one's formulation of the abortion "narrative." I believe that those who decide that the fetus is a "person" do so not solely, and perhaps not even primarily, because they are persuaded that it is a "person" from the instant of fertilization or from some later stage in the pregnancy or because of scientific "proofs" that may be adduced on the subject. Their determination stems, at least in part, from a conscious or unconscious worldview in which women play no more than a supporting role in the drama of life, one whose destiny and purpose are to serve as a vessel for bringing new life into the world. In that view, a woman can never be regarded as the subject, and the fetus will always count for more than she does. To those who embrace a contrary worldview, the woman's purpose is entirely self-directed, the importance of her procreative role is minimized, and she will always count for more than the fetus, which is not regarded as a "person" at all.

In light of the foregoing, I will now turn to the positions reflected in the halakhic sources. I first consider the question of the fetus's personhood and then examine how the halakhic decisors analyze abortion and the likely gender implications of that analysis.

Halakhic Genealogy

The feminist analysis, then, challenges the definition of the fetus's personhood as the central question to be asked in connection with abortion. In what follows, however, we shall see that the principal, if not the exclusive, halakhic approach turns on the fetus's standing as a "life." Accordingly, this chapter will focus on disproving the claim that the rabbinic sources necessarily define the fetus in terms of personhood. From a feminist perspective, proceeding in this manner leaves me vulnerable to the charge that I have bought into the basic halakhic premise instead of dismantling it; it might be argued that I have accepted a halakhic agenda that calls for first defining the fetus's personhood and then allowing that decision to determine all else that follows with respect to abortion. My primary response to that potential criticism is that insofar as one favors (for reasons that need not be discussed here) preserving the "morphology" of halakhic discourse, the attempt to enter into a feminist-halakhic conversation can be fruitful only if halakhic logic is followed to some degree and we are able to show that the halakhah's *own method* allows for interpretations different from the ones that traditionally have been offered. It should be said as well that when we set out to adjust halakhic conclusions in accord with values we regard as just and right, we must forgo any expectation that the halakhic discourse will manifest ideological identification with the values driving those adjustments. Although such identification may sometimes be found, more often we will have to rest content with a practical determination that advances the cause, even though the concepts and values it embodies may be at odds with our goal. For example, I will demonstrate in what follows that even if those who treat abortion as forbidden only by rabbinic law do so for reasons that are problematic from a gender perspective, their views can still advance feminist positions *in practice*.

Background: The Fetus in the Bible

The Bible refers directly to abortion only in the following verses:

> When men fight, and one of them pushes a pregnant women and a miscarriage results [lit. "her children come out"], but no other damage ['*ason*] ensues, the one responsible shall be fined according as the woman's husband may exact from him, the payment to be based on reckoning. But if other damage ensues, the penalty shall be life [*nefesh*] for life. (Ex. 21:22–23)

The abortion described in this verse is involuntary. The pregnant woman happens to be in a place where men are fighting, and, at least according to the plain meaning of the text, the two fighters have no intent to strike her or injure her in any way. It therefore could be argued that the case here described is not at all analogous to deliberate abortion performed for medical or other reasons and thus it has no bearing on the subject at hand. Nevertheless, the passage appears to be instructive with respect to the status of the fetus within its mother's womb: is it to be considered an independent being endowed with personhood, what the rabbis term a "life" (*nefesh*)?

The central exegetical question raised by the verse is the referent of the "damage" that does or does not ensue. Is it damage to the mother or damage to the fetus that is in question? According to one interpretation, "no other damage ensues" means that the woman is not injured but the fetuses "come out," that is, they are harmed or killed. In that case, the woman's husband may demand monetary compensation for the fetuses (which are considered his property), but the act is not deemed murder or even accidental homicide. Should there be "other damage," that is, should the woman die, then the penalty is "life for life." According to a second possible interpretation, "other damage" refers to the fetuses, and the passage may be understood to mean that if the fetuses come out but do not die, the man responsible need only pay compensation, but if there is "damage" and the fetuses die, he is subject to capital punishment because he has killed a "life."

All classic Jewish interpreters follow the *Mekhilta* and reject the second possibility; they take the view that "other damage" refers to the woman and, therefore, that killing a fetus is not a capital offense:

> *No other damage ensues*—Do I take this to mean damage to the woman or damage to the fetuses? It is taught: *He who fatally strikes a man* (v. 12)—[the reference to "man" is] to exclude fetuses. What, then, is the meaning "no other damage ensues"—damage to the woman, not to the fetuses. (*Mekhilta De-Rashbi* 21:22)

The *Mekhilta* raises alternative readings similar to those noted above. The second reading (that is, damage to the fetuses) is definitively rejected[12] because of the word "man" appearing in verse 12. That term is taken by the *midrash* to exclude fetuses that cannot survive outside the womb, and the *Mekhilta* infers on that basis that the word "damage" in our verse refers to the woman and not to the fetuses, for damage cannot apply to one incapable of surviving. In this reading, the verse emphasizes that despite the unique situation, a woman's pregnancy has no practical implications with respect to the crime of striking a person. The only difference the pregnancy makes is that compensation must be paid to the husband for the injured fetuses.[13]

Thus, in rabbinic tradition, the fetus does not have the status of a "life"; the exegesis applied to the verse neutralizes any such suggestion. The word *'ason* refers solely to the mother, and the verse in no way implies that distinctions should be drawn among fetuses at various stages of development. The Hellenistic tradition, in contrast, does draw such distinctions, holding that a fetus whose human form is complete acquires personhood and that one who kills such a fetus has committed a capital offense.[14]

Abortion in Rabbinic Literature

Building on the comments of the *Mekhilta* and its commentators, the first issue we will consider is whether the fetus is a "life" (*nefesh*). If it is, feticide would violate the prohibition on murder or killing; if not, it becomes necessary to ascertain the basis on which it has been argued that feticide is nevertheless forbidden.

I will begin by presenting the sources that relate to the status of the fetus, offering several interpretive options. Because this study treats the rabbinic sources as background for the positions taken by the decisors and is not concerned with the rabbinic sources in and of themselves, it will suffice to note the disagreements that arise and to forgo efforts to harmonize them. Along with presentation of the relevant sources, I will attempt to examine the suitability of the various interpretive options by considering their internal consistency. The analysis will examine the sources chronologically—tannaitic material, amoraic material, medieval authorities, and later authorities.

THE TANNAITIC DISCUSSION

Is the Fetus Considered a "Life"?

> If a woman is having difficulty giving birth, the fetus within her belly is cut up and removed limb by limb, for her life takes precedence over its life. If most of [the fetus] has emerged, it is not touched, for one life is not set aside for another. (M 'Ohal. 7:6)

This *mishnah* deals with a situation in which a woman is already at the point of giving birth and her life is being endangered by the fetus. It rules that an abortion may be performed to save her life, which takes precedence over that of the fetus. Once most of the fetus[15] has emerged, however, its status changes from "fetus" to "life," and its mother no longer takes precedence; its life is not sacrificed to preserve hers.

The *mishnah* lends itself to at least two different understandings, reflecting an ambiguity in the text itself. The first reading leads to the conclusion that although the fetus is not considered a life—as is evident from the final sentence—it may be aborted only in the face of clear and present danger to the mother and only during the birthing process. The premise that such permission to abort is limited to cases of mortal danger is confirmed by the statement that "her life takes precedence over its life," which would be inapt if her life were not in danger. It follows that situations falling short of mortal danger, as where the fetus endangers her health but not her life or places one or more of her limbs at risk, would not provide adequate justification for abortion. On this reading, the fetus is not considered an actual life, but neither is it considered entirely a "nonlife."

The second reading, in contrast, focuses on the final sentence of the *mishnah* to emphasize that the fetus is not considered a "life" at all, not even as it is emerging from its mother's womb; it becomes a "life" only when its head or most of its body has emerged. The wording of the *mishnah* does not necessarily indicate that it is speaking only of a case of mortal danger to the mother or that the fetus may be killed to save the mother's life only during the course of the birthing; if the fetus is not a "life," it is possible that abortion might be permitted before the onset of labor for less grave reasons and, perhaps, for any reason at all. Because the *mishnah* is dealing with a specific situation in which labor has already begun, we cannot conclusively determine how it would rule in other cases; but its assertion that the fetus is not a "life" leaves open the possibility of permissive rulings. Moreover, it may be that the *mishnah* means to emphasize that even after the fetus has begun to emerge from the womb, it does not actually become a life until its head or most of its body has emerged. This interpretation allows for a conclusion that is directly opposed to the one suggested by the first reading: if abortion may be permitted even after the birthing process has begun and the fetus has begun to separate itself from its mother's body, it should be permitted a fortiori at an earlier point in the pregnancy, when the fetus is clearly an integral part of its mother's body.

The Tosefta considers the medical practicalities of the case discussed in the Mishnah:

> If an expert doctor healed with the sanction of the court and caused injury, if it was unintentional, he is not liable; if intentional, he is liable for reasons of sound social policy (*tikkun ha-ʿolam*). If one dismembers a fetus in a woman's belly with the sanction of the court and causes injury, if it was unintentional, he is not liable; if intentional, he is liable for reasons of sound social policy. (T [Zuckermandel] Git. 4, p. 328])

Although the Tosefta speaks of needing a court's authorization to perform an abortion, it does not necessarily imply that abortion as a rule is forbidden except in those specific cases where it is permitted. The situation described in the *mishnah* is one of active labor ("difficulty giving birth"), and court authorization may be needed at that stage because of the greater concern about the personhood of the fetus. In any case, the injury spoken of is injury to the woman,[16] not to the fetus, whose death is assumed to be necessary to save the mother's life.

A *mishnah* in *'Arakhin* seems to bolster the second reading of the *mishnah* in *'Ohalot*:

> If a [pregnant] woman is sentenced to death, execution of the sentence is not delayed until she gives birth. If she is already in labor [lit. "seated on the birthing stool"], imposition of the sentence is delayed until she gives birth. If a woman is put to death, one may derive benefit from her hair. If a beast is put to death, it is forbidden to derive benefit from it. (M 'Arak. 1:4)

The distinction between a woman not yet in labor and a woman in labor may attest to an interest in protecting the fetus once it begins to emerge from its mother's womb. The Mishnah may see the fetus at that stage as a being that is starting to live in its own right, and it therefore permits delaying the execution until after it is born.[17] The principal discussion in the tannaitic literature, then, is whether a fetus is considered a "life." The simple conclusion, it seems to me, is that these sources do not recognize the fetus as a life, at least not until the birthing process begins.

THE AMORAIC DISCUSSION

Is the Fetus Considered a "Life"?

The principal talmudic discussion of abortion appears in the *gemara* on the *mishnah* in *'Arakhin* just discussed. The complete passage follows:

> MISHNAH. If a [pregnant] woman is sentenced to death, execution of the sentence is not delayed until she gives birth. If she is already in labor [lit. "seated on the birthing stool"], imposition of the sentence is delayed until she gives birth. . . .
>
> GEMARA. Is it not self-evident [that execution proceeds without delay]; for it [the fetus] is [part of] her body! No; it is necessary [to state the rule], for I might say: Inasmuch as it is written (Ex. 21:22) "according as the woman's husband may exact from him"—[the fetus] is the husband's property, which he should not be made to lose; therefore, the rule is stated. But we could still say [that execution should be delayed until the birth of the fetus]! Rabbi Abahu said in the name of Rabbi Yoḥanan: Scripture says "then they shall both of them die" [Deut. 22:22 (OJPS)]—["both of them"

is meant] to include the fetus.[18] But [these words] are needed [to teach a different law, namely, the man and the woman are both to be executed] only if they are equally blameworthy, [these being] the words of Rabbi Yoshiah. [No,] what was said [about the fetus being killed] is learned from "both" [leaving "of them" as the basis for Rabbi Yoshiah's rule].

If she is already in labor, etc.—What is the reason for this? Once [the fetus] has moved from its place [and begun to emerge], it is a separate body. Rav Judah said in the name of Samuel: If a woman is taken out to be put to death, she is first struck on the area of the womb, so the fetus is killed first, lest she be disgraced [by having a bloody fetus emerge after she is dead]. (BT 'Arak. 7a)

The *mishnah*, as noted, means to protect the fetus that has begun to move from its place in the womb. That understanding is support by the *gemara*'s comment: "Is it not self-evident; for it is her body"—that is, as long as the fetus has not begun to move, it is clearly part of the mother's body, but once it has begun to move and the woman is in labor, "it is a separate body" entitled to greater concern about its standing. (The amoraic "begun to move" appears to be synonymous with the tannaitic "seated on the birthing stool.")

It seems to me that the *gemara*'s conceptual distinctions are dictated by the discussion in the *mishnah* itself and that the question of the fetus's standing as a "life" is translated in the *gemara*'s terms to seeing it as part of the mother's body ("it is her body") or, in a different formulation appearing at various points, "a fetus is its mother's limb [lit. 'thigh']."[19] There is no logical or jurisprudential necessity to consider the two questions—whether the fetus has standing as a "life" and whether it is "its mother's limb" or "a separate body"—as identical, and there may be no conceptual identity between them (though neither is there any need to distinguish between them halakhically). Nevertheless, it appears that the *gemara* regards the onset of the birthing process as an intermediate stage that warrants delaying the mother's execution. If the *mishnah* in *'Ohalot* is then read in light of the discussion in *'Arakhin*, the following picture emerges: because the fetus is part of its mother's body and is not considered an independent life, aborting it is permissible in various circumstances, such as the mother being subject to capital punishment, the presence of mortal danger (and, perhaps, even nonmortal danger) to the mother, cases of rape or incest, and so forth. If, however, the fetus has begun to emerge—that is, if the birthing process has started—the question of its personhood is of heightened significance, for it has begun to disengage from "its mother's body" (though it is not considered a "life" until its head or most of its body has come out). Given this understanding, the *mishnah* in *'Ohalot* can be read as a specific instance of the principle discussed in *'Arakhin*: One might have thought that once the fetus begins to move, it may not be harmed, but the *mishnah* teaches that it may be aborted even then in order to avoid mortal danger to the mother. The reason is that it is not yet considered a "life," and a full-fledged life (the mother's) takes precedence over what is still only a possible life. This bolsters the second reading of the *mishnah* in *'Ohalot* discussed above, rejecting the idea that abortion is permitted only where the mother is in clear and present danger.

Desecrating the Sabbath to Save a Fetus

Additional light may be shed on the fetus's standing as a "life" by considering whether the Sabbath may be desecrated to save it. The well-known rule is that "saving a life [*nefesh*] supersedes the Sabbath,"[20] and it therefore may be inferred that if the Sabbath can be desecrated to save a fetus, the fetus is considered a life or, at least, partly a life; conversely, if saving a fetus does not warrant desecrating the Sabbath, it is not considered to be a life. Where the mother is in danger along with the fetus, superseding a biblical prohibition to save her is not in question:

> MISHNAH. If a pregnant woman smells [food on Yom Kippur and is seized by a craving for it], she is fed until her mind is at ease. A person who is ill [and needs to eat] is fed in accord with the advice of experts; but if no experts are available, he is fed on his own say-so, until he says "enough."
>
> GEMARA. If a pregnant woman smells sacrificial meat [which may not be eaten] or pig meat [and is seized by a craving for it], a small stick is dipped in its gravy and placed on her mouth. If her mind comes to be at ease, good; if not, she is fed the sauce itself. If her mind comes to be at ease, good; if not, she is fed the fat of the item itself, for nothing stands in the way of protecting life except for [the prohibitions on] idolatry, incest, and bloodshed. (BT Yoma 82a)

The *mishnah* and *gemara* here allow for the conclusion that even a biblical prohibition is waived in a case of mortal danger to the mother, but they provide no guidance regarding a case of danger to the fetus itself.[21]

The *gemara* in *'Arakhin*, in contrast, states explicitly that the Sabbath is to be desecrated if necessary to save a fetus:

> Rav Naḥman said in the name of Samuel: If a woman was in labor ["seated on the birthing stool"] and died on the Sabbath, a knife is brought, her belly is opened, and the fetus is removed. This seems self-evident; what did he do [that violates the Sabbath]? He was simply cutting meat! Rabbah said: No, [the statement] is needed [to teach that it is permissible] to carry the knife through the public domain. Now, what does it teach us? That in a case of doubt [about the danger to life], the Sabbath may be desecrated? [We already know that, for] it was taught: If someone was under a collapsed structure, but it is uncertain if he is there or not, if he is alive or not, if he is a Canaanite or an Israelite—the rubble is searched on his account. But you might say: there [in the case of the collapse] he was alive and is presumed to have remained alive; here [in the case of the fetus] there was no such presumption of life, so it teaches us [that the Sabbath is nevertheless to be desecrated]. (BT 'Arak. 7a–b)

The passage may be understood in two ways. On the one hand, it may be understood to teach explicitly that one may violate the Sabbath to save a fetus even where the risk to life is uncertain because it is not known if the fetus survived the death of its mother. Alternatively, it may be understood to refer specifically to a "woman seated on the birthing stool." According to the second of the readings I have suggested for the passages in *'Ohalot* and *'Arakhin*, that is the stage at which one must begin to be more cautious about the fetus's status, for it has begun to emerge from the womb and acquire independence. Only at that point does the Mishnah (in *'Arakhin*) become interested in protecting the fetus and delaying the mother's execution until after its birth. Similarly, it may be that the duty to desecrate the Sabbath in the present context arises because the fetus has already begun to change its status to one of "life." It may also be inferred that the case here is a special one in which the mother has already died and the fetus is therefore no longer dependent on her for sustenance; it is "as one situated inside a box," as Tosafot put it (at BT Nid. 44b), and only for that reason may the Sabbath be desecrated on its account, since it is partly alive. This interpretive option seems bolstered by the concluding lines of the *gemara*, which take the view that if the mother has died, the fetus is not presumed to be alive, yet the Sabbath nevertheless is desecrated in order to save it, even though it is not yet considered fully a life. The rationale may be that of "desecrate one Sabbath on his behalf so he will [survive to] observe many Sabbaths" (BT Yoma 85b), and there is no necessary link between the two ideas. That is: it is not logically necessary to infer its standing as a "life" from the duty to desecrate the Sabbath on its account.

The *Rodef* (Pursuer)

Rodef (the "pursuer" who chases another with the intention of killing him; as a general matter and subject to various conditions, killing the *rodef* is a permitted act of self-defense) is a third concept that can serve as a lens for examining the personhood of the fetus. A different interpretive turn for the *mishnah* in *'Ohalot* can be found in the *gemara*'s discussion of this *rodef*:

> Rav Huna said: A minor in pursuit (*rodef*) may be saved with his life. Thus he maintains that a *rodef*, whether an adult or a minor, need not be formally admonished. Rav Ḥisda asked Rav Huna: [It was taught in the case of a fetus endangering its mother's life that] if its head has emerged, it is not to be touched, for one life is not set aside for another. But why should that be? It [the fetus] is a *rodef*! No, that case is different because she is pursued by [decree of] Heaven. (BT Sanh. 72b)

The question raised in this passage is whether a minor can be considered a *rodef* and therefore subject to the basic rule that "the blood of one [the targeted victim] may be saved with the blood of the other [the pursuer]." The question has important implications for the *gemara*'s understanding of the *mishnah* in *'Ohalot*: is it permitted to kill the fetus because it is not a life or because it is considered a *rodef*? To say it may be killed because it is a *rodef* bolsters the first of the two interpretive options presented earlier and has a substantial bearing on the prohibition of abortion that we are examining.

Rav Huna takes the view that a minor pursuing another person (according to Rashi, another minor) to kill him may be killed so as to save the life of the person he is pursuing, and we do not reason that he is minor and therefore not subject to punishment. The *gemara* infers from Rav Huna's statement that a *rodef*, whether minor or adult, need not be admonished before being killed, for the main point is to save the life of the person pursued. Rav Ḥisda, on the other hand, believes that killing the *rodef* is an act in the nature of punishment and therefore must be preceded by admonition, just as would any imposition of capital punishment by a court.[22] Rav Ḥisda's question pertains to how the *mishnah* in *'Ohalot* is to be understood. The ruling there is that once its head has emerged, the fetus may not be killed to save its mother's life, because one life is not set aside for another. But, asks Rav Ḥisda, if the infant is, in fact, a *rodef*—as seems reasonable to say, since it is jeopardizing the mother's life—why not kill it, even if its head has already emerged, given R. Huna's view that a minor *rodef* may be killed? The *gemara* resolves his question with the argument that the fetus is not a willful *rodef* and the danger to the mother's life therefore can be considered an act of God; since the fetus is not responsible, its life is not set aside for the mother's. In other words, Rav Ḥisda understands the *mishnah* in *'Ohalot* to be saying that the fetus may be killed as long as it is still in its mother's womb not because it is considered a *rodef* but because it is not considered a "life," for if it were a *rodef*, it could be killed even after emerging. And even though the *gemara* dismisses Rav Ḥisda's challenge to Rav Huna on the grounds that a fetus can never be considered a *rodef*, because it is not aware of its actions, it nevertheless accepts the underlying analysis that the fetus may be killed if it endangers the mother's life because it is not considered a "life."[23]

The Jerusalem Talmud likewise refers to the *mishnah* in *'Ohalot* in the context of the *rodef*:

> *These are saved with their lives, etc.*—If one pursues his fellow intending to kill him, whether in the house or in the field, he is saved with his life. The rule is the same for one pursuing his fellow intending to kill him and one in pursuit of any other offense in the Torah; he is saved with his life. . . . If a *rodef* himself becomes the one pursued, what is the rule? The [former] *rodef* is to be saved with the life of the one [originally] pursued. If an adult becomes a minor, what is the rule? The adult is to be saved with the life of the minor. Rabbi Jeremiah asked: Is it not taught, "If its head or most of its body has emerged, it is not touched, for one life is not set aside for another?" . . . Rabbi Yosi bar Bun said in the name of Rav Ḥisda: That case is different, for you do not know who killed whom. (JT Sanh. 8:9; 27c)[24]

The dilemma posed by the Jerusalem Talmud is identical to that of the Babylonian—can a *rodef* who is a minor be killed? The formulation of the question here is different, though, for the Jerusalem Talmud asks whether in the case of "an adult who has become a minor"[25] the life of the adult may be saved at the expense of the minor's life. The *mishnah* in *'Ohalot* is cited as a source that can be helpful in resolving the dilemma. Rabbi Jeremiah reads the *mishnah* in the same way as does the Babylonian Talmud: according to the *mishnah*, an adult may not be rescued at the cost of the minor's life, for once most of the fetus has emerged, it is considered a life and may not be killed even though it is a *rodef* with respect to its mother. Like the Babylonian Talmud, the Jerusalem Talmud rejects that position, but it does so by denying that the fetus is the sole *rodef* and suggesting the mother is a *rodef* as well, "for you do not know who killed whom." In other words, this may be considered a case of mutual pursuit—the mother is in mortal danger on account of the fetus, but the fetus also is in mortal danger on account of the difficult birth. Accordingly, this is not a classic case of *rodef*, and no conclusions may be drawn from it regarding whether an adult may be saved by killing a pursuer who is a minor.

Thus, neither Talmud applies the category of *rodef* to the *mishnah* in *'Ohalot*, though the term, if at all applicable, would apply to the child already emerging from the womb and not to the fetus during the course of the pregnancy. As a result, we cannot say that the *rodef* discussion bolsters in any way the first interpretive option for the *mishnah*. We can say, however, that the second interpretive option gains support in each Talmud, for it is permitted to kill a fetus threatening its mother while still in her womb not because it is considered a *rodef* but because it is not considered to be a life.

Noahides

An additional perspective on the talmudic attitude toward abortion derives from the discussion of Noahide obligations in tractate *Sanhedrin*.[26] The text seems to imply an absolute prohibition on abortion by a Noahide and suggests the act would be considered bloodshed for which he would be put to death. Most of those who take a nonpermissive position on the issue cite this source as proof that it is biblically prohibited for a Jew to perform and abortion, for there is another passage that rules, in the same context, that nothing prohibited to a Noahide is permitted to a Jew:

Rav Jacob bar Aḥa found written in a book of *aggadah* in Rav's study hall: A Noahide may be sentenced to death by a single judge, on the basis of [testimony by] a single witness, without admonition, on the basis of [testimony by] a man but not by a woman, but even [by a witness who is] a relative. It was said in the name of Rabbi Ishmael: Even for [killing] fetuses. . . . What is Rabbi Ishmael's reason? For it is written (Gen. 9:6), "Whoever sheds the blood of man, by man shall his blood be shed"—Who is a man in a man?[27] A fetus in its mother's womb. . . . (BT Sanh. 57b)

Considering this passage in isolation, it is clear that a Jew is not to be put to death for feticide.[28] The disagreement between Rabbi Ishmael and the unnamed first *tanna* pertains to whether a Noahide is considered a murderer and put to death for feticide. The first *tanna* answers in the negative, for he interprets the verse in question as specifying the manner in which capital punishment is to be imposed on a Noahide when warranted. Rabbi Ishmael, however, interprets the verse as subjecting Noahides to capital punishment for feticide, distinguishing them in that regard from Jews.[29]

As already noted, however, the foregoing passage must be considered in the context of what follows a few pages later:

A teacher said: Every commandment given to the Noahides and repeated at Sinai is given to both [Noahides and Jews]. [One might say, though,] on the contrary; once it was repeated at Sinai, it should be considered as given to Jews only and not to Noahides! No, the prohibition of idolatry was repeated at Sinai, yet we find that a gentile is punished for it as well; it follows that the commandment was given to both. [A commandment] given to Noahides and not repeated at Sinai is given to Jews only and not to Noahides. [One might say, though,] on the contrary; since it was not repeated at Sinai, it was given to Noahides only and not to Israel! No; there is nothing that is permissible for a Jew but forbidden for a gentile. (BT Sanh. 59a)

The Talmud compares the duties imposed on Noahides with those imposed on Jews, and invokes the maxim that "there is nothing that is permissible for a Jew but forbidden for a gentile."[30] (For convenience, I will sometimes abbreviate the maxim to "nothing permissible" [*leika mid'am*].) Although that maxim is not easily reconciled with various prohibitions applied to gentiles but not to Jews, it appears to be the thread that runs through the discussion. Its veiled premise is that the various prohibitions imposed by the commandments are designed to elevate a person spiritually and that it is Jews who are meant to attain that higher spiritual plane. Rabbi Ishmael takes the view that for Noahides, the prohibition on murder includes feticide, and his view thus seems to pose considerable difficulty if Jews are not likewise forbidden, with the same degree of severity, to abort a fetus. It seems to me, however, that the maxim of "nothing permissible" is not so much a formal ruling as a moral lesson, establishing certain premises about the nature of the prohibitions or the characteristics of those who are subject to them. In other words, it is not a neutral principle to be formally and straightforwardly applied in all cases; rather, it calls for examination of the nature of the prohibition, its intended target, and its moral significance. I would posit, therefore, two substantive impediments to treating "there is nothing that is permissible for a Jew but forbidden for a gentile" as meaning that feticide is prohibited for a Jew as a matter of biblical law.

First, the talmudic discussion goes on to raise the question of stealing something of trivial value ("worth less than a *perutah*"), an act forbidden for a gentile but permitted for a Jew. The Talmud explains that because of their easygoing nature, Jews will absolve a petty thief, although Noahides will not; hence, for Noahides, even taking something trivial is considered theft. In other words, the definition of "theft" is socially determined.[31] The same cannot be said of capital cases, of course, and murder cannot be defined by reference to a particular society; still, the Talmud's explanation here suggests that application of the maxim requires an understanding of whom the commandment is directed to. The same commandment may take on different aspects, depending on the community being addressed. It is possible, therefore, that Noahides are warned more severely about feticide because they are known to be steeped in this practice. Not so Jews; accordingly, the maxim "nothing is permissible" is not relevant here, just as it is not relevant in the case of petty theft.

Second, if "nothing is permissible" assumes from the outset that Jews cannot be less moral than Noahides, it becomes necessary to inquire into the moral goal of any given prohibition. That moral quality is not always a given and not always self-evident. An example appears in the words of Isi ben Akiva in the *Mekhilta*:

> *When a man schemes [against another and kills him treacherously]* [Ex. 21:14]—Why is this passage said? Because it says *If anyone kills any human being, [he shall be put to death]* [Lev. 24:17]—I might have thought this includes one who acts deliberately, and one whose act is accidental, and gentiles [lit. "others"], and the healer who [unintentionally] causes death, and one who strikes another under the authority of the court, and one who disciplines his son or his student are all included. Hence it says *schemes* [to exclude one whose act is accidental]; *a man*, to exclude a minor [perpetrator]; *a man*, to include gentile [perpetrators]; *another* [lit. "fellow"] to include a minor [victim]; *another*, to exclude gentile [victims]. Isi ben Akiva says: Before the giving of the Torah, we were admonished with respect to [all] bloodshed; after the giving of the Torah, does the prohibition become less severe rather than more? In truth, they said, he is exempt from the law of a human court, and his judgment is given over to Heaven. (*Mekhilta De-Ri, Masekhta De-Neziqin, Mishpatim*, sec. 4)

It seems to me that Isi ben Akiva's moral outcry can be understood if one assumes at the outset that "you shall not murder" represents a sweeping, universal prohibition that applies equally to Jews and non-Jews alike. But if one were to argue that "you shall not murder" does not apply to all people equally, his outburst is incomprehensible. It follows that the claim of "does the prohibition [for Israel] become less severe rather than more" or "there is nothing that is permissible for a Jew but forbidden for a gentile" necessarily encompasses a particular interpretation of the commandment or the prohibition that gives rise to the moral outburst.

So, too, with respect to abortion. One who believes that the rule of "nothing permissible" means that abortion is biblically forbidden necessarily assumes that abortion is essentially similar to homicide and therefore forbidden except in a case of certain mortal danger to the woman. But that is not a necessary assumption with regard to the prohibition's definition or its moral significance. It may instead be assumed (in accordance with a variety of sources) that inducing an abortion is permissible not only in cases of mortal danger but also in cases of nonmortal risks to health, physical or spiritual humiliation to the woman, or violation of her dignity—all factors to be weighted morally against the abortion of a fetus that is not yet considered a life. In other words, it is possible that Noahides are categorically admonished not to spill the blood of a fetus because they are known to be wanton in that regard. That prohibition, however, does not imply a moral hierarchy that sets a person who would never cause an abortion under any circumstances on a higher plane. On the contrary; given the construct I suggested earlier, abortion may be morally superior to leaving the fetus alive in cases where the value of preserving the woman's life, health, or dignity exceeds that of preserving the fetus's life. Accordingly, to declare abortion committed by a Noahide to be a capital offense does not necessarily mean that it constitutes murder; it may simply be a prohibited act of lesser degree. And if that is so, it is possible that the prohibition will be waived for the sake of the mother's health or other needs, and in such circumstances, it may be that abortion is permitted even for a Noahide. Tosafot offer a reading close to this one:

> If its head has emerged, it is not to be touched, for one life is not set aside for another. But before its head has emerged, the midwife extends her hand and cuts it into limbs and removes it in order to save the mother. Idolaters, however, are forbidden to do so, for they are admonished regarding feticide. But it may be said that for a Jew, it is a commandment to act so as to save the mother, *and it is possible that even for an idolater, it is permitted.* (Tosafot on BT Sanh. 59a, s.v. *leika mid'am*; emphasis mine)

Those who believe that the discussion of Noahides establishes a meta-principle regarding the biblical prohibition of abortion, in light of which all other sources must be interpreted, are thus assuming in advance what they are out to prove. Without an advance understanding (in this case, a nonpermissive one) of the nature and force of the prohibition, the maxim of "nothing permissible" lacks all meaning.

At the same time, I recognize that because Rabbi Ishmael's *midrash* is based on a biblical verse, the same verse that functions as the source for prohibiting murder on the part of Noahides, Rabbi Ishmael's statement can be construed as including feticide in the overall category of murder. In that event, Jews, too, would be subject to the prohibition, and abortion would be permitted only in cases of mortal danger to the mother. It is difficult to reject such a reading entirely; but given that the other sources do not define a fetus as a life and are concerned about its status only at the stage of birth, it seems to me that the two reservations I noted earlier, together with the impression conveyed by the other sources, support the view that the discussion of Noahides must be interpreted in light of those sources rather than the other way around.

There is a further objection to the view that the discussion of Noahides implies a biblical prohibition on abortion. If the prohibition is so severe, why was it never conveyed to Israel directly, and why was it not repeated at Sinai? The tannaitic and amoraic sources already call into question the premise that everything forbidden to a Noahide is necessarily forbidden to a Jew as well and suggest that in some cases (such as the prohibition on eating a limb torn from a living animal) it was necessary to explicitly and directly impose the prohibition on Israel.

In sum, we may say that all the tannaitic sources adopt the view that a fetus is not considered a "life" (*nefesh*); in the amoraic sources, there is a split between the sources that discuss Noahides and the other texts. The overall picture shows a clear inclination to view abortion as, at most, a prohibition having only the force of rabbinic, not biblical, law. If a range of sources teach that the fetus is not a life, the view that the duties imposed on Noahides imply that Jews are subject to a biblical prohibition on abortion is left without any significant support.

Abortion during the First Forty Days of Pregnancy: The Fetus as "Merely Water"

The status of the fetus during the first forty days after its conception poses a question that lies somewhat outside the inquiry into whether the prohibition of abortion is biblical or rabbinic. The questions here are whether abortion at so early a stage of pregnancy is prohibited at all, and, if it is, what is the force of the prohibition and on what is it based? The question of abortion at this stage, then, is not necessarily linked to the question of the fetus's personhood. Some who find abortion to be biblically prohibited include even this early stage within the prohibition, while some who see it as only a rabbinic prohibition do not apply the prohibition to a fetus within the first forty days (though neither the permissive nor the nonpermissive approach necessarily entails a connection between the legal status of the fetus during the first forty days and the force of the prohibition, for one may say the prohibition, whether biblical or rabbinic, applies only after the first forty days). In other words, the sources before us do not logically compel any decision regarding the force of the general prohibition, since they differentiate between the status of the fetus during the first forty days and its status thereafter. The decisors, however, do not always accept that distinction.

The *mishnah* states that a fetus miscarried within its first forty days does not induce birth-related ritual impurity, for there is no concern that a child has already been formed:

> If a woman miscarries on the fortieth day, she has no concern about a child [having emerged and therefore no birth-related impurity]. On the forty-first day, she remains [impure] for [the interval associated with the birth of] a male and for [that associated with the birth] of a female and for [that associated with] menstrual impurity. Rabbi Ishmael says: On the forty-first day, she remains [impure] for [the interval associated with the birth of] a male and for [that associated with] menstrual impurity. On the eighty-first day, she remains [impure] for [the interval associated with the birth of] a male and for [that associated with the birth] of a female and for [that associated with] menstrual impurity. For the male is completed on the forty-first day and the female on the eighty-first. The sages say: Formation of a male and formation for a female are the same; for both, it is on the forty-first day. (M Nid. 3:7)

The talmudic discussion supports the *mishnah*'s determination on the basis of a case involving a priest's daughter. Leviticus 22:13 states that "if the priest's daughter [who married a nonpriest and thereby became disqualified from eating priestly food] is widowed or divorced and without offspring, and is back in her father's house as in her youth, she may eat of her father's food. No lay person may eat of it." The Babylonian Talmud interprets "as in her youth" to exclude one who is pregnant; in other words, the fetus precludes a priest's daughter who is the pregnant widow of a nonpriest from eating her father's priestly food. Later, the talmudic discussion takes a closer look at the meaning of "pregnant," and Rav Ḥisda permits a widow who does not know if she is pregnant to eat priestly food during the first forty days following her wedding, for during that time the fetus is considered to be "merely water." And even if it later turns out that she is pregnant, that status does not apply to the first forty days:

> It was taught: If a priest's daughter was married to a nonpriest and he died, she immerses and may eat priestly food in the evening. Rav Hisda said: She

> immerses and eats until the fortieth day, for if she is not pregnant, she is not pregnant; but if she is pregnant, until the fortieth day it [the fetus] is merely water. Abbaye said to him: If so, consider the later clause: if she turns out to be pregnant, she has sinned retroactively [by eating the priestly food]. [Rav Ḥisda replied:] Retroactively [only] to the fortieth day. (BT Yev. 69b)

THE DISCUSSION AMONG THE MEDIEVAL AUTHORITIES

Desecrating the Sabbath for a Fetus

One important context in which the medieval authorities consider a fetus to be a "life" is with regard to protecting it, when necessary, by desecrating the Sabbath or eating on a fast day. As we have seen, the rabbinic sources do not draw an absolute connection between the duty in certain circumstances to desecrate the Sabbath for the sake of a fetus and its standing as a life. Indeed, one may say the opposite: even though a fetus is not considered a "life," one may nevertheless be obligated, for other reasons, to desecrate the Sabbath on its behalf. The medieval authorities develop and expand the discussion.

As discussed earlier, the tannaitic and amoraic texts in BT *Yoma* do not cite a case in which the fetus alone is in danger. The directive there to desecrate the Sabbath or the fast when there is danger or potential danger to a pregnant woman proves nothing about the fetus's status. However, Rashi's comments on that passage suggest that it is possible to draw inferences about the fetus, whose condition is directly tied to the mother's, but he does not clearly address a situation in which the fetus alone is endangered and the mother is not:

> *If a pregnant woman has smelled* [*food on Yom Kippur*]—The fetus smells the food and craves it, and if she does not eat it, both are endangered.
>
> *In accord with the advice of experts*—If two physicians say he is in danger if he does not eat. (Rashi on BT Yoma 82a)

Some of the medieval authorities argued that danger to the mother and danger to the fetus could not be separated; accordingly, their views would seem to be irrelevant to any discussion of the fetus's standing as an independent life. This was the explicitly stated view of Rosh[32] and Ran.[33] The wording of the *Halakhot Gedolot* is a bit obscure. Naḥmanides understood the author to be referring directly to the fetus. But one could understand "protection of life" as used at the end of the passage to refer to the life of the woman:

> And it need not be an ill person; it could be a pregnant woman whose child would move from its place in her womb if she did not eat. And even though we say there is doubt about whether it will survive or be a stillbirth,[34] it seems better to give her [food], for it was taught, "if a pregnant woman smells sacrificial meat or pig meat. . . . , for nothing stands in the way of protecting life except for [the prohibitions on] idolatry, incest, and bloodshed." (*Halakhot Gedolot*, end of the laws of Yom Kippur, p. 188)

Naḥmanides drew several conclusions based on this passage in *Halakhot Gedolot*:[35]

1. Even if there is danger solely to the fetus,[36] the mother is fed because of concern about a miscarriage.
2. Even though a fetus in principle does not invoke the concept of saving a life, with regard to observance of the commandments, the Sabbath is desecrated on its behalf on the grounds of "desecrate one Sabbath on his behalf so he will [survive to] observe many Sabbaths."
3. The Sabbath is to be desecrated even where the pregnancy is within its first forty days.[37]

According to Naḥmanides's reading of *Sefer Halakhot Gedolot*, the principle of saving lives does not pertain to a fetus, for it is not a life. The Sabbath is to be desecrated on its behalf because it is nonetheless a potential life, but that rule has no implications regarding the fetus's personhood.[38]

In his novellae on *Niddah*, Naḥmanides himself explicitly raises, *but then rejects*, the possibility of drawing a connection between the fetus not being a life and the duty to desecrate the Sabbath on its behalf.[39]

Is Naḥmanides referring to a fetus in the special circumstances described in *'Arakhin* or to a fetus in general? The answer depends on how one understands his position. Does he believe (as he suggests in his interpretation of *Halakhot Gedolot*) that the Sabbath is to be desecrated even for a fetus less than forty days after conception; or only for a fetus more than forty days after conception; or only for a fetus that is no longer considered "its mother's limb"? Later in his discussion in *Torat Ha-'Adam*, Naḥmanides cites an opinion that the Sabbath is not desecrated for a miscarried fetus unless there is concern about the mother's life. The case in *'Arakhin* is a special one in which the mother has already died and the fetus is considered already born and no longer "its mother's limb." Only in such a case is the Sabbath to be desecrated on the fetus's behalf:

> Now, some take the view that the Sabbath is not to be desecrated for a miscarried fetus, and that in the case of the pregnant woman who smells [food], the concern is that she might die, for anyone who miscarries is presumed to be endangered. And the case of the woman in labor who dies on the Sabbath has a different rationale, for since she has died, it is as if the fetus has been born, and is no longer its mother's limb; for it is not dependent upon her . . . and it has the presumption of being alive, and cases of doubt about life are to be resolved leniently [that is, in favor of suspending the halakhic requirement that might endanger the life]. (*Torat Ha-'Adam, 'Inyan Ha-Sakanah,* pp. 28–29)

What is Naḥmanides's own position? Does he agree with "some [who] take the view," or does he share the opinion of the author of *Halakhot Gedolot*? The author of *Minḥat Ḥinukh* understood that Naḥmanides differed from the author of *Halakhot Gedolot* and took the view that the Sabbath should not be desecrated for a fetus, except where its mother died and it is considered to have been born in all respects.[40] R. Abraham Ha-Levi Gombiner, author of *Magen 'Avraham*, takes a similar position.[41] In sum, however, Naḥmanides's position remains unclear.[42]

The Tosafists treat the question of desecrating the Sabbath for the sake of a fetus in the context of the sources in *'Ohalot* and *'Arakhin* discussed earlier:

> *It dies first*—But it may be that only when its mother is still living is [the fetus's killer] not liable until its head emerges, for it is somewhat dependent on its mother's life; but where she has died, [the killer of the fetus] is liable, for it is as if simply situated inside a box. You might ask: Should you want to say it is permitted to kill it in the womb even if its mother has died, and do not treat it as simply situated inside a box, why then can the Sabbath be desecrated for its sake by bringing a knife through the public way to tear the mother, as is shown in the first chapter of *'Arakhin* (7b)? The answer would

> be: For the sake of preserving life the Sabbath may in any case be desecrated on its behalf, *even though it is permissible to kill it*; for if one is moribund as a result of human action, one who kills him is not liable, as is said in the chapter *Ha-Nisrafin* (BT Sanh.78a). Most of those who are moribund go on to die, yet the Sabbath is still desecrated on their behalf, as is said in the final chapter of *Yoma* (84b)—when preservation of life is at stake, one does not assume that the situation will necessarily turn out as most similar situations do. (Tosafot on BT Nid. 44a–b; emphasis mine)

In other words, the Tosafists themselves distinguish between a case in which the mother is alive and the fetus, still dependent on her for its nourishment, is not yet an independent life, and a case in which the mother has already died and the fetus is no longer dependent on her. In the former case, one is not liable for killing the fetus, but in the latter case one is, for the fetus is "as if simply situated inside a box." But they add that even if one were to say it is permitted to kill the fetus in utero after its mother dies, the Sabbath is nonetheless desecrated for its sake. Tosafot's line of reasoning has several implications:

1. The Tosafists understand the *mishnah* in *'Ohalot* in a manner consistent with the second interpretive option described earlier; that is, the fetus has no independent standing as a life and, accordingly, no legal standing by dint of which it can create legal facts in civil cases. The *mishnah* in *'Ohalot* corresponds to the treatment of the matter in *'Arakhin*, which sees no contradiction between executing a pregnant woman unless she is "seated on the birthing stool" and desecrating the Sabbath for the sake of the fetus once its mother has died.
2. The Tosafists determine that it is *permissible* to kill the fetus. This is an unambiguous statement that is highly significant in analyzing the force of the prohibition. At first blush, it appears inconsistent with statements by Tosafot elsewhere to the effect that though a Jew is not punished for feticide, it nevertheless is "not permitted." The Tosafists may believe that it is permissible to kill the fetus where necessary to save a life or in other cases where something is in play that trumps the prohibition on feticide (such as the mother being subject to capital punishment). But even if we take "it is permissible" to mean only that one who kills a fetus is not

> liable, they are referring even to a situation in which the mother has died and the fetus is considered to be living in its own right. A fortiori, then, when the mother is alive (and the fetus is dependent on her) feticide should certainly incur no liability and may even be permitted.

No manuscripts are extant of Tosafot on this part of tractate *Niddah*, so it is impossible to know with certainty whether this is an authentic version or whether it contains a scribal error, as argued by R. Moses Feinstein (whose position will be discussed fully below). Tosafot *Ha-Rosh* does not treat the paragraph tag-lined "It dies first," and R. Tam's *Sefer Ha-Yashar* does not cite alternative readings of the paragraph. In the first printed edition of tractate *Niddah* (Venice), the reading is identical to that in our printings.

To summarize the treatment of the issue by the medieval authorities, we can say it is unclear whether logical inferences may be drawn regarding the fetus's status as a life—and, correspondingly, regarding the existence of a formal prohibition on feticide and its biblical or rabbinic force—from the rules regarding desecration of the Sabbath in order to save a fetus. Some authorities believe danger to the fetus cannot be isolated from danger to the mother, a position that precludes drawing the inferences in question; and those who focus on danger to the fetus itself disagree about whether the Sabbath is desecrated to protect the life of the fetus. And even those who believe the Sabbath is to be desecrated for the sake of a fetus do not determine on that basis whether or not the fetus has standing as a life (according to Tosafot, it may even be permitted to kill a fetus a priori); accordingly, the issue of desecrating the Sabbath for the sake of a fetus is not determinative with regard to the existence of a biblical prohibition on feticide.

Rodef

As we have seen, both Talmuds conclude that a fetus should not be classified as a *rodef*. It follows that the permissibility of feticide in the *mishnah* in *'Ohalot* cannot be grounded in the fetus's status as a *rodef* and must reflect the determination that a fetus is not considered a "life." That seems to be the position of Rashi, who writes:

> *Its head has emerged*—In the case of a woman in danger because of a difficult delivery. The earlier statement taught: the midwife extends her hand and

> cuts the fetus, removing it limb by limb; for as long as it has not emerged into the world, it is not a life and it may be killed to save its mother. But once its head has emerged, it is not to be touched and killed, for it is as if born, and one life is not set aside for another. (BT Sanh. 72b)

Consistent with the first interpretive option presented earlier, however, this does not necessarily mean that Rashi believes abortion is permitted in circumstances in which there is a clash between the fetus and the interests of the mother (as one might have thought, given that the fetus is not a life). It is possible, rather, to read him as permitting feticide *only* to save the mother, because the fetus is not a life.

Maimonides, notwithstanding the conclusion reached by both Talmuds, determines that a fetus jeopardizing its mother's life may be killed because it is considered a *rodef*:

> Now, it is a negative commandment to not spare the life of a *rodef*. Accordingly, the sages taught that if a pregnant woman is having difficulty delivering, it is permitted to cut up the fetus in her belly, whether by drug or by hand, because it is like a *rodef*, pursuing her to kill her. But once its head has emerged it is not to be touched, for one life is not set aside for another, and this is the nature of the world. (*Mishneh Torah*, *Hilkhot Roẓeiaḥ U-Shemirat Ha-Nefesh* 1:9)

What Maimonides says here raises several questions:

1. What could be the rationale for regarding the fetus as a *rodef* while it remains in its mother's womb but removing it from that category as soon as its head has emerged? Why is the argument that "this is the nature of the world" (which seems a paraphrase of the talmudic comment that "she is pursued by [decree of] Heaven") relevant only when the fetus has emerged, but not while it remains in its mother's womb?
2. Does Maimonides here disagree with all other medieval authorities and take the view that the fetus is considered a life and therefore may be killed only if it is pursuing its mother to kill her? The practical significance of this distinction pertains to the force of the prohibition. Taking his words at face value, it would appear that the fetus may be killed only

if it is an actual *rodef*; otherwise, feticide would be murder. But if his words are understood in accordance with the premise that a fetus is not a life, feticide would be permissible even in non-*rodef* situations, that is, not only when it is posing a definite mortal danger to the woman.

Maimonides's substantial new departure in understanding the *mishnah* in *'Ohalot* may be illuminated further by his general understanding of the *rodef*. He treats the issue in *Hilkhot Roẓeiaḥ* (Laws of the Murderer); for our purposes, the following passage is relevant:

> If they admonished him and he is pursuing [another], even if he did not accept the warning, because he is continuing to pursue, he may be killed, but if they can rescue the pursued at the cost of one of the pursuer's limbs, such as by hitting him with an arrow or a stone or a sword and cutting off his hand or breaking his leg or blinding his eye, they should do so. But if they cannot aim [well enough to do so] and cannot rescue [the pursued] without killing the pursuer, they kill him even though he has not yet killed. (*Mishneh Torah, Hilkhot Roẓeiḥ* 1:7)

In light of this, it may be said that Maimonides meant to treat the fetus as a *rodef* for purposes of determining the *manner* in which the mother is to be rescued. If she can be rescued at the cost of one of the fetus's limbs alone, the fetus is not to be killed, and that is what the *mishnah* means when it says "limb by limb." Maimonides does not mean to treat the fetus conceptually as *rodef*; if he did, he would have no reason to distinguish a fetus in the womb from one in the process of emerging. Rather, he meant to say that the entire birthing situation "is the nature of the world," and that is why he is careful to say the fetus is "like a *rodef*" and not a *rodef* in actuality.

The author of *Sefer Miẓvot Gadol* cites Maimonides verbatim,[43] not mentioning the questions posed by his comments, and R. Beḥye b. Asher ibn Halawa likewise seems to accept that position without reservations.[44] Moreover, Maimonides's commentators are silent on the matter—oddly so, given its problematic nature. The later authorities, in contrast, engage in an intense and wide-ranging exposition of Maimonides's position (see the discussion below). In general, I agree with Feldman that discussion of the fetus as a *rodef* would have ended with the resolution of the matter in the two Talmuds, had not Maimonides's comments on the matter and the various interpretations given them forged a new way of understanding the *mishnah* in *'Ohalot*. That understanding set the stage for more restrictive rulings regarding abortion.

Noahides

Of the medieval authorities, only the Tosafists considered the Noahide aspect of the prohibition on abortion:

> *Nothing* [*that is forbidden for a gentile*] *is permissible for a Jew*—We do not say this regarding something that is commanded for Jews; an idolater who rests [on the Sabbath] is liable, yet for Israel, it is a commandment. And with respect to feticide, for which an idolater is liable and a Jew is not liable, it nevertheless is not permitted. But a difficulty is posed by what is said in the chapter *Ben Sorer U-Moreh* (BT Sanh. 72b), that once its head has emerged, it is not touched, for one life is not displaced for another, but before its head has emerged, the midwife extends her hand and cuts it into limbs and removes it to save the mother. But it is forbidden for an idolater to act in that way, for they are admonished with respect to feticide. We may say in response that here, too, it is a commandment for Jews to save [the mother] and it may be that even for an idolater, it is permitted. (Tosafot on BT Sanh. 59a)

Tosafot analyze the nature of the prohibition on abortion, determining that one must consider not only the saving of the fetus but also the duty to save the mother, for otherwise the rule of "nothing permissible" would contradict the *mishnah* in *'Ohalot*. This determination has important implications related, among other things, to the status of the fetus. If we say there is an absolute prohibition on feticide, it follows that that fetus has the status of a life; but if it may be killed, for example, to save the mother's life, it cannot have that status, since "one life is not displaced for another." (It is possible, of course, that Tosafot would agree that for purposes of saving the mother's life, the fetus should be regarded as a *rodef* and may therefore be killed even though it is a life.)

In their commentary on tractate *Ḥulin*, the Tosafists reiterate the distinction between prohibition and commandment; where there is a positive commandment involved for Jews, the rule of "nothing is permissible" does not apply:

It is permitted for both an idolater and a Jew—For regarding something with respect to which a Jew is commanded, we do not say "is there anything that is permissible for a Jew [that is forbidden for a gentile]." . . . And even though a Noahide is put to death for feticide, as is said there, a Jew is not put to death, but it nevertheless is forbidden. (Tosafot on BT Ḥul. 33a)

To resolve the difficulty posed by the rule of "nothing permissible," Tosafot here draw an interpretive distinction between the positive commandment to save the woman and the negative prohibition against aborting the fetus. In doing so, this commentary is consistent with the other sources that treat the subject of abortion and, as it turns out, with the Tosafists' approach in tractate *Niddah*, which, as I see it, does not imply a biblical prohibition. The commentary on *Niddah* suggests that the rule of "nothing permissible" cannot be applied in this case, because Jews are commanded to save the mother; accordingly, there is no moral tension between the duties imposed on the Noahide and those imposed on the Jew. On the other hand, those who see discussion of Noahides as clearly establishing a biblical prohibition on abortion for Jews will need intricate argumentation to resolve the problem posed by the gulf between the treatment of Noahides and the many other sources that do adopt that interpretation.

The Fetus as "Merely Water"

The medieval authorities considered two questions pertaining to the status of the fetus, one related to the circumstances under which a woman may eat priestly food (*terumah*) and the other to when, if at all, a father may bequeath property to an unborn son.

With respect to eating priestly food (for clarification, see earlier discussion of the talmudic sources), no one disagrees with the view that until forty days into the pregnancy, the fetus is "merely water." As Maimonides sums it up, "throughout the [first] forty days, it is not a fetus but is considered merely water" (*Mishneh Torah, Hilkhot Terumah* 8:3).

Regarding bequests, opinions are divided; but the lines are drawn not over the status of the fetus but over the intentions of the testator. The question posed is whether it may be said of the fetus, during its first forty days, that the father's "mind is on it"—is he aware that his wife is carrying a fetus or is it not really present in his consciousness? Ritva believes that during the first forty days, the father's state of mind precludes saying that property can be bequeathed to the fetus, for "his mind is not on it." And according to Me'iri, even after forty days one cannot say the father's mind is on the fetus, for the fetus remains "something unknown." Nevertheless, the situation changes somewhat with respect to bequests, for "with regard to bequests, a person's mind is on anything whose arrival he pays attention to, and once something is formed, the mind encompasses it."[45]

We have already encountered Naḥmanides's position on this matter in his comments on the *Halakhot Gedolot* regarding desecration of the Sabbath for the sake of a fetus less than forty days old.[46] Naḥmanides interprets the author of *Halakhot Gedolot* as allowing Sabbath desecration in such a case "so that he may observe many Sabbaths" (though the author of *Halakhot Gedolot* himself does not say that). But I have already shown that Naḥmanides does not draw a connection between the fact that the fetus is not a "life" and the duty to violate the Sabbath on its behalf—though there is no need to take that as Naḥmanides's halakhic determination. In any event, even if Naḥmanides meant to adopt the approach of the *Halakhot Gedolot*, we still find a division of opinions among the medieval authorities, for Rosh and Ran do not share Naḥmanides's understanding of *Halakhot Gedolot*, nor do they make any mention of the duty to desecrate the Sabbath for the sake of a fetus less than forty days old.

It seems to me that on the whole, the medieval sources allow one to conclude that an embryo during the first forty days of pregnancy is not classified as a fetus and that there is no prohibition at all on aborting it at that stage.

THE DISCUSSION AMONG THE LATER AUTHORITIES

When one traces the halakhic exegesis that appears in the rabbinic literature and in the writings of the medieval authorities with respect to the array of issues related to abortion, one can draw several conclusions regarding the personhood of the fetus and its relationship to the woman carrying it. The intertwining of these interpretive threads will enable us to present the picture in its entirety, so that we might reach a general conclusion regarding whether, when, and under what circumstances (if any) abortion is permissible. Therefore, I have organized my discussion of the later authorities not around the specific issues presented to this point but with reference to the key responsa written on the subject. By their nature, those responsa produce a synthesis of the various sources in accord with each decisor's understanding of the situation that confronted him and the conflicting moral values it posed.

I cannot, of course, discuss every one of the later authorities who took up the question. Instead, I will examine those responsa that figure extensively in the findings of the leading contemporary decisors or that I regard as particularly important. Because the halakhic discussion in the responsa literature tends to be marked by synthesis and analysis of earlier sources, I will present the issues in the sequence used in the responsa themselves, assigning them to categories only if the decisor himself does so.

The Sixteenth Century

RADBAZ Two important sixteenth-century decisions by R. David b. Solomon Ibn Zimra (Radbaz) hold that the prohibition on abortion is a matter only of rabbinic, not biblical, law. Radbaz was asked about the practice, accepted among midwives, of killing a fetus still in utero when the mother was dying in childbirth. Radbaz replied that the practice should certainly be protested, and that it was even permitted on the Sabbath to bring a knife and extract the fetus in an attempt to save it, but, nonetheless:

> there is no act of murder involved and, yet, no violation of the Sabbath. . . . And should you say there is at least uncertainty about whether there is human life here, for the Sabbath is violated on account of it, one may respond that since it has not yet come out into the world, and it lacks the presumption of survival, one who kills it is not considered to have taken a possible human life. (Radbaz, 2, 695)

Radbaz was addressing the seeming contradiction between the fact that the Sabbath may be desecrated to save a fetus and the fact that one who kills a fetus is not guilty of murder. His explanation bolsters the argument that there is no necessary linkage between the issues. The Sabbath may be desecrated to save a fetus because the fetus is considered "a possible life"; but that does not necessarily imply that killing a fetus is murder. His position is further clarified by another responsum on whether a priest who struck a woman deliberately, causing her to miscarry, is disqualified on that account from reciting the priestly blessing:

> In our case, he is not disqualified [even if he acted deliberately], for this is not the killing of a human life; it has not yet attained the presumption of survival, since it has not yet come out into the world. Know that if a woman is having difficulty giving birth, the fetus *in utero* is to be cut up, because of the danger to its mother (M 'Ohal. 7:6); and why should that be, given that one soul is not to be set aside for the sake of another? The reason is that the fetus does not yet have a presumption of survival; and even though some have said the reason is that [the fetus] is a *rodef*... it is, in any event, the first reason that is true. And conclusive proof for this [view of the] law is the verse "If men should fight...." Accordingly, it is clear that [this priest] is [only] liable to the woman's husband or his heirs for the value of the fetus, and why should he be disqualified from priestly service [and the priestly blessing] [merely] on account of monetary liability[?]. (Radbaz, letter 14, *'Oraḥ Ḥayyim* 22)

It appears that Radbaz shares Rashi's view that the fetus is not considered a life and that the priest in this case may go on reciting the priestly blessing because he has not committed murder. That conclusion is bolstered by the fact that the punishment for killing a fetus is monetary (that is, civil), not criminal, and it rounds out the view according to which abortion is not to be seen as violating a biblical prohibition.

The Sixteenth and Seventeenth Centuries

MAHARIT R. Joseph Trani (Maharit) wrote two detailed responsa concerning abortion; at first glance, they appear to contradict each other.[47] Contemporary decisors make extensive use of these responsa, and I therefore will attempt to clarify his position by reconstructing his original response.

The first of the two documents is marked by several oddities. Contrary to usual practice, the question posed to the decisor does not appear at the beginning of the responsum, though the context allows us to infer that the author was asked whether a Jewish physician is permitted to assist in aborting a non-Jewish fetus. Immediately following his conclusion regarding that question, there appears an additional and entirely unrelated passage dealing with the afternoon prayer. Finally, unlike Maharit's other responsa, this one does not conclude with his signature. These facts call into question the authenticity of the text, as we shall see.

An examination of the responsum shows that it considers the personhood of the fetus and the force of the prohibition on aborting it; Maharit examines the contradictions among the sources and attempts to resolve them. As he reads the *mishnah* in *'Ohalot*, the rationale of "her life takes precedence over its life" implies that in the most severe case of danger to the mother's life, her life is to be favored; but if we are not dealing with such a case, we must be concerned about the status of the fetus. As he puts it, "the life of the fetus provides a basis for concern and uncertainty." But he immediately directs our attention to the contradiction between this reading of the situation and that of the passage in *'Arakhin* holding that the mother's life is to be favored not only in a case of risk to life but also in a case of disgrace. It further follows from the passage in *'Arakhin* that the fetus is considered to have the status of uncertain (that is, potential) life for purposes of desecrating the Sabbath to save it, and that the Sabbath is therefore to be desecrated in the case of a woman seated on the birthing stool. If that is so, he asks, how can the mother and the fetus be put to death together? And, in addition to everything else, the consideration of Noahides suggests that a Jew is prohibited from killing fetuses.

Maharit's effort to derive a coherent reading of all these sources suggests that one truly should be concerned about the life of the fetus and that the case of the woman about to be executed is distinct, in that the fetus there is considered to be a limb of its mother destined to die with her. But where a woman is dying a natural death, the fetus is considered to have already come into the world, with only "a door locked before it"; accordingly, the Sabbath is violated to save it. There is a difference of opinion regarding saving the life of a prematurely delivered fetus, but Maharit rules that uncertainty with regard to human life is to be resolved leniently, and it follows, in his view, that it is forbidden to put a gentile's premature fetus to death as well. He concludes, in the end, that the Jewish physician is forbidden to assist in aborting a non-Jewish fetus because of the prohibition on "placing an obstacle in the path of the blind," given that gentiles are forbidden to kill fetuses and doing so is a capital offense. The responsum suggests that Maharit considers the fetus to have the status of "uncertain [that is, possible] life," and that his overall inclination with respect to abortion is to forbid it.

The second responsum follows an entirely different course. For one thing, it begins with a clearly stated question: "Is it permitted to assist a gentile woman wanting to become pregnant or to abort? Is there any prohibition on account of loss of gentile life?" In the responsum, Maharit makes no reference at all to the issue of "placing an obstacle in the path of the blind"; instead, he determines that if this is an expert physician who has assisted Jewish women, the principle of not treating non-Jews in a discriminatory fashion, lest doing so generate hatred of Jews, might well be invoked if he declined to assist the gentile patient. Moreover, if he deceived her by taking a fee and not attempting to heal her (by aborting the pregnancy), he would violate the prohibition on stealing from a gentile. In his view, no issue of loss of life is presented here, for Jews do not consider fetuses to be lives at all, or even partial lives, and one who causes an abortion is liable only for the value of the child-to-have-been, to be paid to the woman's husband. Moreover, lest one think execution of a condemned pregnant woman should be delayed until after the fetus is born so that the husband does not lose the fetus's value, the explanation given in *'Arakhin* that "it is plain that it is part of her body" implies, according to Maharit, that "concerns about loss of life do not drive [this issue]." At the end of his responsum, he determines that with respect to a Jewish woman, "for the sake of its mother, it appears to be permitted to become involved in helping her abort, since it is her medical treatment." That is, he certainly does not infer the existence of a prohibition based on biblical law; rather, inasmuch as the fetus is not considered a person, it is permissible to abort it for the sake of any need of the mother, including the avoidance of disgrace, as specified in the passage in *'Arakhin*. Maharit signs the responsum in his usual fashion.

This responsum, too, has a number of surprising elements. First, the question posed concerns a gentile woman, but Maharit devotes only a few words to that aspect of the matter and does not sum up his conclusion; at the end of the responsum, he considers only the case of a Jewish woman. Moreover, he refers not at all to the fact that a Noahide who kills a fetus is subject to the death penalty, nor does he mention the *mishnah* in *'Ohalot*. And, of course, how can we account for the major difference between the two responsa regarding the force of the prohibition?

Because of these difficulties, R. Feinstein suggested that the responsum is a forgery, and he declined to consider it.[48] R. Waldenberg, in contrast, attempted to reconcile the two responsa, arguing that Maharit wrote a single responsum that, "for some organizational reason," the copyist divided into two parts. After reconstructing the original version of the responsum, R. Waldenberg concludes that Maharit began by presenting the contradictory talmudic passages, as a result of which he had some doubts about the actual halakhah. By the end, however, Maharit decided the matter in accord with the view that a fetus is not considered a person and, accordingly, that "concerns about loss of life do not drive [this issue]."[49]

Support for R. Waldenberg's view can be found in the comments of R. Elijah Ben-Ḥaim.[50] He does not say if he is familiar with R. Waldenberg's responsum (published in 1967), but he, too, believes, contrary to R. Feinstein, that Maharit's responsum is not a forgery and that there is reason to believe we are dealing with a single responsum. It seems likely that part 1 of Maharit's responsa (in which the responsa on abortion are contained) was published in Salonika but that his sons later transferred the printing to Venice, evidently because they were dissatisfied with the Salonika printing. In his introduction to part 2 of Maharit's responsa, the author's son writes as follows:

> Almost immediately after this book of divine Torah reached the hands of diligent students, it became readily evident to those who examined it that the craftsmanship of the engravers [that is, printers] was deficient, with respect to the paper and the printing . . . in some places the letters are seen and not seen, printed in ink on erased paper. From beginning to end they reversed law and made Torah into two Torahs. . . . And after I saw that, I decided to go to preeminent craftsmen, who engrave properly in the famed city of Venice. (Introduction of Maharit's son to *Maharit*, part 2)

Ben-Ḥaim notes as well that R. Ḥaim Benvenisti, a student of Maharit, wrote about the confusion in the responsa and said that Maharit himself was blameless in that regard.[51] Accordingly, Ben-Ḥaim believes that the first responsum dealt with the afternoon prayer, the subject treated in its final passage, and that the two responsa should be combined so that the entire first part of the first responsum, up to the point where the subject changes to the afternoon prayer, is placed at the end of what is now the second responsum.

In that event, it seems likely that the question posed to Maharit was whether a Jewish physician could abort a gentile woman's pregnancy. He responded that a fetus is not considered a life; that with respect to a gentile, the principle of "desecrate one Sabbath so he may observe many Sabbaths" does not apply; and that the only prohibition is that against "placing an obstacle in the path of the blind" if no other physicians are present. If other physicians are present, there is no prohibition. This suggestion is consistent with R. Waldenberg's reconstruction. R. Waldenberg himself, in his dispute with R. Feinstein over whether the responsum is a forgery,[52] notes that the author of *Ha-Kenesset Ha-Gedolah* cites these responsa by Maharit regarding abortion without expressing any concern about internal contradictions or possible forgery.

All of the foregoing suggests it is quite likely that Maharit does not take the view that abortion is biblically forbidden. His position is a more lenient one, allowing for abortion even in cases where there is no clear mortal danger to the woman, inasmuch as the only concern is over monetary loss to the husband. Accordingly, "We say there that a woman about to be executed is struck opposite her womb, so the fetus dies first and the woman is not brought to a state of disgrace. From this we see that the fetus is killed directly in order to avoid disgrace to the mother, and they were not concerned about this entailing a loss of life."[53]

'EMUNAT SHEMU'EL During the seventeenth century, R. Samuel Kaidenower wrote what is almost certainly the most lenient responsum written by any of the later authorities on the subject of abortion. The question deals with the extent, if any, to which a Jewish physician asked to assist in the abortion of a gentile woman's pregnancy is forbidden to do so. From an examination of the *mishnah* in *'Ohalot*, he concludes that there is no prohibition on feticide, since it is permitted, even a priori, to set aside the life of the fetus for the sake of its mother. Not only is there no biblical prohibition, but it is hard to say with any certainty that there is any rabbinic prohibition: "there is no biblical-law prohibition, *only a bit of a rabbinic prohibition*" (emphasis mine).[54]

ḤAVVOT YA'IR A responsum by R. Yair Bachrach deals with whether a fetus that is a *mamzer*[55] may be aborted.[56] He finds no distinction in principle between a fetus that is a *mamzer* and one that is not—not as a matter of legal status and not as a matter of social treatment—and the halakhic question turns out to be whether it is permitted to abort (any) fetus in a situation that does not involve mortal danger to the mother. His responsum has two distinct parts.

The first part of his analysis rests primarily on the second interpretive construct applied earlier to the *mishnah* in *'Ohalot*, which is based on the distinction between a fetus that has started emerging and one that has not yet begun the birthing process. He concludes that once the fetus has started emerging, it may not be aborted except to save the mother—the position implied by the *mishnah* in *'Ohalot* and strengthened by the passage in *'Arakhin*. Before that point, however, "it appears, according to all opinions, to be permitted."[57] Nor, in his view, is there any basis for questioning that conclusion on the grounds that the Sabbath is desecrated to save a fetus or that the mother is fed on Yom Kippur to avoid endangering it, for in both cases the permissive ruling is meant to protect the mother from danger, not only the fetus. If there were danger to the fetus alone, we would not desecrate the Sabbath to save it nor would we relieve the mother from fasting, for if it is *permitted* to kill it, it is impossible to say the Sabbath is violated to save it.

In his view, the statements of the Tosafists, who permit both killing the fetus and desecrating the Sabbath on its behalf, lack any foundation and are worded imprecisely. Rather, they should have said that even though the Sabbath is desecrated on a fetus's behalf, one who kills it is not liable (and the action may even be permissible), for the Sabbath is desecrated, in essence, for the sake of the mother, not the fetus. On the basis of the formal halakhic assessment in the first part of his responsum, he concludes that the ruling in the case at issue should be permissive. In the second part of his responsum, however, he expresses a different opinion regarding the halakhic constructs of the first part and clearly does so for reasons of "public policy" or to justify existing custom and endow it with legal force. Invoking the importance of deterring forbidden sexual relations, he takes a different halakhic tack and suggests that abortion is forbidden on account of wasteful emission of seed.

Most of R. Bachrach's discussion, though, is directed to Maimonides's view of the fetus as a *rodef*. He is troubled primarily by Maimonides's justification of the feticide on the grounds that the fetus is a *rodef*, contrary to the words of the Mishnah, though Maimonides himself goes on to agree with the conclusion in the *gemara* that once the fetus's head has emerged it cannot be seen as a *rodef*, for that is the nature of the world. R. Bachrach argues that it makes no sense to adopt the claim of *rodef* with respect to the fetus even prior to the emergence of its head, for is it not the "nature of the world" that a pregnancy entails risks when the fetus is in the mother's womb as well? His response is grounded on the fact that while the fetus is not considered a "life" and killing it is not a capital offense, doing so certainly entails a sin. According to R. Bachrach, Maimonides thought so as well, which is why he wrote that the fetus is "*like* a *rodef*": even though it is not a "life," it may not be killed gratuitously, that is, it may be aborted only when it subjects its mother to mortal danger.

The *Ḥavvot Ya'ir*'s ultimate conclusion is that aborting a fetus is not permitted, even if it is a *mamzer*, and, accordingly, that no abortion is permitted unless it is necessary to save the mother's life. However, this conclusion is not necessarily dictated by R. Bachrach's halakhic analyses.

We see from this responsum that the rationale for a strict line of interpretation is grounded in pedagogic considerations, primarily deterrence of promiscuity ("in order to erect a barrier against promiscuity and those who pursue it"). The halakhic analysis is consciously and openly rejected, and the responsum therefore cannot be seen solely as a "formal" halakhic analysis. In what follows, I will support my argument that, from a woman's perspective, this is a one-sided assessment (both because is cannot deter an adulterous man to the same degree as an adulterous woman and because it fails to take account of the effects on a woman's life) and that this one-sidedness is a recurring feature of contemporary rulings.

The Eighteenth and Nineteenth Centuries

The eighteenth century produced three principal responsa on our subject. Two of them are widely considered in the contemporary decisional literature; the third is considered primarily by R. Waldenberg and R. Ovadia Yosef.

SHE'EILAT YA'AVEẒ The question posed to R. Jacob Emden (*Ya'aveẓ*) dealt with the possibility of permitting abortion for a woman, unmarried or married, who had engaged in promiscuous sex.[58] He believed that aborting a kosher (that is, non-*mamzer*) fetus was forbidden, but that a *mamzer* could be aborted on the premise that its adulterous mother had engaged in sexual relations that constituted a capital offense and, were the community authorized to try capital cases, they would execute her and kill her fetus as part of that process. Although the Jewish community in R. Emden's day did not try capital cases, such a woman was still subject to a heavenly imposed death penalty. Accordingly, the situation is precisely the one discussed in *'Arakhin*. The fetus is considered "a limb of its mother," and as long as it retains that quality, it has a role in the sin she committed and she may abort it. Beyond that, R. Emden argues, suicide on the part of the woman would be considered a meritorious act, and she would not be punished for it. But he immediately adds:

> Even in the case of a kosher fetus there would be a basis for ruling leniently in a case of great need, as long as it had not begun to move [toward emerging]. [That is so] even if it is not a case of mortal danger to its mother, but only to save her from its bad effects, for it causes her great pain. But this requires further inquiry.[59]

This is a fairly surprising conclusion, for if it is permitted in principle to abort a fetus to save the mother from disgrace, it is not clear why there should be a distinction between a *mamzer* and a kosher fetus. But despite those comments, and even though he discusses the *Ḥavvot Ya'ir*'s rationale and concludes that the prohibition on wasting seed is waived for the sake of fulfilling a commandment, R. Emden nevertheless concludes that aborting a kosher fetus is considered unnecessary destruction: "in our view, in an ordinary case [that is, a case of a kosher fetus], there is a prohibition on wasting a fetus."[60]

In other words, R. Emden concedes that a fetus may be aborted to spare its mother "great pain," and it appears from context that he is not necessarily speaking of danger to her physical health but emotional suffering as well. Nevertheless, he hesitates to follow that principle to its conclusion and ultimately permits abortion only if the fetus is a *mamzer*. His difficulty seems to hinge on how "great pain" is to be interpreted. Still, we should emphasize his central interpretive posture: he accepts the distinction between a fetus that has begun to emerge and one that has not yet done so, and he assumes that abortion would be permitted, even if not needed to save the mother, *before* the birthing process begins. That determination is consistent with the second interpretive option we suggested earlier for the *mishnah* in *'Ohalot* and for the passage in *'Arakhin*. In any case, the difficulties he himself notes with respect to the distinctions between a married woman and an unmarried one remain unresolved.

HA-NODA BI-YEHUDAH According to R. Ezekiel b. Judah Landau (*Ha-Noda Bi-Yehudah*), the principal problem in Maimonides's treatment of abortion is that according to the *mishnah* in *'Ohalot*, a fetus may be aborted to save the mother even if it is not a *rodef*, because killing a fetus is not a capital offense but killing the mother is. Nevertheless, R. Landau himself believes it is forbidden to kill the fetus: "Is it permitted to kill one who is mortally wounded [*tereifah*[61]] in order to save who is whole? We have never heard of such a thing!"[62] To be sure, the Sabbath is not violated to save the fetus alone if its mother is not in danger; but because it is nevertheless forbidden to kill the fetus, one might think that even if the mother is endangered, it is best to adopt a passive stance and not actively rescue her at the expense of the fetus. Maimonides therefore had to attribute to the fetus a status similar to that of the *rodef* in order to teach that it may be killed.

R. Landau's comments here are quite surprising. If the life of the fetus is not important enough to warrant desecration of the Sabbath, how can one sit passively by and not save the mother at its expense?

Although he reaches a contrary conclusion, the R. Landau's comments support the second possible reading of the *mishnah* in *'Ohalot*. Initially, it would seem that one should have more reservations about feticide when the woman is seated on the birthing stool, for the fetus has already begun to emerge; nevertheless, the *mishnah* says it is permitted to kill the fetus to save the mother. The need to emphasize that the fetus's resemblance to a *rodef* is what makes the feticide permissible arises from the preconception that feticide is forbidden; and the *mishnah* overall is interpreted in that light though its plain meaning does not require that reading. Accordingly, Maimonides's position, which considers the fetus to be a *rodef* before it begins to emerge from the womb but not after, is problematic. But at the end of his responsum, R. Landau acknowledges that he has not resolved this difficulty: "I still do not see this clearly, and far-fetched resolutions have already been offered in previous generations."[63] These remarks may weaken his overall interpretation of Maimonides's position with respect to *rodef*.

As for a Noahide, there is no problem from R. Landau's perspective, and the rule of "nothing permissible" is not pertinent, for he believes that Jews, too, are forbidden to kill a fetus. To sum up his position, we may say that he believes the prohibition on abortion to be of biblical force even though a fetus is not regarded as a life. It may be killed only if it is considered a *rodef* and killing it is necessary to save the mother's life.

BEIT YEHUDAH The responsum by R. Judah Ayyash deals with a surprising and striking question, one in which we hear quite explicitly about situations in which women want to terminate a pregnancy for reasons unrelated to adultery or promiscuity:

> Some women become pregnant *and do not want to bear more children and do not want to be pregnant at that time*, and some become pregnant while nursing and are concerned about the evil eye or about the danger to the nursling. They prepare potions and drugs that they know about in order to abort the fetus so it becomes a stillbirth. (*Beit Yehudah, 'Even Ha-'Ezer* 14; emphasis mine)[64]

The first part of the responsum considers whether capital punishment applies to the killing of a fetus that is essentially a stillbirth; R. Ayyash concludes that feticide is forbidden but does not explain whether the prohibition is biblical or rabbinic. In the second part, he considers the matter from a different perspective—the woman's exemption from the commandment to procreate and her consequent authorization to drink "a sterilizing potion." He cautions against erroneously concluding that a woman's authorization to drink a sterilizing drug implies permission to do so in order to abort a fetus, for the cases are distinct. She may drink the sterilizing drug to avoid pregnancy because she is not commanded to procreate and, therefore, is not commanded to avoid sterilization; in the case of abortion, however, the prohibition arises because feticide is like taking a life. His use of the term "like taking a life" (lit. "like killing a life") might lead one to expect him to conclude that abortion is prohibited as a matter of biblical law, but in summation he writes: "Accordingly, drinking a medicinal potion to abort a fetus is forbidden, but as a matter of rabbinic law."

R. Ayyash, however, does not deal at all with women who want to abort fetuses because they do not want to be pregnant at a given time. According to his reasoning, there is still a rabbinic prohibition, which precludes abortion simply to comply with the circumstances of one's life. There is a distinction, however, if the woman is a nursing mother and there is risk to an existing child: "But a woman who becomes pregnant while nursing is permitted to do what she can to abort, for there is danger to the child."[65]

In summary, the general tendency of halakhic rulings issued through the eighteenth century (at least from the principal responsa, which we have reviewed) was to consider abortion as prohibited solely by rabbinic law.

During the nineteenth century, a range of decisions appeared on the issue of abortion, some strict and some lenient, too numerous to allow for full discussion.[66] Yet, for the most part, even those who viewed abortion as a biblical violation did not take that to mean abortion was permitted only where there was certain mortal danger to the mother, that is, where the fetus was a genuine *rodef*. Rather, they identified a variety of circumstances involving harm to the woman's health, danger to one of her limbs, or pregnancy at a very young age, in which abortion was permissible.

Accordingly, the remainder of our discussion will focus on a number of key twentieth-century decisors, analyzing their interpretive approaches with respect to the original sources and the rulings that preceded them as well as their own conclusions. The twentieth-century rulings seem to manifest a clear inclination to rule strictly, ranging from the high number of decisors who find the prohibition to be biblically based (and the correspondingly low number who find it to be rabbinic) to the issuance of rulings that permit abortion only when there is mortal danger to the mother, that is, when the fetus can be considered an actual *rodef*. In that context, and before moving to an analysis of contemporary decisional trends, we need to consider how Maimonides's comments regarding the fetus as *rodef* have been understood.

The Issue of *Rodef* as Treated by the Later Authorities

Given what I believe to be the importance of the issue of *rodef* in connection with the moral positions expressed in contemporary rulings, let me digress briefly and consider some of the ways the later authorities have responded to the difficulty posed by Maimonides's presentation of the fetus as *rodef*.

As we have seen, both Talmuds conclude that the fetus should not be seen under the rubric of *rodef*. Accordingly, there is no basis for questioning the determination (in the *mishnah* in *'Ohalot*) that the reason it may be aborted is that it is not considered a "life." Nevertheless, Maimonides held it permissible to kill a fetus jeopardizing its mother's life because it is "like a *rodef*," and that determination raised some difficulties. First, does it make logical sense to regard the fetus as like a *rodef* while it remains in utero but as no longer a *rodef* once its head has emerged? And, second, does Maimonides adopt a position at odds with that of all the other medieval authorities and treat the fetus as a "life," ruling on that account that it may be killed only when it poses a mortal threat to its mother? As we saw in *Sefer Mizvot Gadol*, the codifications that followed Maimonides do not consider the problematic nature of what he says and simply cite it verbatim.[67]

Many have attempted to explain Maimonides's position and the substantially new direction he takes in understanding the *mishnah* in *'Ohalot*, and the scope of this work does not allow for detailed presentation of the literature in its entirety.[68] We can say, however, that while a few of the suggested explanations offer a stringent interpretation according to which feticide may be permitted only if the fetus is seen as a *rodef*, most of the later authorities do not adopt that reading and instead follow the second interpretive option set out earlier with regard to the *mishnah*. Denying that Maimonides disagrees with Rashi's view that the fetus is not a life, they thereby render redundant the *rodef* rationale for permitted feticide. In what follows, I will consider several interpretations.

R. Isaac Schor (*Koaḥ Shor*) claims that Maimonides in fact accepts Rashi's view and believes that the fetus is not a life.[69] Classifying the fetus as a *rodef* is meant to emphasize *how* it is to be treated. Just as efforts are made not to kill a *rodef* immediately and instead to rescue the person pursued by disabling one of the *rodef*'s limbs, so, too, is it forbidden to kill a fetus if the mother can be saved by merely injuring one of its limbs. That is what the *mishnah* intends when it says "limb by limb."

R. Jacob (called Zalman) ben Ephraim Schor of Lutsk (one of the authors of *Ge'onei Batra'i*)[70] suggests that Maimonides believed that feticide is permitted a priori because the fetus is not yet considered a life, just as Rashi wrote, and that the *rodef* rationale accordingly is unnecessary (as is evident from the case of the man who strikes a pregnant woman, causing a miscarriage; he is liable only for the value of the fetus and is not considered a murderer, as he would be had he taken a life). The fetus is classed as a *rodef* to teach that feticide is permissible by any means, not only by one or another abortifacient drug: "One need not pity him by selecting an easy death or killing him specifically by a drug; rather he may be killed directly [lit. 'by hand'] in any matter he wishes" (*Ge'onei Batra'i* 45). According to this explanation, Maimonides referred to *rodef* not to permit the feticide but to teach the *form* it could take.

R. Shneur Zalman of Lublin (*Torat Ḥesed*) determines that Maimonides believed the fetus to be a limb of its mother and that the notion of *rodef* cannot be literally applied to the *mishnah* in *'Ohalot*; for just as she can be saved at the cost of one of her limbs, she can be saved at the cost of the fetus, which has the status of one of her limbs.[71] In his view, therefore, the fetus can be considered a *rodef* only if it has begun to emerge, for it is then considered a separate body (though still not a life), and it may be killed only because it is a *rodef*. The author of *Torat Ḥesed* adds that the rationale for allowing the killing of a *rodef* (according to Maimonides) is to rescue the person being pursued; accordingly, even though a fetus in the process of emerging is a *rodef* without intending to be, it may be killed (for it is not yet a life, even though at this stage one must be more careful about its standing). Once its head has emerged, however, it is considered a life, and since it is not pursuing its mother deliberately or maliciously, and what is happening is merely the nature of the world, it may not be harmed.

The response of R. Ḥayyim Ozer Grodzinsky (*'Aḥi'ezer*) closely resembles that of the author of *Torat Ḥesed*; he, too, believes Maimonides rules that a fetus has the status of one of its mother's limbs.[72] Accordingly, the law of the *rodef* should be applied only when the mother is seated on the birthing stool and the fetus is already considered a separate body, though not a "life." Only at that stage is recourse to the rule of *rodef* needed to justify the feticide.

In *Ohel Mosheh*, R. Moshe Zweig argues that Maimonides resorted to the law of *rodef* to teach that one is *obligated* to kill a fetus jeopardizing its mother; that one is *permitted* to do so is self-evident, since the fetus is not considered a life. The distinction matters in cases where there is no agreement on carrying out an abortion, as when the mother wants to allow the child to be born despite the danger to herself or, alternatively, where the husband wants the child to be born despite the danger to his wife. In such cases, R. Zweig believes, the abortion is not only permitted; it is required.[73]

R. Ḥayyim Soloveitchik (of Brisk) is among the few to adopt an extremely strict interpretive stance and take Maimonides's words at face value; that is, he regards the fetus as a *rodef* at every stage, and therefore permits feticide.[74] His reasoning can be summarized as follows: Acting to save human life, on account of which the entire Torah may be set aside, applies with respect to a fetus, as a potential life, just as it applies to its mother. Accordingly, one may save its mother not because her life intrinsically has priority over the fetus, but only because of the law of the *rodef*, a special provision. (The proof that R. Ḥayyim Soloveitchik considered the fetus to be a life lies in the law applicable to a pregnant woman who smells food on Yom Kippur and develops a craving. She is fed until her mind is at rest, and the medieval authorities disagree over whether the reason she is fed is the danger to her own life or to that of her fetus. Those who maintain it is the danger to the fetus believe that the fetus, too, is within the rubric of "you shall live by them [the commandments]" and that preservation of its life, too, warrants displacement of the other commandments, if necessary. It follows that protection of a fetus cannot be displaced by protection of the life of another.)[75] Accordingly, the life of the fetus yields to the life of the mother only because the duty to stop a *rodef* is invoked. Once the fetus's head has emerged, however, that obligation no longer applies to it (even though, as a practical matter, it continues to "pursue" her), because she is considered to be pursued by heavenly decree.[76] This interpretation, though, is problematic—why should "pursuit" (that is, the status of being a *rodef*) be attributed to the fetus while it is within its mother's womb but to "the heavens" or "the nature of the world" only after the fetus's head has emerged?

To sum up the discussion thus far, we can say that two approaches form the axis around which the many interpretations of Maimonides's position revolve. One approach believes that Maimonides does not dispute Rashi's view and that he, too, does not consider the fetus to be a "life." He nevertheless introduces the category of *rodef* in order to teach the manner in which it is to be put to death (directly or not, limb by limb, etc.); alternatively, the category is pertinent only where the fetus has already begun to emerge, in which case we become more concerned about its status as a "separate body." These interpretations are consistent with the second option we offered at the outset for understanding the *mishnah* in *'Ohalot*. The other approach (which is adopted only by a small minority of decisors) strives to take Maimonides's words at face value and read the *mishnah* in *'Ohalot* in light of his statement that only when the fetus endangers its mother's life as an actual *rodef* may it be killed; no other reason can suffice.

The question of *rodef* and the intensive discussion devoted to it provide a striking instance of the deployment of moral considerations in halakhic interpretation, as we shall see when we turn to the contemporary decisors. Maimonides's statement, interpreted as authorizing feticide only where the fetus puts its mother's life in jeopardy, has become the platform for today's stringent rulings with respect to abortion—notwithstanding the many difficulties in taking Maimonides at face value and contrary to the interpretive tradition of the early modern authorities. In general, I believe that but for Maimonides's introduction of the concept of *rodef* into our understanding of the *mishnah* in *'Ohalot,* the discussion would not have developed to the point of regarding the fetus as a "life," a position contrary to the entire interpretive tradition of the medieval authorities. At the same time, his words provide an excellent source for those who maintain a stringent view to use in claiming that abortion is a biblical prohibition. Adoption of the more stringent understanding of Maimonides's view thus serves as a sort of litmus test for a decisor's moral perspective with regard to the issue of abortion.

CHAPTER FOUR

Abortion in Contemporary Halakhic Rulings

As we have seen, the sources cited above allow for a variety of interpretive courses. Moreover, we have seen that some readings of the texts are more reasonable than others and are more in line with other parallel sources. Halakhic decisors must issue a halakhic determination and, therefore, must make a series of interpretive choices that will support their final ruling. It seems to me that these interpretive choices are likely to reflect the application of various factors, including implicit moral and gender-based considerations regarding the role and nature of women.

Our review of rulings by the authorities who wrote during the fifteenth to nineteenth centuries conveys the impression that many decisors were inclined to rule leniently and to regard the prohibition on abortion as only a rabbinic one. The rulings of contemporary decisors, in contrast, seem to shift course, for a majority of them hold abortion to be biblically forbidden. One also finds extremely severe rulings (more severe than any in the earlier literature) according to which abortion is not permitted even during the first forty days of pregnancy or, alternatively, is permitted only in cases of substantial mortal danger to the woman.

In what follows, I will consider in detail only the rulings of rabbis Unterman and Feinstein, but they reflect to a substantial degree the similar interpretations adopted by the other decisors who rule stringently. I have selected them because they place in clearest focus the principal arguments and interpretive courses used to ground their position and represent the limiting case of the most stringent decisions on the subject.

The Stringent Position

RABBI I. J. UNTERMAN

R. Isser Judah Unterman, chief rabbi of Tel Aviv and later of the state of Israel, is well known for his forceful opposition to abortion, including his (unsuccessful) efforts to persuade government ministers and other influential people to tighten the legal prohibition on such procedures.[1] In a halakhic essay on the subject,[2] he considers the permissibility of abortion *during the first forty days* of a pregnancy in a case where a woman contracted rubella and physicians feared that the fetus would suffer a defect. I will argue that the form and content of his essay are linked.

R. Unterman begins with a very brief discussion of Sabbath desecration for the sake of a fetus, advancing an opinion and then basing it on a reading of the sources. The very form of the presentation thus makes it evident that it is the opinion that drives his argument and that the halakhic analysis rests primarily upon it. This opening discussion would seem to provide a clear route to considering the fetus's status as a "life," but R. Unterman does not cite the talmudic sources on the issue nor does he refer to the dispute among the medieval authorities over whether the Sabbath is to be desecrated when only the fetus is endangered. Instead, he relies primarily on the opinion of the author of *Halakhot Gedolot,* who, as construed by Naḥmanides, does not differentiate between the first forty days and a more advanced stage of pregnancy. The tendentiousness in choosing this interpretive approach is readily evident. Would it not be more reasonable to begin the discussion with the question of the fetus's standing as a "life" in the *mishnah* in *'Ohalot,* where the issue is dealt with directly and explicitly? Is there no need to present the comments of other medieval authorities, who maintain that risk to the fetus cannot be isolated from risk to its mother and that one therefore cannot infer anything about the fetus's personhood from the question of Sabbath desecration? R. Unterman's exegetical choices are illuminated by what he goes on to write after presenting the argument based on Sabbath desecration:

> It seems logically obvious that it is forbidden to kill it [the fetus] as a matter of Torah law. And even though doing so is not a capital offense, to cut off the life of a fetus is an appurtenance of murder.[3]

R. Unterman first resorts to reason and only after, and in a manner consistent with his opinion, devises a course of analysis and reading of the sources that prove his point. His opinion is an express statement of moral judgment. Even were one to say that the discussion of Sabbath desecration that precedes his opinion is what dictates the direction of the ruling, I have already shown that the matter is one on which the medieval authorities disagree and that a stringent conclusion is far from inevitable; accordingly, even his reliance on the proof derived from the matter of Sabbath desecration entails a moral determination consistent with his opinion.[4] In the same vein, R. Unterman concludes that even if feticide is not actually murder subject to its full penalty, it still entails, in a real sense, an injury to human life, in a way that "is an appurtenance of murder." He supports that claim on the basis of a discussion of Noahides, in which he concludes that the prohibition applies to Jews as well, given the maxim of "nothing permissible."[5]

R. Unterman's ensuing reading of the sources is meant to support the stance initially presented, and it is in that light that he understands Maimonides's invocation of the law of *rodef*. As noted, Maimonides's comments give rise to two central questions: (1) why is it necessary to invoke the rationale of *rodef* to justify feticide, given that killing the fetus to save the mother is permitted in any event because the fetus is not considered a life; and (2) why is the fetus considered a *rodef* only until it has begun to emerge, at which point the danger to the mother comes to be seen as "the nature of the world"? To answer the first question, R. Unterman assumes that Maimonides believes the law of saving a life applies to a fetus; the Sabbath, therefore, is desecrated on its behalf.[6] Accordingly, if the Sabbath is desecrated on account of the fetus's life, how could it be permissible to kill the fetus to save the mother's life? Saving its life is as much a biblically imposed obligation as saving the mother's life, and how could one life be saved at the expense of the other? That is why Maimonides needed the rationale of *rodef*, for saving the fetus's life yields to saving the mother's only if it is considered a *rodef*, and in that case alone is the mother to be saved at the fetus's expense. As for the second question, R. Unterman responds that "the birth itself, in which the fetus emerges from the mother's womb, is not considered an act of pursuit, for that is the way of the world."[7] This explanation suggests that most natural births are free of complications and the emergence of the fetus is normal and expected; accordingly, if there are complications, they should be attributed to God and not to the fetus. But still unanswered is why the complications should not be attributed to "the heavens" while the fetus remains in utero and why only then should the fetus be regarded as a *rodef*. Why does the rationale of "it is the way of the world" apply to delivery but not to pregnancy?

The practical consequences of R. Unterman's comments are as follows:

1. It is permitted to perform an abortion only in a case of clear mortal danger to the mother and not for any other reason.
2. It is forbidden to perform an abortion even if the pregnancy is still in its first forty days; that follows from Naḥmanides's understanding of *Halakhot Gedolot*, according to which the Sabbath is desecrated on behalf of a fetus even at so early a stage of the pregnancy.

Despite the broad discussion of many varied sources in the talmudic literature, nowhere in R. Unterman's consideration of abortion is there express and detailed treatment of the *mishnah* and *gemara* in tractate *ʿArakhin*, which raise, as I have shown, other interpretive options for both the *mishnah* in *'Ohalot* and the issue of *rodef*, thereby allowing for various halakhic determinations.[8]

As for the determination that an early-stage fetus is "merely water," R. Unterman believes it irrelevant to the question at hand, for he maintains that the Sabbath is to be desecrated for the sake of a fetus during the first forty days of pregnancy. In other words, the fetus must be viewed through "the lens of the future": even though it now is "merely water," a living being that must not be harmed will develop from it in the future. In that regard, he reverses matters: it is specifically Noahides who are not warned against feticide during the first forty days while Jews are so warned; accordingly, abortion may not be permitted even at so early a stage in the pregnancy.

R. Unterman's analysis has two principal foci. The first is the issue of desecrating the Sabbath on behalf of a fetus (as we have seen, a matter disputed among the medieval authorities). The argument that the fetus is a "potential life" completely vitiates what we have seen to be the widespread determination that the fetus is not a life at all, for treating it as a "potential life" requires treating it as an actual life in almost all respects. Accounting for the concept of *rodef* in this way simply intensifies the contradiction between the assumptions. The practical effects of the halakhic ruling are clear. One who believes the fetus is not a life will find it easier to permit abortion not only in cases of clear mortal danger to the mother but also when it is known that the fetus will suffer severe birth defects (contrary to R. Unterman's ruling that a mother who contracted rubella could not abort her fetus even during the first forty days of the pregnancy), when there is non-life-threatening physical danger to the woman, when the fetus is a *mamzer*, or in other cases. The second focal point in R. Unterman's analysis is the issue of the Noahide, which serves as the source for the determination that a Jew may not perform an abortion because it is an appurtenance of murder, though that determination entirely disregards the passage in *'Arakhin*. R. Unterman's manipulation of the sources is evident. Sources that do not address the issue directly become central to his discussion, and other, pertinent, sources are not considered at all. His following remarks may explain that choice:

> And it is worth publicizing the matter and explaining it to the public in our time, when induced abortions have become so common and this affliction has spread in many families. I have already told ministers and influential people that it is urgent that the law be strengthened and violators punished in order to remove this blight from among us. The matter has thus far not been corrected, and the evil impulse uses empty rationales to mislead people into committing these disgusting actions that are subject to the sixth of the Ten Commandments, "You shall not murder."[9]

These words bolster the view that this is a case in which ideology drives halakhic determinations.

RABBI M. FEINSTEIN

R. Moses Feinstein takes a view very close to that of R. Unterman. He, too, infers the existence of a biblical-law prohibition from the passage dealing with Noahides, from the maxim of "nothing permissible," and, primarily, from his understanding of Tosafot on the relevant texts. The Tosafists' argument is that where a Jew is subject to some obligation (in this case, saving the mother), the rule of "nothing permissible" does not apply. R. Feinstein thinks they resorted to that answer because they believed the prohibition of feticide is biblically imposed and therefore had to deal with the question of why it is not forbidden for a Jew to kill the fetus in order to save its mother. Their response is that a Jew is subject to a separate commandment to save the mother and that the rule of "nothing permissible" therefore does not govern.[10] That understanding of the Tosafists, of course, would seem to contradict what they say in tractate *Niddah* (BT Nid. 44b, s.v. *ihu mayyit bereisha*). Tosafot there adopt the wording "it is permitted to kill it," and, as I have shown, it is reasonable to believe that to be the authentic reading.[11] R. Feinstein, however, believes it to be a scribal error:

> One should not be misled by the wording of Tosafot in *Niddah* . . . which twice says "it is permitted to kill it" . . . for it is obvious and clear that it is a scribal error and it should be read, if you will, that "one who kills it in utero is exempt" . . . and it is an evident scribal error. (*'Iggerot Mosheh, Ḥoshen Mishpat* 2:69)[12]

As for the law of *rodef*, R. Feinstein understands the *mishnah* in *'Ohalot* to support a stringent understanding of Maimonides's position, namely, that abortion can be legitimated only if the fetus is regarded as a *rodef*. In his view, feticide is permitted to save the mother only when the fetus poses a clear and present mortal danger to her. Once its head has emerged, each is considered a *rodef* with respect to the other (as the Jerusalem Talmud says), and neither life is to be preferred over the other; prior to that point, the fetus is not considered fully a life while the mother is, and so she has preference and the fetus may be killed. In other words, the preference she enjoys over the fetus is purely a temporal one, not a substantive one.[13] But once its head has emerged, it, too, is a full-fledged life. At that point, the fetus is still a *rodef* pursuing its mother, and for that reason it might be justifiable to kill it even after its head has emerged; but since it is not known who is pursuing whom, the mother's earlier preferred status is vitiated.

R. Feinstein's interpretation of Rashi is consistent with that position; in his view, Rashi holds that the prohibition on murder applies to the fetus (though the murderer is not subject to capital punishment), and the authorization to abort it to save the mother is solely because the fetus is not yet a full-fledged life. Thus, when Rashi says "it is not a life," he means it is not *yet* a life, not that it is not a life at all:

> But while it is still a fetus in its mother's belly, not yet entirely a life, the mother's advantage over the fetus—she is entirely a life but it is not yet entirely a life—suggests that only the fetus is a *rodef* but the mother is not a *rodefet*; and for that reason, the fetus may be killed under the law of *rodef* because of that advantage [possessed by the mother]. . . . And so as a matter of law, according to Tosafot, according to Maimonides, and even according to Rashi, the prohibition of murder, from "you shall not commit murder," applies to feticide as well, though one who kills it is not put to death. And it is forbidden to kill it even where there is danger to others; the authorization [to kill it] extends only to saving its mother from dying while giving birth *and not to any other of the mother's needs*; that is obviously forbidden. (Ibid.; emphasis mine)

From the discussion of Sabbath desecration for the sake of a fetus, R. Feinstein concludes that if one is obligated to save a fetus at the cost of desecrating the Sabbath, one cannot say that there is no prohibition on killing it. He understands Naḥmanides's statement in a manner consistent with that, seeing no basis whatsoever for the view that Naḥmanides believes the prohibition on feticide to be rabbinic only. That Naḥmanides permits desecration of the Sabbath for the sake of a fetus (and even for a fetus during its first forty days) attests conclusively, in his view, that one is obligated to save the fetus and that it is certainly forbidden, as a matter of biblical law, to kill it—were that not the case, Sabbath desecration would not be permitted for its sake. In other words, R. Feinstein finds a causal, substantive connection between the authorization to desecrate the Sabbath for the sake of a fetus and the fetus's standing as a life, and he rejects all the efforts to interpret Naḥmanides differently.[14]

R. Feinstein dismisses the passage in *'Arakhin* as a special case of "scriptural decree," according to which both the woman and the fetus are to be put to death; accordingly, in his view, one may not infer from it the absence of a biblical-law prohibition against feticide. And, in fact, Rabbi Yoḥanan there treats the seemingly extraneous scriptural word "both" ("If a man is found lying with another man's wife, both of them—the man and the woman with whom he lay—shall die. Thus you will sweep away evil from Israel" [Deut. 22:22]) as the basis for inferring that if the woman is pregnant, her fetus is to die as well.[15] In other words, we have here a sort of special "scriptural decree" unique to this case, precluding, it would seem, any inference that the prohibition of murder does not encompass feticide. But the explanation that it is "scriptural decree" does not address the earlier portion of the passage and its question about the matters being "obvious." The basic premise is that the fetus is considered a part of its mother's body and that there is no reason at all to delay the mother's execution until after it is born. The only rationale for delaying execution of the judgment pertains to the father's property interest in the fetus and his consequent monetary loss if execution is not delayed. If one follows the course and internal logic of the talmudic passage, one sees that the reference to "scriptural decree" is meant to teach that despite the father's *monetary* loss, execution of the judgment is not to be deferred; that is scripture's decree. If one assumes the existence of a biblical prohibition against feticide, as R. Feinstein argues, could one say that the scriptural decree is meant to overcome concern about the husband's monetary loss?[16]

R. Feinstein refers to Maharit's responsum as well. As we saw, Maharit wrote what seem to be two contradictory responsa, the first a strict one that forbids abortions and the second very much the contrary.[17] Our examination of the texts showed the first responsum to be the one of questionable authenticity, inasmuch as it does not bear his signature and encompasses unrelated matters. It seems to me that this is a printer's error and that the original text can be reconstructed with a reasonable degree of confidence.[18] But R. Feinstein dismisses the second, more lenient responsum as a forgery: "It therefore is obvious that no attention at all should be given to this responsum, for it certainly is a forgery by some misguided student who wrote it in his name."[19]

In sum, the interpretive moves used by R. Feinstein to support and advance his stringent position seem to be quite problematic. First, it is evident that he structures his argument in a way that transforms sources that do not deal directly with the issue (such as passages on Sabbath desecration for the sake of the fetus[20] or on feticide by Noahides) into central texts and marginalizes or entirely disregards the more pertinent sources. Similarly, he relies on one individual's opinion (Naḥmanides's interpretation of the author of *Halakhot Gedolot*, to the exclusion of the other medieval authorities) and adopts a fairly forced interpretation of Naḥmanides's words even though a more straightforward understanding of them would imply that the obligation to desecrate the Sabbath for the sake of a fetus is unconnected to its status as a life.

Second, R. Feinstein applies the rationale of "scriptural decree" to the passage in *'Arakhin*, the purpose of which seems to be to isolate a halakhic statement and prevent it from being treated as precedent. And there, too, he does not deal adequately with the issues—not with the argument that it is "obvious" and the response to it, and certainly not with Samuel's comment, according to which one must actively verify that the fetus has been killed before executing judgment on the woman, in order to prevent her degradation. ("Scriptural decree" teaches only that both are killed together.)

Third, R. Feinstein resorts to arguments of "scribal error" and "forged responsum" that do not properly grapple with the sources.[21]

From all the foregoing, it appears that R. Feinstein's interpretive decisions are quite forced and likely attest to his difficulty with reading the sources in a manner consistent with his preconceived moral stance. It seems to me that this suffices to prove that his rulings reflect a moral judgment (to which he adhered consistently throughout his life); indeed, he does not conceal his position with respect to performing abortions:

> I have written all this with regard to the great breach in the world, as the governments of many states have permitted killing fetuses, and among them are the heads of the government of the state of Israel. Uncounted fetuses have already been killed, and in times like these it is necessary to erect a fence around the Torah and certainly to avoid leniencies with respect to the most serious prohibition of murder. (*'Iggerot Mosheh, Ḥoshen Mishpat* 2:69)

Once again, we find that it is ideology that dictates interpretive decisions.

In what follows, I will consider the gender-based implications of that ideology.

ADDITIONAL AUTHORITIES WHO RULE STRICTLY

Most of the decisors who believe abortion to be biblically forbidden employ similar exegetical strategies, inferring the force of the prohibition from the discussion of Noahides and setting aside the *mishnah* in *'Arakhin* as a special case in which the mother is sentenced to death and execution is not delayed. But I have found no one who takes as stringent a view as R. Unterman—who declines even to distinguish between the first forty days and later stages of a pregnancy and treats abortion as outright murder from the very start of the pregnancy—and R. Feinstein, who acknowledges the need for "further inquiry" regarding the first forty days but certainly forbids abortion after that for any reason at all other than certain mortal danger to the mother.

R. Ovadia Yosef, for example, who rules that abortion is biblically forbidden, nevertheless distinguishes between the first trimester and the later stages of a pregnancy, asserting that even a Noahide is not put to death for performing an abortion during the first trimester, when the fetus is not yet recognizable as such. Accordingly, the first-trimester prohibition is solely rabbinic, and abortion may be permitted even in cases of nonfatal illness. After the first trimester, abortion is permitted only if two physicians independently attest that the fetus is a *rodef* jeopardizing the mother's life.[22]

R. Solomon Zalman Auerbach likewise infers the existence of a biblical prohibition from the discussion of Noahides. He therefore rules that abortion is forbidden even if the fetus is found to suffer from Tay-Sachs disease, and he forbids amniocentesis to clarify the matter. Nor does he permit abortion when the woman will develop depression following the birth. He does, however, allow a woman who was raped to try to prevent a pregnancy by using a "morning-after pill" or an IUD within seventy-two hours of the rape. He also allows abortion where the fetus is diagnosed as anencephalic, a condition that proves fatal within days or weeks of birth.[23]

R. Samuel Ha-Levi Wosner believes abortion to be biblically forbidden even though it is not considered actual murder. He permits abortion, however, if the fetus is hopelessly defective and there is possible danger to the mother.[24]

R. Josef Shalom Elyashiv believes abortion to be forbidden by biblical law but interprets Maharit as saying that because the fetus cannot live independently of its mother, she is not obligated to provide it with life if by doing so she will remain ill all her life. For example, one may treat a cancer patient to extend her life, even briefly, though doing so would be fatal to her fetus.[25]

Also worthy of attention is the position of R. Aaron Lichtenstein on abortion, even though it is not cast as a halakhic ruling.[26] R. Lichtenstein distinguishes between the force of the prohibition and its basis and scope. Its force is biblical, in accord with the discussion of Noahides, and it therefore is based on the prohibition of actual murder, even though one who commits feticide is not punished as a murderer. With regard to the scope of the prohibition, however, his position differs significantly from that of R. Unterman and R. Feinstein. R. Lichtenstein believes that the prohibition of murder per se applies only during the final trimester of a pregnancy, for even a Noahide who aborts a fetus would be liable for murder only if the fetus had developed to the point of being independently viable were it to be born. Like R. Unterman, R. Lichtenstein does not consider the passage in *'Arakhin*, and he dismisses the view that the prohibition on abortion is only rabbinic: "that opinion should not be taken seriously as one worthy of much consideration, not only because it is morally alarming but because it runs contrary to clear halakhah."[27] Notwithstanding his strict position, R. Lichtenstein distinguishes between the various stages of a pregnancy and the severity of the prohibition associated with each stage. R. Unterman and R. Feinstein, as noted, draw no such distinctions.[28]

The picture that emerges from the foregoing shows that even among the majority of contemporary decisors who believe abortion to be biblically forbidden, the positions taken by R. Unterman and R. Feinstein are especially strict and make use of problematic and forced interpretations. But all the decisors who view abortion as biblically forbidden confine their recognition of women's needs to physical needs, and even that recognition is afforded with reservations, as in the case of those who forbid abortion where the danger to the mother is nonmortal. No account is taken of the circumstances of the woman's life, and no consideration is given to interests extending beyond those of physical (or mental) health. Their positions thus maintain, indirectly and unconsciously, the image of a woman as a material, physical being lacking independent human value. We cannot say whether the decisors' concept of a woman's image or value shapes their view of the force of the prohibition (biblical or rabbinic) or whether the vector points in the opposite direction and the determination that the prohibition is biblical lends further support to their view of women. Be that as it may, the social and gender consequences of these rulings make it impossible to free oneself of this social construct. That point gains added force when we consider the positions of the more lenient decisors who argue explicitly for consideration of matters that go beyond the material or physical construct of a woman's image. It is to those decisors that we now turn.

The More Lenient Decisors

RABBI B. M. H. UZIEL

R. Benzion Meir Hai Uziel deals with the question of whether a woman may abort a fetus when her physicians are certain that if she does not do so, she will become totally deaf in both ears.[29] He begins with those sources that deny the existence of a biblical ban on abortion. From the *mishnah* in *Niddah*,[30] he concludes that the fetus lacks any "life whatsoever" and is entirely dependent on its mother's vitality; and he goes on to infer from the passage in *'Arakhin* that feticide is permissible (for otherwise how could one respond to the *gemara*'s question "Is it not obvious? It is her body?"). If one believes it forbidden to kill the fetus, then the mother should not be executed until after the fetus has been born, for it is preferable to withhold one's hand and delay imposition of the sentence (something normally impermissible) than to actively cause the death of the fetus. He therefore rejects the explanation given by *Ḥavvot Ya'ir*, who argued that but for the rationale of "it is her body" it would, in fact, be necessary to wait and save the fetus, of course not causing its death; rather, "we certainly say that since the fetus is like the woman's body, killing it is nothing more than cutting a piece of flesh."[31]

As for the sources from which the opposite may be proven, such as the discussion of Noahides, R. Uziel adopts the Tosafists' distinction between the commandment to save the mother and the prohibition against performing an abortion for no reason at all; but "saving the mother" is understood quite broadly, consistent with the passage in *'Arakhin*: "even if it is a slight need, such as [avoiding] disgrace to the mother."[32] Accordingly, there is no need to posit a contradiction between what the Tosafists say regarding Noahides and their statement in *Niddah* that "it is permissible to kill it." In *Niddah* ("it is put to death first"), they considered the *mishnah* in *'Ohalot* and the passage in *'Arakhin*, which speak of a woman already in the process of giving birth, and even though at that stage one must be more concerned about the status of the fetus, it is still permissible to kill it, for it is endangering the mother's life.

Elsewhere, however, they wrote that it is forbidden to kill it if doing so is unnecessary to save the mother, because of the law regarding willful destruction and injury.

Regarding Maimonides's introduction of the *rodef* concept into his understanding of the *mishnah* in *'Ohalot*, R. Uziel believes Maimonides took the *mishnah* to be speaking of a fetus that had already begun to emerge (as implied by the wording with which the *mishnah* begins: "If a woman is having difficulty in giving birth"), giving rise, in his mind, to two questions:

1. If we say that the fetus is not a life even though is has already begun to emerge (that is, the birthing process has begun), why is it necessary to state that her life has precedence over its life, for it is not a life; and if we say that even though it is not a life, it nevertheless is forbidden to kill it (that is, feticide is not murder but is a prohibited act), why should that be so here, given that halakhah allows for the taking of otherwise prohibited actions where necessary to cure a dangerous illness?
2. If we say the converse—since the fetus has begun to move toward emergence, it is a body in its own right and considered a life—why does the rationale of "her life has precedence over its life" trump the rationale of "why would you say [your blood is redder]"?[33]

Applying the status of *rodef* to a fetus that has begun to emerge resolves these problems, for even if the fetus is considered a "life," the rationale of "why do you say [your blood is redder]" does not apply to a *rodef*. And it therefore is necessary to say that the life of the mother takes precedence over that of the fetus, for were it not a *rodef*, that would not be the case, since the fetus, too, has the status of a life. But once its head emerges, it stops being a *rodef*: "For on the contrary, since it wants to emerge entirely in order to breathe new life and escape strangulation . . . it is clear that it is not the fetus that is causing the birthing difficulty; it is, rather, natural causes not dependent on the fetus."[34]

R. Uziel does not see the discussion of desecrating the Sabbath on behalf of a fetus as posing any particular difficulty. The Tosafists expressly say[35] that because of risk to life, Sabbath is desecrated on behalf of the fetus even though it is permissible to kill it, but the desecration is permitted only for the need—even a slight need—to the mother. Where there is no such need at all, feticide is forbidden on account of "waste and denying the possibility of life to a Jewish soul."[36]

From the foregoing, one can conclude that the prohibition on abortion is rabbinic only; and when one weighs a rabbinic prohibition against the anticipated misery of becoming deaf, it is permitted to avoid that result by performing an abortion.

RABBI E. WALDENBERG

The most prominent decisor of the last generation to deal with the subject of abortion was R. Eliezer Waldenberg. He ruled that abortion is forbidden only as a matter of rabbinic law, which generated a line of permissive rulings that allowed, in some situations, for abortion to be performed even at the latest stages of a pregnancy. In order to consider his responsa in relation to the pertinent talmudic passages and responsa, I will describe the course of his argument in his principal responsum, referring to other writings as needed.[37]

From a formal perspective, it is striking that R. Waldenberg begins his responsum with a discussion of the Noahide issue. It appears that R. Waldenberg, well aware of the stringent tendency in contemporary halakhic rulings, chose to use this source as his point of departure in order to highlight his fundamental view that Jews are biblically exempt from punishment for abortion and to clear the path to setting forth the principal halakhic arguments that show the prohibition to be rabbinic only. To confirm the distinction between Noahides and Jews, he considers at length the question of the fetus's status as a life and argues, on the basis of a variety of sources, that fetuses are not considered lives until they emerge into to the world. It is noteworthy that R. Waldenberg, in contrast to other decisors, considers the biblical text and its exegesis in the *Mekhilta* with respect to the status of the fetus and demonstrates that the position of the medieval authorities, according to whom the fetus is not a life, is well grounded in those sources.

In the context of clarifying the fetus's status as a life, R. Waldenberg deals with Maimonides's characterization of the fetus as a *rodef*. In his view, Maimonides—like Rashi and the other medieval authorities—believed that the fetus was not a life. Maimonides nevertheless resorted to the *rodef* rationale for authorizing feticide because even though the fetus is not considered a life, it is still forbidden (though not by biblical law) to kill it; and one therefore might have thought that in a case of danger to the mother, the principle of "sit passively and do nothing" should prevail and bar saving the mother at the cost of harming the fetus. To avoid that inference, he rules that the fetus is *like* a *rodef.* That also resolves the question of why it becomes forbidden to kill the fetus as it is emerging from the womb on the grounds that the danger to the mother at that point is "in the nature of the world"; it is because the fetus is not fully a *rodef* in the sense that would permit "saving the life of one by taking the life of the other." In other words, the rationale for allowing the fetus to be killed while it is still in its mother's womb is the same as the rationale for forbidding the killing once it has emerged; the underlying variable is whether the fetus has the status of a life. While it is in its mother's womb, it is not considered a life, but there is still no plenary authorization to kill it; hence, to authorize feticide, it must be considered "something of a *rodef.*" Once it is emerging, killing it would be permitted were the law of *rodef* fully applicable, for it is in all ways considered a life; but since its status as only "something of a *rodef*" has not changed, it may not be killed. R. Waldenberg believes that none of the leading decisors ever thought of interpreting Maimonides to mean that were the fetus not a *rodef,* Jews would be subject to capital punishment for feticide just as Noahides are.[38]

As we have seen, Tosafot in *Niddah* say "it is permitted to kill it," and some interpreters take the view that this is either idiomatic usage or a scribal error. R. Waldenberg believes Tosafot here is following a view that rejects the maxim of "nothing permissible" and therefore sees no basis for saying feticide is forbidden to a Jew. There may be a rabbinic prohibition, meant to "erect a fence around [proper conduct] in the world," but there is certainly no biblical prohibition. (The *Ḥatam Sofer* interprets Maimonides's position in that way, as already noted, and so does the author of *'Arukh La-Ner*, who writes that Maimonides believes the *mishnah* in *'Ohalot* does not accept the maxim of "nothing permissible."[39])

As for the problems seemingly posed by the issue of Sabbath desecration for the sake of a fetus—particularly the statement of Tosafot in *Niddah* that it is permitted to kill a fetus, at odds with the authorization to desecrate the Sabbath to save it—R. Waldenberg sees their solution as grounded in severance of the causal relationship between the two rules. I have already discussed at length how this position is the more likely one given what the

Tosafists and other medieval authorities say on the matter. R. Waldenberg sums up the issue of Sabbath desecration for the sake of a fetus in these terms:

> And the explanation of the Tosafot appears to be that they believed the authorization to desecrate the Sabbath [on behalf of a fetus] depends not on whether or not it is forbidden to kill it but on whether by doing so, it will be able to observe many Sabbaths. (*Ẓiẓ 'Eli'ezer* 9, 51, *sha'ar* 3, chap. 2, par. 5)

R. Waldenberg thus believes that the prohibition on a Jew performing an abortion is rabbinic only, though it is not clear whether he agrees with Maharit that the source of the prohibition lies in the prohibition of wounding another or in the principle of "erect a fence around [proper conduct] in the world."[40] He therefore believes that the decision to abort may take account of such matters as family dignity, the status of the fetus as a *mamzer*, rape, or disgrace. In all cases, however, it requires the consent of the husband, inasmuch as his property is involved.[41]

RABBI S. YISRAELI

The responsum of R. Saul Yisraeli is striking in its treatment of a range of factors and considerations related to a woman's life. R. Yisraeli holds that the fetus is not a life and that the prohibition against killing it is solely a matter of rabbinic law, derived from the prohibition on wounding or on waste; accordingly, abortion may be permitted "to ease the suffering and burden of others, as in the case of the suffering associated with delaying execution." In other words, if it is permitted to execute a pregnant woman without waiting for her to give birth in order to avoid increasing her suffering, there is a powerful rationale for permitting abortion in those cases falling within the broad category analogous to the suffering caused by delayed execution. As he says:

> In conclusion: the fetus is not considered a life. . . . And it has nothing to do with the dispute over [Sabbath desecration] in cases of danger to the fetus. . . . Accordingly, where its survival entails suffering for another, analogous to suffering caused by delaying the mother's execution, even though [the fetus] is not the responsible agent, its existence is what precludes

removal of the suffering and it is permissible to kill it on that account. (*'Amud Ha-Yemini*, 32, par. 9)

One may infer from R. Yisraeli's responsum that his lenient opinion relies primarily on the passage in *'Arakhin*, which is dismissed as "irrelevant" to the question of abortion by those who rule stringently. Here, too, one can see the extent to which decisors structure the sources in a manner that serves the moral position they support.

Moral and Gender-Based Concepts Related to Abortion

In light of all the foregoing, we can say with reasonable certainty that the interpretive stance supporting the view that abortion is biblically forbidden is far from self-evident. Indeed, analysis of the sources suggests that the contrary view, that the prohibition is rabbinic only, is the more reasonable one. The decisors who take that view, though they are fewer than those who take the more stringent one, have no need for forced explanations and disregard of sources that are at odds with their moral judgments. In contrast, the responsa of the stricter decisors raise numerous difficulties, beginning with their emphasis on sources that deal only indirectly with the issue and their corresponding marginalization or total disregard of sources that deal with it directly and explicitly. Moreover, these responsa are marked by forced interpretations and problematic arguments. Accordingly, I believe the dominant tendency among the leading contemporary decisors, who see abortion as a biblical prohibition, embodies a particular moral stance and that a careful examination of their arguments and their treatment of the basic sources shows that their conclusions grow out of a process involving something more than formal halakhic reasoning.

Given that, several questions arise: To what extent does that moral stance take account of a woman's perspective? What exactly is that perspective? Is that perspective routinely displaced, in the analysis that leads to a halakhic conclusion, in favor of other values or considerations? My central argument in this chapter is that the vast gulf between the various rulings on abortion—and, specifically, the dominance of a strict tendency that does not necessarily follow from the original sources (and, indeed, is problematic in light of those sources, as I have tried to show at length)—exposes a series of hidden, gender-based preconceptions. These ideas sometimes are garbed in the mantle of moral neutrality (such as the argument regarding the need to deal with the personhood of the fetus), but they suggest that women are seen as objects rather than subjects, that there is little if any understanding that femininity extends beyond the reproductive function, and that there is minimal sensitivity to the woman's physical and psychological needs beyond the context of mortal danger.

THE STRINGENT POSITION

As we have seen, many of the responsa that deem abortion biblically prohibited treat the woman as "present but absent"; that is, her presence is self-evident, but she is considered only in terms of her *physical* state during the course of pregnancy and birth. Almost no attention is given to the array of other perspectives likely to be raised by an unwanted pregnancy or by circumstances that will cause her disgrace or dishonor.

That, I believe, is how the responsum of *Ḥavvot Ya'ir* should be read when it draws no distinction between a fetus that is a *mamzer* and one that is not. R. Bachrach considers the matter solely from the perspective of the fetus:

> There is no distinction between a case in which the pregnant woman is his duly married wife and the most kosher of women and a case in which the fetus is a *mamzer* from an adulterous relationship; for it is no surprise to you that the law treats a *mamzer* the same in all respects as a kosher Jew, and he is fit to be a great judge . . . ; he is forbidden only to enter the congregation [that is, to marry a non-*mamzer*] and to sit on the Sanhedrin; and we have already seen that with regard to redeeming someone from captivity, a *mamzer* who is a scholar takes precedence over a High Priest. (*Ḥavvot Ya'ir* 31)

Which is to say, the halakhic discussion flows entirely from the question of the fetus's status. It does not occur to the writer to analyze the question from the woman's perspective as well and to relate to her psychological and social state once the calumny of her adultery becomes public, to her future relations with her husband, or even to the complex set of relationships they are likely to have as parents of the child once it is born. The woman as subject disappears entirely from the array of halakhic considerations.[42]

Even R. Jacob Emden, whose comments open the door to recognizing shame to the woman as a relevant issue and who permits aborting a fetus that is a *mamzer*, nevertheless hesitates to do so directly for the purpose of sparing the woman disgrace—even though the passage in *'Arakhin* speaks expressly and unhesitatingly about avoiding disgrace to a woman who has committed a terrible crime for which she is about to be executed![43] He distinguishes in principle between a fetus that is a *mamzer* and one that is not in a manner that would allow abortion where there is "great need," but he is uncertain whether the pregnancy of an unmarried woman (whose child is not a *mamzer*) entails "great need":

> Even in the case of a kosher [that is, non-*mamzer*] fetus there would be a basis for ruling leniently in a case of great need, as long as it had not begun to move [toward emerging]. [That is so] even if it is not a case of mortal danger to its mother, but only to save her from its bad effects (*me-ra'ato*), for it causes her great pain. But this requires further inquiry. (*She'eilat Ya'aveẓ* 1:43)

Yet, given this ruling, R. Waldenberg suggests that R. Emden laid the groundwork for permitting the abortion of a fetus that is a *mamzer* "for the need of its mother, in order to save her thereby from the embarrassment and disgrace she would suffer and that would remain her lot, once it was born, throughout her life."[44] That rationale, R. Waldenberg believes, applies similarly to a woman who was raped (and the logic may be extendable to a pregnancy resulting from consensual sexual relations by an unmarried woman).[45]

In this context, it is interesting to note R. Uziel's position regarding abortion of a fetus that is a *mamzer*. He believes that a *mamzer* may be aborted, but only by its adulterous parents, and that it is forbidden to abort the fetus of an unmarried woman, since that fetus, when born, will not be an actual *mamzer*.[46] In other words, even R. Uziel, who considers a mother's suffering under other circumstances, looks at the matter of *mamzerut* from the fetus's perspective, not taking account of the psychological or social state likely to ensue for the mother following the birth of a *mamzer* or out-of-wedlock child.[47] R. Yonah Zweig, like R. Feinstein, does not distinguish among various sorts of fetuses and the circumstances in which they were conceived:

> For if we permit it in a case where it causes her great pain, you have left things open to interpretation, for who can estimate or assess whether the

> fetus causes her great pain or slight pain. Moreover, in that case there will [always] be a permissive ruling if the woman says she will feel shame on account of the fetus, for there is no suffering greater than shame.[48]

In other words, any effort to draw distinctions between one fetus and another and among the circumstances in which they were conceived sacrifices the standard of objectivity. Accordingly, the mother's words cannot be treated as reliable in such cases.

The picture that emerges is that the strict position allows no room for leniency where the fetus is a *mamzer* or in cases of extramarital relations or even of rape, for the law is grounded in the status of the fetus and not at all in factors related to the woman.

All that notwithstanding, it is widely believed that where there is a conflict between the mother's life, or even her health, and the life of the fetus, the halakhah clearly favors the life of the mother. However, although that is indeed the general rule, the following comments by R. Feinstein show that even that basic principle can be narrowly interpreted:

> And for this reason, I have taught that even if the physicians say there is concern that the mother might die if the fetus is not killed . . . it would still be forbidden to kill the fetus unless the physician's assessment is that it is *nearly certain* that the mother would die; for since it is because [the fetus] is considered a *rodef*, it must be virtually certain that it is a *rodef*. (*'Iggerot Mosheh*, *Ḥoshen Mishpat* 2:69; emphasis mine)

According to R. Feinstein, if there is no clear and immediate mortal danger to the mother, the mother may not defend herself—not against the possibility of mortal danger, not against nonmortal physical danger, and certainly not against danger to her psychological stability. R. Feinstein's ruling, which permits abortion only to avoid the mother's *certain* death, seems to me to indicate a concealed gender preconception that sees nearly total correspondence between a woman's reproductive role and her personhood, which is defined primarily in biological terms of preserving life. R. Feinstein reduces a woman's value to that of an instrument for the advancement of reproduction, even at the cost of her health and the quality of her life.

Because his understanding may seem unduly extreme, let me clarify. R. Feinstein's interpretive choices left him no alternative but to see the fetus as a "life" (albeit not a full-fledged one); it therefore may be aborted only if it is a *rodef*. Given that conclusion, there is no basis for considering the woman's physical or nonphysical needs, for killing a *rodef* would be murder were it not necessary to save the life of the person being "pursued." But the important questions are whether R. Feinstein's interpretive choices are reasonable (in my view, as explained earlier, they are problematic) and, more significantly, whether they are driven, perhaps only semiconsciously, by preconceptions regarding women and their exclusively (or at least primarily) procreative role. Defining the value of a woman's life in exclusively functional or biological terms can be problematic even for those who regard women as "different but equal." Difference itself does not contradict substantive equality, but valuing a woman's life solely in functional terms imports a substantive inferiority into that evaluation. It is also worth noting that when R. Feinstein first voiced his views on abortion in the 1930s, he was still living in Russia, and the newborn Soviet Union had just become the first country in the world to recognize women's right to free and legal abortion. We should not discount the possibility that R. Feinstein's strikingly restrictive stance on abortion was in some sense reactionary.

Albeit to a lesser degree, R. 'Aharon Lichtenstein adopts a similar approach to the appropriate balance between consideration of the fetus's interests and those of the mother. This is best expressed in a halakhic position paper written by R. Lichtenstein for the Committee to Consider Prohibitions Applicable to Artificially Induced Abortions established by the Israeli Minister of Health in 1972 for the purpose of examining the law that until then had regulated abortion. True to his view that the halakhah recognizes an axiological system independent of its own ethics, R. Lichtenstein believes that halakhah itself demands an accounting of meta-legal considerations relevant to the practical world."[49]

Accordingly, R. Lichtenstein adopts an extremely strict attitude toward abortion, in the spirit of rulings by R. Feinstein and R. Unterman. As I explained earlier, however, his position is more complex than theirs, and he regards abortion as subject to the prohibition of murder only during the final trimester. He avoids establishing absolute benchmarks, because there is room, and even a need, to apply decisions to concrete situations in an effort to find the optimal halakhic and moral balance among all the factors arising in each case. But despite that emphasis, he concludes as follows:

> It is worth making clear, certainly to those who, in seeking a humane approach, are liable to adopt slavishly an overly liberal attitude in this area, that from the perspective of the fetus and those concerned with its welfare, liberality in this direction comes at the expense of humanity. . . . It is not only the honor of God which obligates us, regardless of the cost, to avoid what is prohibited and to obey the commands of the Holy One Blessed be He that are expressed in this Halakhah. It is also the honor of man in Halakhah, the humane and ethical element which insists on the preservation of human dignity and concern for human welfare, that rises up in indignation against the torrent of abortions.[50]

This formulation resounds with R. Lichtenstein's moral pronouncements: "from the perspective of the fetus and those concerned with its welfare"; "the humane and ethical element which insists on the preservation of human dignity and concern for human welfare." But R. Lichtenstein chooses to formulate the question solely from the perspective of the fetus. To view the woman as a legitimately interested party with a position or a say regarding pregnancy or abortion is branded as "overly liberal," while concern for the fetus and its interests is deemed the concern of "humanity." Moreover, "human dignity . . . and human welfare" in this context refer to the dignity and welfare of the fetus but not of the woman. A claim like "liberality comes at the expense of humanity" can be advanced only if "liberality" is not valued at all or is regarded as having no humane aspects of its own.

Can liberality working on behalf of women's existential interests never be regarded as humane? It is precisely the liberal approach that freed women from the need for secret abortions that jeopardized and sometimes claimed their lives. And it is that approach that placed on the public and ethical agenda the voices of women who had been raped, sometimes by their partners, or who became pregnant, despite the precautions they took, at a time in their lives when bearing a child would be impossible from their perspective. The inability to obtain abortions placed these women in extremely harsh psychological, economic, and day-to-day situations, and the liberality that changed all that should be seen as no less humane than the approach that takes account only of the moral aspects associated with the fetus.

It can certainly be argued that R. Lichtenstein's words are meant as a counterweight, an antithesis, to the one-sided feminist claim that a woman's rights over her body allow her to abort at will, and it is true that he is speaking out against the "torrent of abortions," but does that mean that every abortion is unjustified? In other words, what is revealed here is that the halakhic ruling in this case is motivated by clear considerations of "public policy"; and while it is not unique in that regard and other halakhic decisions proceed in that manner as well, the difference here lies in the ruling's harsh effects on the lives of women.

It seems to me that R. Lichtenstein acknowledges the reasonableness of the claim that abortion is forbidden only rabbinically; for were the prohibition unequivocally biblical, he would not need to garner the universal moral arguments that he does not appear to find in the earlier sources. As I demonstrated earlier, R. Lichtenstein believes the passage in *'Arakhin* should be rejected, as should attempts to use it as a source for the halakhic view regarding the fetus, first and foremost because it is "morally alarming" and only secondarily because it runs counter to another express halakhah. In other words, R. Lichtenstein seems not only to sense the ethical inadequacy of his halakhic sources in this case, as he suggests in other contexts,[51] but also to imply criticism of the halakhic stance suggested by the passage in *'Arakhin*. I certainly do not believe that a decisor must suppress his ethical commitments when he sets out to decide a halakhic matter; but I believe, as I have said, that the position here taken is not *balanced*, in that it fails to take account of women as part of the "story" of the abortion situation in all its complexity. Accordingly, the "morality" of the "humane" position, as presented in R. Lichtenstein's essay, is one-sided and gender-biased. The problem becomes more severe when, as here, we are dealing with a position paper submitted to a governmental body and its rhetoric adopts a normative-educational tone even though R. Lichtenstein, in issuing a personal ruling, might take account of the questioner's particular circumstances and be led by them to take a more lenient stance.

Believing, as I do, that neither the strict decisions nor the lenient ones derive exclusively from formal analysis, let me clarify the problem further by suggesting that modern decisors[52] are caught in the clash between two developments of great moral importance.

On the one hand, rapid progress in science and medicine has advanced our understanding and perception of the fetus as a human entity. Especially meaningful in that regard has been the ability to hear the fetal heartbeat and to use ultrasound to observe its form and movement, as well as the capacity to sustain premature infants born as early as the sixth month of pregnancy. These developments make it much harder to accept the Torah's statement that one who strikes a pregnant woman and causes her to miscarry is liable only for monetary compensation to her husband or some of the rabbinic notions that see the fetus as nothing more than a limb of its mother, having no independent status. Meanwhile, the very recent and ongoing enhancement of our ability to identify birth defects in utero has allowed for more specific and better-informed consideration of the quality of the fetus's future life.

On the other hand, human consciousness has developed a more nuanced regard for women, who are now seen not only as bestowers of life but also as persons in their own right, possessed of independent destinies and rights. These rights include the basic right not to become pregnant and not to raise children at all (recall that under halakhah, women are not subject to the commandment to procreate) or, at least, not to see that role as women's exclusive or primary function.

The problem faced by the decisors is not posed specifically by the halakhic sources, which allow ample room for interpretation and for consideration of leniencies. It is more one of striking the proper balance between these moral developments and the halakhic sources. The decisors, however, do not share that understanding of the question posed to them; to put it differently, they do not generally consider the woman's needs (other than her physical ones) as a legitimate aspect of the moral analysis of the problem. The moral dilemma, as a rule, is understood as one involving only the fetus's personhood or, more recently, the quality of its future life in the event of severe birth defects.

With some hesitancy, I would suggest that there may be an additional factor contributing to the complexity of this situation: the battle of women around the world for legalized abortion and the resultant hardening of the Roman Catholic Church's position on the matter. In the past, the Church's canon law distinguished between a fully formed fetus and one that had not yet attained that stage of development; the boundary was generally set at about forty days into the pregnancy. But that distinction was eliminated in 1869 by Pope Pius IX, partly in an effort to fight growing promiscuity. That period also saw the start of the movement for "voluntary motherhood" or for reproductive freedom. Since 1917, canon law has drawn no distinction between fetuses at different stages of development.[53] It is entirely possible that canon law drew halakhah in the same direction,[54] as R. Zweig writes:

> Moreover, it is not only leading physicians and legal scholars who oppose permitting artificial abortion even in a case such as the one we are considering. The [Catholic] clergy and its leader have expressly declared that it is forbidden according to their faith to kill a fetus even if it will be born with defects or abnormalities. If so, there is an additional prohibition here, related to the desecration of God's name if we permit it. . . . Such an act would, God forbid, cause a desecration of God's name throughout the world, and of that it is certainly said "for you are a holy nation"—do not allow another nation to be holier than you.[55]

His words, it seems to me, provide considerable support for my view regarding the imbalance between the fetus and the mother. Allowing the abortion would entail "desecration of God's name" because the woman's perspective on this issue is not taken as a moral one and is therefore regarded as irrelevant. But it is easy to argue that if concern for a woman's health, dignity, wishes, and various needs is regarded as a moral consideration, the claim regarding desecration of God's name is blunted and maybe even reversed.

One may ask whether or to what extent there is a correlation between the halakhic tendency to rule strictly regarding abortion and the development of a woman's movement pursuing that right and the church's position. It seems to me that the comments of R. Feinstein[56] and R. Zweig strengthen the case for such a correlation. Studies in similar areas have shown that when women organize as a group to secure their rights by arguing in principle about discrimination, the establishment turns them away. When, however, they press their claims on an individual basis, they are received with greater responsiveness. Particularly instructive is a study by Chaves arguing that as long as women sought to be accepted as clergy on an individual basis, their requests were not seen as a gender-based challenge and were accepted, but when they organized politically, on a gender basis, it was almost certain that church authorities would reject their requests.[57] In other words, he demonstrates a correlation between women's efforts to be recognized as legitimate members of the clergy and their churches' refusal to recognize them.[58]

THE LENIENT POSITION

To this point, we have focused on the gender biases inherent in the rulings that deem the prohibition on abortion to be biblically based. However, I do not mean to suggest that those who see the prohibition on abortion as only rabbinic have freed themselves of gender biases; I am certain that their inclination to rule leniently cannot be attributed to their adoption of the feminist challenge to the existing gender order. Indeed, the position that understands the prohibition to be rabbinic may well embody to an even greater extent the preconceptions that stress a woman's procreative function and treat her primarily in that light, as is evident in the distinction between the circumstances that may or may not be legitimately taken into account in deciding whether an abortion is justified. A clear illustration of this lack of balance is provided by a halakhic article published some years ago by R. Moses Tzuriel.[59] R. Tzuriel in effect offers a summary of precontemporary and contemporary halakhic rulings on abortion, and I am convinced that his conclusions bolster my sense that they entail gender biases.

R. Tzuriel argues that until our time, when decisors considered the prohibition on abortion, they generally mentioned no factor other than mortal danger to the mother as a potential justification for abortion. Nowadays, however, technological and medical advances have made it possible to examine the health of the fetus, and questions arise regarding whether and when the fetus's health might justify abortion.[60] Here, once again, note that the discussion emphasizes the perspective of the fetus. That emphasis is reinforced in what follows:

> It is clear that there is no authorization to abort a healthy fetus when there is no evident mortal danger to its mother. All other rationales for abortion—economic conditions, a desire not to interfere with one's "career," preservation of one's appearance, limited living space, etc.—are unacceptable. In this article, we consider only the abortion of a fetus that we know in advance will be born with a severe illness, physical or mental.[61]

In the remainder of the article, R. Tzuriel goes on to present an extremely lenient position (derived from understanding the prohibition on abortion as rabbinic only) that does not consider the fetus to have the status of a "life," and he quotes a long line of decisors who permitted abortion in the absence of danger to the mother. But he rejects rationales for abortion that do not pertain to the fetus itself and serve, instead, the non-health-related interests of the mother.[62]

I would argue that it makes no sense, at least not analytically, to distinguish between aborting a physically or mentally defective fetus and aborting a healthy fetus because of needs that are not the fetus's own. If the fetus is not a "life" and its abortion therefore may be permitted in some circumstances, forbidding that abortion in other circumstances demands a good explanation. What categorical difference among circumstances warrants such a distinction? The question resounds even more forcefully given R. Immanuel Jakobovits's firm determination that all authoritative halakhists agree that physical or mental defects do not in themselves negate a person's right to life, whether before or after birth.[63] The handicapped and infirm are entitled to the same human rights as others. Human life is of infinite value and its sanctity is not conditioned on having one or another ability. One may question, to be sure, Rabbi Jakobovits's remark that "some children may be born unwanted, but there are no unwanted children aged five or ten years,"[64] but his position is certainly a coherent one. The distinction that has been drawn, however, between the fetal-health-related circumstances said to justify abortion, and the circumstances in which abortion has been found unwarranted, which are typically tied to the mother's life situation, accentuates one's sense that recent decisions on the subject have been grounded in gender biases.

One might argue that the distinction being drawn is between abortions that challenge the value of the "sanctity of human life" and those that do not challenge that value. But that distinction is questionable. Why does aborting a defective fetus do less violence to the sanctity of human life than aborting a healthy fetus whose birth would harm its mother's dignity or life plans? And what of the value of preserving the dignity of the woman and her ability to lead her life in a way that is consistent with her intellectual, professional, or emotional needs? Dworkin's analysis, discussed in chapter 3, is extremely pertinent in this context. Does "sanctity of life" refer only to physical, biological life? That would seem to be the case, at least with respect to women, if they are not permitted to abort pregnancies for reasons that do not necessarily entail physical limitations or flaws.

As noted, I believe the distinctions that are drawn among these sets of circumstances are not neutral and that gender considerations play a significant role in defining them. R. Tzuriel does not enumerate all the considerations I have listed, but his placement of the word "career" in quotation marks in the Hebrew original is enough to give the impression that he regards it as a shady rationale at best. The point I wish to emphasize is that even lenient decisors limit the range of permitted abortions in accordance with preexisting worldviews that do not necessarily reflect respect for women as subjects with independent interests and needs. Even if more than a few contemporary decisors deem the prohibition of abortion to be only rabbinic in force, that still does not mean that the human needs of women, beyond the purely physical ones, are regarded as factors that legitimately bear on the decision of whether or not to abort. Even according to these decisors, the principal function of women was and remains procreation and birth. As a general rule, it seems to me that a position that focuses only on the personhood of the fetus is not necessarily one that honors the "sanctity of life," for it avoids, consciously and unconsciously, recognizing women as subjects to be valued in and of themselves.

In this context, let us revisit the position of R. Waldenberg, who takes a lenient position, regarding abortion as forbidden by rabbinic law only, but whose decisions are nevertheless problematic from a gender-based perspective. I am referring to R. Waldenberg, who occupied an unusual position as a decisor by virtue of his (unofficial) role as rabbi of Shaarei Zedek Hospital in Jerusalem.[65] The formulations of his responsa demonstrate that he was close to the medical staff there and discussed matters with them orally and in writing; in other words, he was involved on the front lines and did not deal with these issues in academic isolation. In any event, one can see even R. Waldenberg's lenient position as reflecting his desire to preserve the existing gender order. Abortion, or related diagnostic procedures, are permitted in order to enable a woman to maintain marital relations with her husband or to bring additional children into the world.[66] This is not a matter of placing her interests center stage or of seeing her as a subject, though those might be the long-range effect of such decisions. He gives clear voice to his perspective on a woman's purpose and place in relation to her husband, and it is evident that he does not adhere to any egalitarian ideas in that regard:

> And so the Creator, may He be blessed, saw man's needs and pleasures and created him alone and took one of his ribs and formed the woman from it. He brought her to the man to be his wife and his helper and supporter, for she was considered to be as one of his limbs that serve him and he was to rule over her as he rules over his limbs. She was to desire him as his limbs desire to please his body. . . . And this idea brings about true household peace and sets the man and the woman each in his or her proper place, knowing his or her duties in the shared and united household. (*Ẓiẓ 'Eli'ezer* 19, 35)

The hierarchal concept expressed in this responsum is unambiguous, but does it appear elsewhere in R. Waldenberg's responsa? In his main responsum on abortion, R. Waldenberg addresses the case of a pregnant woman who has been diagnosed with cancer but does not want to abort her fetus although doctors have warned that continuing the pregnancy will cost her her life. R. Waldenberg rules that the woman's preference is to be honored:

> A woman is afflicted with cancer, God protect us, and she will die of it sooner or later. She is pregnant, and the physicians say that continuing the pregnancy will shorten her life, but the woman says she does not care about that and that she wants to continue the pregnancy and bear the child so as to leave a memory. In this instance, if we were to follow the opinion that the prohibition on aborting a feticide is not considered murder, and certainly if we follow the opinion that the prohibition is only a matter of rabbinic law and that one should rule leniently to allow abortion to help heal the mother or to spare her great suffering, then we should not heed the mother's pleas in this case and we should set aside the fetus's life in order to prolong that of the mother. For when it comes to protecting human life, even a brief prolongation of life warrants setting aside all the prohibitions in the Torah. But if, in this unique and tragic case, we rely on the *Bayit Sheleimah* and the *'Avnei Ẓedeq* and those who rule stringently that abortion should not be performed even where danger is present, we can rule that her pleas should be heeded and we should withhold our hand and do nothing, relying on divine mercy and allowing her to complete the pregnancy. (*Ẓiẓ 'Eli'ezer* 9, 51, *sha'ar* 3, chap. 3, sec. 13)

R. Waldenberg's views here are surprising in several respects. Throughout his halakhic discussion, he emphasizes that the prohibition is rabbinic, thereby permitting abortion even in the latest stages of a pregnancy and even when there is no mortal danger to the mother. One might therefore expect that in a case of such clear mortal danger to the mother, abortion would be required, as R. Waldenberg himself suggests when he writes initially that "we should not heed the mother's pleas in this case." What, then, is the meaning of the turnaround that leads him to rely here on strict decisors who forbid abortion even in cases of danger?

One can interpret R. Waldenberg's comments in either of two ways. On the one hand, he shows great sensitivity to the woman's wishes and respect for her decisive stance. The woman is seen as a subject, and she makes her own decisions about her body, her life, and her future. But we must ask whether R. Waldenberg would allow the woman to die or to shorten her life if she were suffering from a horrible illness or severe pain but was not pregnant—that is, what would happen if the issue arose *outside the procreative context*? Is the life of a woman valued in terms as absolute as that of a man, or might her ability to bring children into the world muddy those waters? R. Waldenberg's treatment of euthanasia is clear; he takes a very strict view not only of active but even of passive euthanasia.[67] Euthanasia is forbidden in all situations, and the patient must continue to be treated by all the means at the physician's disposal. According to the description of the abortion case described, continuing the pregnancy will shorten the woman's life, that is, hasten her death; conversely, one may conclude, terminating the pregnancy will prolong her life. If so, terminating the pregnancy should be regarded as any other treatment likely to extend the life of a moribund patient even briefly.

In one case, R. Waldenberg considered a moribund boy enduring intense pain. His mother objected to further treatment, but his father argued for continuing to try all possible ways of saving him, even if the likelihood of success was very small and the treatment would prolong his suffering. R. Waldenberg ruled as follows:

> Moreover, extending a life as short and hard as this one is not only so that he will observe many Sabbaths [the rationale, it should be recalled, for desecrating the Sabbath on behalf of an ill person] nor is to allow him time to repent and confess and so forth. *It is, rather, because there is an obligation, as an end in and of itself, to maintain the life of a Jew, however briefly, and it is a*

> *scriptural decree* [*inferred from a verse regarding the return of lost property*] *"you shall return it to him"—the loss of his body*. . . . And if that is the case on the Sabbath, it is a fortiori obligatory during the week to strive to save even those in this state, and to return their lives to them, even for a brief time, and it includes a case in which suffering is involved. (*Ẓiẓ 'Eli'ezer* 18, 62; emphasis mine)

This example leaves no room for doubt as to R. Waldenberg's position on the need to do everything possible to extend the life of a sick person. It also explains why human life is regarded as an end in itself and must be extended by whatever means are available, even when doing so entails terrible suffering. It is possible that the suffering of the woman in the abortion case under discussion is even greater, for saving her life would entail losing the fetus; but do the halakhic categories with which he is dealing allow for differences between one form of suffering and another? Moreover, what has become of his concern about the "slippery slope," so clearly cited in his responsa in this area? Can the suffering of a pregnant woman about to lose her child be so clearly differentiated from other forms of suffering as to obviate that concern?

From a gender perspective, two opposing observations may be offered. On the one hand, R. Waldenberg honors the woman's wishes. On the other hand, given a halakhic worldview that denies personal autonomy in matters of life and death, it is difficult to see his position as a genuine endorsement of her independence in these matters. I would argue that this seeming clash of values derives from R. Waldenberg's belief that a woman's primary function is procreative; accordingly, if she believes her still unborn progeny is more important than her own life, she should be heeded—not because she has a sovereign right to decide but, perhaps, because her life is seen not as an end in itself but only as a means for creating new life. I cannot make that assertion unequivocally, but it seems clear that the procreative context leads him to take a different halakhic position—one that contradicts his categorical prohibition on active or even passive euthanasia.[68]

A further risk inherent in this responsum is that is sets a high halakhic bar for women who may find themselves pregnant and suffering from incurable or terminal disease. They may sense that even though there is no actual halakhic obligation to carry on with the pregnancy, they are expected to do so, under the rubric of doing more than the law requires. In that sense, R. Waldenberg's words may become a normative standard rather than merely a theoretical observation.

A halakhic analysis focused on uncovering the decisors' guiding values thus demonstrates, through critical reading, the place occupied by gender considerations and the extent to which they shape the corpus of halakhic rulings. Uncovering the gender preconceptions inherent in these responsa allows for critical judgment of those halakhic rulings that open a door—either in their structuring of the sources or in their actual content—to an ethical and moral conversation about their underlying premises. The criticism is sometimes "internal," conducted in light of the tradition itself or the modus operandi of decisors in general (as we have seen in the case of R. Waldenberg) and sometimes "external," in accord with general moral values and ideas of justice and, in particular, with how they are understood and applied in connection with women. It is that criticism and conversation to which I turn next.

Halakhic Discourse and Feminist Discourse

In many ways, a feminist-halakhic discourse would seem impossible. As two very different worldviews, one drawing on the secular-liberal tradition and the other shaped by a religious tradition, feminism and halakhah rest on diametrically opposed premises: fundamental liberal ideas such as autonomy, ownership of one's body,[69] and reproductive freedom are seen in the religious tradition as contradicting human subservience to divine authority and to a binding normative system. It may be possible, within the religious tradition, to speak of freedom of thought or action, but only within the value system of that tradition.

For example, halakhah asserts the theological-juridical principle that a human being does not possess total ownership of his body, which is "property of God." As Maimonides writes in explaining the Torah's ban on monetary compensation to atone for a murder: "for the soul of the one who was killed is not the property of the blood redeemer [the family member entitled to vengeance]; it is, rather, the property of the Holy One blessed be He."[70] Specific laws follow from this principle, such as the prohibitions against suicide or placing oneself in unnecessary danger and the requirement to compel a reluctant patient to undergo lifesaving medical treatment. Most importantly, the principle serves as the primary rationale for a sweeping ban on euthanasia (with the exception of passive euthanasia, which some permit under certain circumstances).[71] The rationale recurs in the halakhic literature and is virtually unchallenged.[72] The ideal of personal autonomy, including autonomy over one's body, appears to be directly at odds with the idea of divine ownership.

There are, of course, respected voices and sources within the halakhic tradition that support personal autonomy; for even if it does not deal with autonomy in the modern sense of the word, halakhah recognizes that human beings have interests—particularly, in relation to their bodies—that are well worth defending. While halakhah does not join in espousing the total autonomy of the individual and one's absolute sovereignty over one's body, neither does it reject those values outright, at least not according to all authorities.[73] Still, it appears that the idea of reproductive freedom contradicts a man's religious duty to fulfill the commandment of "be fertile and multiply" and his wife's religious duty to help him do so. Accordingly, if reproductive freedom means, among other things, the freedom to choose not to bring children into the world, it stands at odds with the religious commandment to procreate.

Let me, therefore, place reproductive freedom at the center of our discussion, for it is the most significant concern from a feminist perspective—and especially so in light of the insights presented in chapter 1. I am referring to the reproductive freedom of a woman, who, as explained earlier, is not herself subject to the commandment to procreate but whose life is the one primarily affected by bringing a new child into the world.

According to halakhah, a man would appear to lack all reproductive freedom, for he is subject to the commandment to procreate; as a practical matter, however, he enjoys considerable maneuverability within the framework of that obligation. For example, if "his soul craves [only] Torah," he is entirely exempt from the obligation. As a matter of biblical law he is obligated only to father one son and one daughter, and once he fulfills that basic obligation, economic or family difficulties are sufficient reason to avoid or delay fulfillment of, the commandment of "in the evening" (that is of continuing to procreate even late in life). As noted in the previous chapter, the Talmud tells of sages who leave their homes for extended periods to study

Torah, and Ritva later writes that he heard of great scholars who drank a libido-suppressing potion after fulfilling the biblical commandment because the religious-intellectual obligation of Torah study supersedes expansion of the family with its attendant difficulties.

The contrast between the halakhic leeway afforded a man in the realm of procreation and the restriction of a woman's reproductive freedom is instructive. A man is fully obligated to procreate; however, his personal interests (Torah study; overcoming difficulties in earning a livelihood) are balanced against the obligation in a way that allows for fairly broad freedom, to the point that his ability to shape his life as he sees fit within the context of his religious obligations is almost unimpaired. A woman, in contrast, is not bound by the commandment to procreate or by the commandment to study Torah and is certainly not regarded as the primary, or even secondary, breadwinner. At first glance, her freedom would appear to be absolute, and there would appear to be no need even to balance various interests or conflicting obligations. In practice, however, she is bound by cultural presumptions that take an unfavorable view of her remaining unmarried; she is subordinated to her husband's obligation to procreate, to the point of being subject to severe limitations on her use of birth control; and, finally, she is denied almost all recognition of her presence as a subject in situations where abortion is a relevant consideration—even though the process is taking place inside her body and is likely to exert a profound influence on the course of her life. All, then, is topsy-turvy: the man, who is subject to obligations, can navigate them in a way that avoids interfering with his desires and wishes; but the woman, who is free of those obligations, nevertheless faces constraints and limitations in whichever direction she turns. In this context, is it truly possible to speak of halakhic justice?

In contrast, feminist and liberal discourse regarding abortion treats bodily autonomy and, especially, reproductive freedom as fundamental principles. But before I begin to outline the potential contribution of philosophical-feminist analysis to halakhic discourse, let me stress that even though we are speaking of different moral and conceptual frameworks, we need not dismiss out of hand the possibility that feminist analysis may have something to contribute to the halakhic discussion. As I shall explain below, the distinction between philosophical-feminist analysis and feminist criticism serves as a point of departure for considering the possibility of a common discourse.

The goal of philosophical-feminist analysis, in the halakhic context, is to clarify interpretive processes and halakhic statements and to uncover their conceptual underpinnings. The use of gender as an interpretive criterion will contribute to an examination of the relationship between the modern cultural framework, founded on such values as liberty and equality, which is the framework within which the decisor dwells, and his halakhic positions.

Feminist criticism plays an important role in pointing out the extent to which egalitarian values are acceptable within the framework of halakhah. Because my perspective is that of a person committed to the ideal of equality between the sexes, what I mean to do in this book is to confront the challenge of applying egalitarian values within the world of halakhah. Where halakhic decisors systematically dismiss those values, I point that out and note the interpretive alternatives they might have adopted in lieu of those that support their conclusions. When I speak of a possible "halakhic-feminist discourse," then, I mean, primarily, the process of pointing out the places where traditional theological and halakhic positions can be expanded so as to reflect the perspective of women in the modern world.

The dilemma of abortion starts with the clash between two values that appear at first glance to be moral absolutes. In feminist-liberal discourse, the matter is generally formulated as follows: The fetus is a being with a measure of personhood (in that it is an actual person, a potential person, or a being having symbolic value), and killing it is therefore forbidden. On the other hand, a woman has an absolute right to autonomy and to reproductive freedom, and she therefore possesses the right to decide what will become of her body and whether or not she wants to bear this child. Robertson puts it this way:

> Abortion has been an intractable issue because of the clash of moral absolutes it presents. On one side are pregnant women who want to be free of the burdens of unwanted pregnancy. To deny them the right to terminate pregnancy effectively denies them the right to avoid reproduction, because birth control may be unavailable or ineffective. On the other hand, abortion destroys an embryo or fetus, and thus displays a willingness to take human life. How is such a fierce conflict to be resolved?[74]

Resolution of the moral dilemma requires denying underlying assumptions: either the fetus's status as a moral being having a right to life or the woman's autonomy and freedom. Intermediate positions on abortion deny neither assumption but blunt both; accordingly, abortion will not always be permitted but will always be considered in a way that balances the various interests at stake.

When we consider the dilemma from a halakhic perspective, we must ask whether these two fundamental premises of the dilemma are, in fact, valid in the conceptual world of halakhah. Initially, the feminist-liberal presentation of the issue does not seem to accord with a halakhic worldview. Inasmuch as a woman is not regarded as a subject with autonomy over her body and free control of her procreative capacity, the moral dilemma from a halakhic viewpoint should be formulated in these terms: Whose personhood takes precedence—the woman's or the fetus's? Does the fact that the fetus is a potential person mean that the woman's interests should be considered only when her very life is at risk?

The sweepingly permissive liberal position takes the view, as discussed earlier, that the fetus is not a "person" in any respect and therefore the termination of its life can be justified for any reason whatsoever. But if we probe this position more deeply, we find that it is not derived directly or exclusively from the fetus's supposed lack of personhood; it is also, and perhaps primarily, the result of assigning weight to the woman's interest in the moral dilemma. Even those who rule permissively do not deny the fetus's potential personhood and will not allow it to be aborted in the absence of some interest on the part of its mother that runs counter to its existence.[75] But adherents of this position, though they acknowledge the fact of the fetus's potential personhood, do not really take it into account; for the interests of the woman as an actual person will always overcome the interests of one whose "personhood" is only potential.

I would argue that because the halakhic analysis takes account *only* of the fetus's status, even the decision that a fetus is not a "life" will not allow for consideration of the woman's interests beyond the very narrow one of remaining alive. The dilemma is always one of "life" in the narrow sense of the word; that is, it arises only when one life is balanced against the other. To put it differently, because the woman is not conceived of as an autonomous subject, no interests of hers beyond her continued existence enter into the picture (at least according to the strictest halakhic interpretations); no dilemmas are posed with respect to her welfare, the quality of her life, her desire to raise the child, and so forth. That, at least, is the position that seems to be held by the large majority of contemporary decisors who regard the prohibition on abortion as one of biblical law, as I have shown at length above. Their halakhic stance can be reformulated in terms of a moral dilemma as follows: We are obligated to protect the life of the fetus (A) and we are obligated to protect the life of the woman (B). A and B are inconsistent. The dilemma is resolved, as we have said, by preferring the life of the woman. But putting the dilemma in these narrow terms excludes the preponderance of struggles over abortion and the bulk of women's experiences in this area. The unavoidable conclusion is that in every instance that does not involve mortal danger to the mother, the status of the fetus as a potential person will trump that of the woman as an actual person (the opposite of Robertson's intermediate position).

It seems to me that to pose the moral dilemma in this way is to predetermine the degree of maneuverability that can be used in reaching halakhic solutions; more precisely, it reduces women and femaleness to mere biological entities whose personhood is coextensive with their femaleness, that is, their procreative function. This analysis confirms MacKinnon's comment that woman are defined as women from a functional perspective, as objects for sexuality and procreation, and that the goal of men is to structure a woman's identity in that way. It seems to me that a position that justifies abortion only in a case of mortal danger to the woman necessarily incorporates such a presumption, even if it is kept under wraps.

Dworkin's comments shed additional light on the point: Halakhic rulings that posit the existence of a biblical prohibition on abortion necessarily assume that the sanctity of life flows from the very fact of its having been granted by the Creator; accordingly, only deprivation of life itself can annul that sanctity. It follows unavoidably that there is no room for other considerations that might warrant preferring the woman's life over that of the fetus. One who sees the importance of life as residing solely in its very existence will find it easy to argue that the fetus's claim on potential life overcomes any interest of the woman other than her own right to remain alive.

I recognize that nothing in the foregoing analysis provides a basis for distinguishing the question of abortion from of that euthanasia. There, too, those who maintain the "conservative" position with regard to the sanctity of life will not permit euthanasia *for men or for women*; and that would appear to contradict my view of the gender bias with respect to abortion. But there is a significant difference: a large majority of the halakhic positions on euthanasia are expressed in the same sweepingly prohibitory style, a uniformity that is lacking in connection with abortion. In the latter case, we find a wide gap between the analysis of the halakhic sources and the sweeping conclusion of contemporary decisors that abortion is a biblically based prohibition. I would argue that the prohibitory tendency in contemporary rulings is the product of a conscious choice, a choice that becomes evident when we consider that those rulings interpret the earlier sources in a way that is anything but inevitable. Other interpretations can be (and have been) offered, as I have shown; and the deliberate choice made by the contemporary decisors can be seen as reflecting a gender bias.

The moral dilemma from a halakhic perspective could have been formulated very differently, in a way that takes seriously the woman's standing as a subject and assigns it weight; and that could have been done without buying into the liberal ideology of bodily autonomy or reproductive freedom. It is enough to mention Samuel's comment in the passage in *'Arakhin* expressing concern about the woman's disgrace and taking account, not only of the fetus's life vis-à-vis the woman's life, but also of the fetus's life vis-à-vis the woman's posthumous disgrace. In that balancing, the fetus's life is outweighed. If the prohibition on "disgracing the deceased" overcomes the life of the fetus, avoiding disgrace to the living should do so a fortiori! Without risking anachronism, I believe that in Dworkin's terms, this position is close to the liberal one that holds the sanctity of life to flow not only from the fact of its existence but also from its nature and quality, matters that depend, of course, on human actions, preferences, and choices. In that sense, Dworkin's analysis nicely illuminates the extent to which formulating the moral dilemma as "life versus life" falls short of conveying the full scope of the problem.

The uniqueness of feminist ethics lies in its directing primary attention to the interests and experiences of women.[76] According to feminists, it is self-evident that the woman is the subject when it comes to abortion. Their analysis suggests, as we have seen, a series of substantive considerations that can justify abortion. These justifications become apparent when one examines the question of abortion through the prism of gender relations within society, with regard both to the *circumstances that give rise* to unwanted pregnancy and the *effects* of those pregnancies on the lives of women. Taken at face value, the passage in *'Arakhin* likewise views the woman as the subject when it comes to abortion. This is evident in both the Mishnah's unwillingness to delay execution of judgment until the fetus is born—that is, its treatment of the anguish an extended delay would cause the woman as the decisive factor—and in Samuel's concern, cited in the *gemara*, about sparing her posthumous disgrace. On the other hand, when we examine the halakhic rationales (if any) offered by the decisors for allowing abortion in cases not entailing mortal danger to the mother, references to sparing the woman disgrace or shame—that is, rationales that treat the woman as the central subject of the abortion dilemma and take account of the effects on her life of unwanted pregnancy—are prominently absent. Even if, when all is said and done, R. Jacob Emden or R. Uziel permit the abortion of a fetus that is a *mamzer*, the analysis is always centered on the status of the fetus.

But the matter does not end there. As I stressed earlier, if what is at issue involves conflicting interests or obligations that shape a person's life, we find a prominent gap between the relative ease with which a man is allowed to take account of his needs and the almost insuperable burdens imposed on a woman wanting to do so, even when halakhic precedent would allow it. Even among those who sound the rhetorical note of subservience to God or of "great commandment" with respect to all matters procreative, we find, as a practical matter, considerable weight being given to the interests and projects of the standard halakhic "person," that is, a man. The interests of women, however, are not considered. If a woman at a particular stage of life is uninterested in bearing any child, or an additional child, she is considered "spoiled," "selfish," or led astray by the perverse values of Western culture, for how can a woman not want to bear children? The effects of an undesired pregnancy on women's lives, well-being, and personal and professional development are entirely absent from the halakhic rulings. In R. Isaac Aramah's terms, "Eve" has attained total ascendancy over "woman."[77] Accordingly, I believe that to the extent the halakhists disregard factors that may ease the lives of women and continue to choose interpretive and halakhic options that aggrandize the standing of the fetus—especially when these interpretations are quite forced—their position can be said to manifest gender bias.

The premise of the foregoing discussion is that under the veil of concisely worded formalism there lurks a hidden world of values that, once uncovered, has much to say about religious and moral integrity. I have argued that to see the fetus as "not a life" does not necessarily imply a permissive position on abortion. Adopting such a position depends on more fundamental beliefs regarding the nature and value of life. A halakhic position that regards the prohibition on abortion as biblical confines the idea of sanctity of life exclusively to biological terms and thereby highlights its treatment of woman as a procreative entity. To state it differently, the difference between liberal positions and the prohibitory religious position pertains to the exclusivity of the claim regarding the fetus's personhood: is it or is it not balanced against the needs and desires of the woman as a subject and the effects of an undesired pregnancy on her life? As MacKinnon writes, the problem is not whether the fetus is a human being; the problem is that if the question is so worded, the fetus's interests will also trump the woman's:

> The abortion choice should be available and must be women's, but not because the fetus is not a form of life. . . . The problem has been that if the fetus has *any* standing in the debate, it has more weight than women do.[78]

To conclude this chapter let me quote Blu Greenberg, who has done a good job of describing my own feelings and of dealing with so emotional an issue from both a halakhic and a moral perspective:

> My stomach tightens at the thought of getting involved in a controversy over abortion, even with myself. Emotionally, theologically, as a Jew, and most of all as a mother who is daily nurtured by the sights and sounds of her children, I am opposed to abortion. And yet, the other facets of unwanted pregnancy are inescapable—fatigue and harassed parents, the shame of rape, the premature end of youth because of a foolish mistake, the degradation and danger of coat-hanger abortion, and not the least, the overwhelming and exclusive claim that a child makes on a woman's life for many of her strongest years.[79]

Adopting a liberal position (even if not a sweepingly permissive one) is not something I do casually. As a woman, as the mother of five children, as one who is faithful to the halakhah, I might have been expected to take a different view. But precisely because of the factors just noted, the opposite is true. Children have tremendous importance for women, but they cannot comprise their entire being or human totality. I believe that the halakhah, from its own perspective, does not reject the criticism I have presented here; on the contrary, it has ample room to incorporate it if the halakhic decisors so wish. As a practical matter, this critique can contribute to a more balanced view on the part of halakhists regarding women's needs and to greater understanding and empathy with respect to their ability to shape their own lives, choices, and preferences in a proper and dignified manner—all within the context of the considerations that must be taken into account in reaching decisions as difficult as those required in the matter of abortion.

PART TWO

Procreation without Sex

CHAPTER FIVE

Artificial Insemination, In Vitro Fertilization, and Surrogacy in Liberal and Radical Feminist Approaches

Artificial insemination as a technique for effectuating conception without sexual relations has been known in modern medicine since the second half of the nineteenth century, and the long-term storage of frozen semen in sperm banks began in 1940. Of all the fertilization methods created by modern technology, artificial insemination is the simplest and longest used.

Artificial insemination can take three forms:

1. Artificial insemination with sperm from the husband (AIH)
2. Artificial insemination with sperm from a donor (AID)
3. Artificial insemination with sperm from the husband and a donor together (AIHD)

AIH is used when natural fertilization cannot take place because of physiological infirmities in the woman or the man, such as impotence, damage to the genital organs, or a high percentage of defective sperm. AID is used when the man is infertile but the female's procreative organs are healthy.

In vitro fertilization (IVF) is a fertility technique in which a woman's ovum is fertilized by a man's sperm outside her uterus. The technology was first used successfully in 1978, following about a century of study, with the birth of the world's first "test-tube baby" to the Brown family in England.

It has generally been assumed that artificial insemination is used when the male partner suffers infertility, while in vitro fertilization is required when the problem is the woman's (such as blockage or absence of the Fallopian tubes). Recently, however, IVF has begun to be used in cases when a man's fertility is impaired as well—when, for example, there is a congenital absence of sperm vessels, the sperm count is low, mobility is impaired, or a high percentage of sperm are defective. IVF can be effective in those cases because it requires a relatively small number of sperm cells.

New Reproductive Technologies (NRT) have been earth-shattering in their effect on thinking about human fertility overall. They offer a range of possibilities for solving problems associated with pregnancy and birth and for overcoming genetic or chromosomal obstacles to the birth of healthier children. These technologies also confirm the image of science as possessed of an unlimited ability to bring about progress, enabling humans to triumph over natural limitations and impediments to fulfilling their desires. But this unbounded progress necessarily entails numerous risks. By extending the scope of human control over the creation of life, it exposes humans to unforeseeable dangers—dangers both to those who are aided by the new technologies and to the offspring born through their use. For example, it permits the introduction of eugenics policies that assign higher value to some human lives than to others,[1] and it reduces the natural process of creating new life to something that can be purchased for money. Questions have been raised regarding the boundaries between the natural and the artificial, the problematic aspects of imposing a human program on a reality whose origins are nonhuman, and the limits of human control over nature.[2] Some believe that artificial procreation shatters all the classical models and that the natural reservations about human involvement in the act of creation rests on the concern that humans are unequipped to anticipate the results of such profound control over procreation; these critics are especially frightened by the irreversibility of some of these genetic interventions.[3] Blurring the boundaries between the biological and the sociological in areas previously controlled by biological fate can politicize issues related to sexuality, childbearing, parenthood, and family. When the New Reproductive Technologies are seen in this way, they raise the specter of "mad science," of a Frankensteinian world in which scientists engage in manipulations having unforeseeable effects on the very fundamentals of life.[4]

One might have imagined that the religious-halakhic system would be particularly vocal in raising reservations of this sort, but that has not been the case; these concerns have been relegated to the margins of halakhic discourse and go almost unheard. One gets the sense that halakhic decisors, with only a few exceptions, are not particularly interested in the weighty theological or moral implications of reproductive technologies. It appears that the wonderful opportunities these technologies offer to infertile men and women have nearly blinded the decisors' eyes to their problematic aspects. But the desire to march hand-in-hand with science and to thereby enable widespread fulfillment of the commandment to procreate may not always be consistent with broader human and, especially, female interests, and it produces weighty human and halakhic dilemmas.

In this chapter, I will examine the positions of feminist ethicists and critics on a range of issues related to artificial insemination, in vitro fertilization, and surrogacy. This chapter is distinct from others in the book, insofar as it focuses exclusively on the discussion of reproductive technologies in general feminist literature rather than on the related halakhic discourse. The ideas will be presented at some length, to provide a sense of the depth and scope of the problems that could result from uncritical and unbalanced use of these technologies as well as to highlight the striking permissiveness of most halakhic rulings on this issue, which reflects a lack of such considerations in the mainstream halakhic discourse.

Feminist Positions on Reproductive Technologies and Surrogacy

The technological innovations at issue give rise to questions of two sorts:

1. *Questions focused on the ethical and practical problems raised by the extra-bodily manipulation of ova, sperm, and fetuses.* For example, does scientific study of these matters undermine the dignity and sanctity of human life? Should fetuses be protected from commercial or scientific

exploitation? What is the status of "pre-fetuses"—fertilized eggs that have not yet matured into fetuses?

2. *Questions related to parenthood.* Who has the right to demand custody of the child produced through egg or sperm donation and who has the duty to care for the child? Who is the parent of a child who is born neither to its genetic mother nor to its social mother? Does surrogacy undermine the very concept of motherhood?

Feminist writers have raised a third group of questions: In contemporary societies in which women do not merely bear children but are defined primarily with reference to their reproductive potential, how do these technologies affect the lives of women? What effects can be anticipated on their health, their security, and their reproductive choices—especially given that it is primarily women whose bodies are being used to develop the new technologies and primarily men who study, plan for, and apply those technologies?[5]

Feminists want to undo the essential connection between motherhood and feminine identity and the associated gender-based expectations—expectations that add substantially to the suffering of infertile women. In that sense, one may speak of the paradox posed, from a feminist perspective, by infertility: on the one hand, understanding and empathy for the intense suffering of barren women; on the other hand, ambivalence regarding their desire for fertility treatment, which can be seen as silent acquiescence to conventional gender roles and gender-based social stratification.[6] The traditional assumption was that women were naturally limited by the role of bearing and raising children and therefore could not take part in social life on the same terms as men. Feminists such as Simone de Beauvoir[7] and Shulamith Firestone[8] therefore took the view that the liberation of women largely depended on their escaping that trap. Firestone maintained that technology had great potential to liberate women from the biological tyranny to which they were subjected. Her book, which was quite influential during the 1970s, left the impression that radical feminism would welcome the new reproductive technologies as an increasingly powerful catalyst for the liberation of women from the burden of procreation and, concomitantly, from the inequality and social inferiority that women experienced. As it turned out, however, feminist critics cited her naïve faith in technological progress while themselves believing it more likely that these new mechanisms would remain under male control and, indeed, augment the social domination of women by men.

And so, radical feminists of the 1980s took a position intensely opposed to all the new technologies, aligning themselves, surprisingly, with the naturalistic and conservative position of the Catholic Church. This opposition was grounded in a perspective that analyzed power relationships between the sexes in terms of domination. Most if not all of these technologies, it was argued, were controlled by men and therefore contributed to men's domination and exploitation of women. In addition to this fundamental argument, one can find several key themes in radical feminist discourse on reproductive technologies, and I will consider the most important of them in what follows.

Artificial Fertilization and Insemination: Radical Feminist Approaches

CONTROL OVER WOMEN'S BODIES

In radical feminist thought, the new reproductive technologies were seen as part of the overall medicalizing of pregnancy and birth, a process meant to control women and their procreative powers for the benefit of men.[9] Indeed, the process brought about the gradual decline in the role of the female midwife as medical involvement in pregnancy and birth grew. With respect to pregnancy and birth, women were transformed from subjects to objects, and their bodies came more and more under the control of physicians. As men became less alienated from procreation, women became more so.[10]

Arguing that birth and motherhood are the basis for female identity, radical feminists see the new birthing technologies as destroying the concept of motherhood, as a means by which men rob women not only of control over birthing but of birthing itself.[11] Men, it is argued, are removed from procreation and distant from their offspring during the course of pregnancy and birth; as a result, they aspire to control nature, to build social institutions and cultural structures that will afford them the illusion of power and continuity. The new reproductive technologies are a way to transform the male illusion regarding procreative power into reality. By manipulating ova and fetuses, men can make themselves into the fathers of humanity, and by implanting ova from one woman into another, they can attain unprecedented control over motherhood itself. Motherhood as a single biological process will unravel; instead of "Mommy" there will be women with a supply of ova to create children, women with uteruses for rent to bear the children, and social mothers to raise them. Once an artificial womb is developed, biological motherhood will become superfluous.

On the other hand, it is argued as well that control over procreation strengthens the ideology that embraces the importance of motherhood. According to this ideology, motherhood (in the context of the traditional family) is the ultimate, natural, and desired goal of every "normal" woman, and a woman who denies her motherly instinct is seen as selfish or "disturbed." The "ideology of motherhood" is an obstacle to women's autonomous motherhood (that is, unconnected, or at least not permanently connected, to a man), for it takes the view that all women want to have children but that single women, and lesbians, are expected to forgo motherhood "for the good of the child." Moreover, the promotion of this ideology causes barren women to be "blinded" by science and manipulated in a way that causes them to lend full support to any technology that will grant them the children they crave.[12]

Andrea Dworkin offers the most radical and scathing formulation of the critique linking reproductive technologies to the oppressive patriarchal regime and to men's desire to control women.[13] She offers two models to describe how women are socially controlled and sexually exploited: the brothel and the farm. Under the former, women are assembled and held for the purpose of sexual relations with men. They cannot come and go freely and are bought and sold as sexual merchandise having no individual or personal worth. Their function is defined in terms that are expressly nonprocreative; they are almost antiprocreative. A woman sells sex; she is not meant to make babies. The farming model, in contrast, pertains to motherhood. Women as a social group are seen as real estate or cattle, and men treat them as a farmer treats his land or his cow. They are sowed with the man's seed, and it is he who harvests the crop of children. This was the principal way to exploit women, treating them as mothers and baby makers. Metaphorically, men treat their land as if it were a woman—a giant, fertile woman. But the farming model is "slippery," and a woman has ways of saying no. She can exercise a bit of control over the intervals between children; moreover, the man's control over the nature of the "crop" is limited. The model therefore requires the constant exercise of power. Recognizing the limitations of the model, men imposed it on all women (other than harlots) in order to control procreation and "administer women's wombs" to bring children into being and leave women subject to men's procreative desires. Men use social and economic sanctions to punish women who try to live outside the model, particularly lesbians and unmarried women.

In Dworkin's view, the new reproductive technologies represent "the new prostitution of procreation." The physician or scientist is the new pimp, and the hospitals and research institutes are the brothels in which women are sold to men, who use their wombs in exchange for money. Before the invention of the new technologies, the farming model was distinct from the brothel model. Even though a woman was regarded as nonhuman, like land, or as subhuman, the farm had symbolic overtones of agrarian romanticism: to sow the soil means to love it; to feed the cattle means to protect, worry about, and care for them. In the farming model, the woman was at least privately owned, and friendly relations could develop between the farm owner and his land, that is, his wife. But reproductive technologies change the terms under which men control procreation. The social control of the farming model is replaced by medical control—more precise and closer to the efficiency of the brothel model. The new reproductive technologies transform the womb into the "province" of the physicians, thereby detaching it from the woman's body, just as the sexual organs are detached from the body of the prostitute:

> These two reproductive technologies—artificial insemination and in vitro fertilization—enable women to sell their wombs within the terms of the brothel model. Motherhood is becoming a new branch of female prostitution with the help of scientists who want access to the womb for experimentation and for power.[14]

In Dworkin's view, therefore, the main problem is not whether the technology in and of itself is substantively good; it is how the technology will be used within a social system in which women already are exploited, already are treated as sexual or procreative merchandise whose lives have no real value if they do not serve the specific purpose of sex or procreation. With the increasing use of reproductive technologies, men will ultimately gain the means to create and control the sort of women they always wanted: diminished as women but "improved"—harlots for sex and harlots for procreation.[15]

Gena Corea offers an example of how Dworkin's "brothel model" already exists with regard to animals in the form of the breeding ranch.[16] Many animals held on ranches are considered genetically inferior and serve as surrogates for the fetuses of superior animals. This distinction between genetically superior and genetically inferior is becoming progressively more pronounced, and Corea fears it may make its way to the human field as well. It is easy enough to dismiss the fate of animals as different from that of women, but, Corea believes, in a world of male superiority, the attitude toward women is not all that distinct. For centuries in patriarchal societies, women and animals shared the same legal status, as chattel.[17] Men owned slaves, cattle, and women. Accordingly, it is not inconceivable, she argues, that a class of professional surrogates might emerge, analogous to what happens on a cattle-breeding farm. In a class-based society, for example, women of color might be considered "less valuable," and therefore sterilized and used as surrogates to carry the children of "more valuable" white women, who would be used to produce fetuses.[18]

CONSTRUCTING A WOMAN'S DESIRE FOR CHILDREN: THE MEANING OF "CHOICE"

According to radical feminists, new reproductive technologies not only control women's procreative function but also affect their reproductive desires and, consequently, their reproductive choices. Christine Overall argues that an infertile woman who wants to undergo fertility treatments should not be blamed, for the desire to become a mother is created, in our pro-natalist culture, by social forces.[19] Susan Sherwin, meanwhile, emphasizes that women are persuaded that their most important goal in life is to raise children and that their lives are incomplete without them. This is because many women have no contact with meaningful work, many do not find themselves in solid heterosexual relationships, and often they are unable to form social connections other than with their partners. As a result, children are their only opportunity for true intimacy and a certain sense of accomplishment, resulting from having done something considered worthwhile.[20]

The claim that a woman's desire to bear and raise children is socially constructed challenges the idea that women have and exercise free choice or free will. Robyn Rowland[21] and Barbara Katz-Rothman[22] note that since the late 1970s, when poor and minority women, whose reproductive choices were severely influenced and limited by economic and social realities, indeed began to challenge the notion that women have free choice, feminists have recognized that the idea needs to be rethought. Can one truly speak of free choice in the context of abortion, for example, if a woman aborts a female fetus because of the higher value assigned in her society to male children? Can one truly speak of free choice in a case of a fetus with Down's syndrome if society does not provide support for raising children with special needs? What of a case in which a woman aborts her (desired) fetus because she lacks the economic means to sustain it? In all these cases, Rowland believes that the concept of "freedom" fails.[23] In her view, the firmest basis on which the right to abortion can be asserted is the ability and the right of women to control their lives and their bodies. When feminists say "the right to choose," they really mean the right to control. Rowland maintains that men in positions of power create the dominant ideas and shape the belief in a world in which free choice supposedly exists—a world in which individuals make choices with regard to their lives and are not limited by social responsibilities to others. Through the illusion of free choice, however (as in the case of fertility treatments), men strengthen their control over women even more: "The illusion of freedom is a powerful control mechanism."[24]

Rowland recognizes that the women's movement has set, as its foremost concern, the demand that women have the right to choose and thus to control their sexuality and procreativity. The new fertility mechanisms likewise have generated slogans along the lines of "a right to choose." But do women choose fertility treatments freely, or does their supposed choice really grow out of social pressure and a cultural construct regarding the importance of biological motherhood? The choices considered in the past opened opportunities to women as a social class, but, she argues, the concept of "choice," in the context of reproductive technologies, closes off opportunities to women (as a social class), and thus it is necessary to limit even the basic right to choose. Certainly, feminists have always sought the freedom to choose. But because procreative technologies allow men to reinforce their control and diminish their alienation from the procreative process (by increasing the alienation of women), freedom of choice becomes secondary, even at the cost of injuring the infertile.[25] Ruth Hubbard believes that when "choices" become possible, they are quickly transformed into pressures or even social obligations to choose the alternative that society prefers.[26] And so, in a pronatalist society, modern reproductive technologies impose a new burden on the infertile, denying them almost any ability to decline to subject themselves to those treatments or to discontinue them once begun. It will always be possible for others to tell them "You did not try hard enough."

BIOLOGICAL PARENTHOOD VS. ADOPTION

The critique of biological parenthood is presented most expansively by Overall. She questions the value placed on genetic connections between parents and children, suggesting that the emphasis on that connection reveals a widespread concept of children as "merchandise." As she sees it, infertility involves primarily the loss of the ability to bear a child of one's own; that is, infertility means an inability to own children, not a lack of opportunities to be with them. That a parent wants to have a child that belongs to him genetically is not necessarily for the good of the child; it is more for the benefit of the parent, just as purchased merchandise brings pleasure to its owner. The genetic link appears to be more important to the man, for he invests less in raising the child—that is, in his sociological paternity—and what makes him truly the child's father is primarily the genetics. The question to be asked, therefore, is whether the desire for a child of one's own warrants a medical response. Is the genetic link so strong as to warrant using invasive therapies? Is it as important to the woman as it is to the man? Women may be more interested in experiencing pregnancy, birth, and child rearing than they are in any genetic link, and it is only cultural and social conditioning that leads people to assign a preference to raising a child who is genetically theirs. According to Overall, the genetic tie is simply not important enough in itself to warrant use of artificial fertilization.

POSSIBLE FLAWS IN THE RADICAL POSITION

Radical feminist writing is focused primarily on the concepts of control and free choice and on a critique of the prevailing patriarchal notion that understands the primary purpose of women to be related to the bearing and raising of children. I believe the radical theory to be problematic in (at least) two ways.

First, the radical theory criticizes patriarchal thought for refusing to see women as subjects and instead making them and their bodies into objects. But despite that criticism, it seems to me to do precisely the same thing in its argument about "construction of will." It reduces women's consciousness (albeit not their bodies) to an object that lends itself to ideological manipulation to attain the goals of the oppressive, controlling force. If the dominant patriarchal culture has in fact planted a "false consciousness" in the minds of women so that it can continue to control their procreative powers and their lives overall, it is unclear how women can continue to practice motherhood—even without fertility therapy—without falling prey to that same ideology that enslaves and oppresses them. In other words, how does the radical feminist critique that speaks of a "constructed will" and of a consequent inability to freely choose fertility treatments pertain specifically to modern procreative technologies? How does a woman who chooses IVF differ from any other woman who chooses to become pregnant in the natural way? I see no need to question whether a woman who believes that the sole, or primary, purpose of women is to bear children has arrived at that belief autonomously or has been led to it by a false consciousness that has been imposed on her; it is enough to criticize the belief itself, for an attack on the autonomy of one's consciousness can be a two-edged sword. If women in fact suffer from a "false consciousness," it is unclear where it begins and ends and who determines that it in fact is false. It could well be argued that the very attack on the autonomy of the consciousness is itself paternalistic and overreaching, demeaning to women in general.

Second, it is hard to make a coherent argument that "freedom of choice" provides the moral basis for allowing abortion or birth control but is disqualified from doing so with respect to reproductive therapy. And if we accept Rowland's argument that the legitimate basis for abortion is not freedom of choice so much as freedom to control one's body, that same argument should apply as well with regard to fertility therapy. These therapies make it possible for women to control their bodies, primarily if that control means becoming a mother by overcoming their bodies' biological limitations.

This is not to say that I reject out of hand the arguments of the radical theoreticians. There is a place for suspicions about the medical establishment's control over matters related to procreation and its increasing control over women's bodies, but it must be accompanied by respect for the desire of infertile women to bear children and must not dismiss these technologies at the cost of giving up a more important principle in the name of freedom of choice.

Artificial Fertilization and Insemination: Liberal Feminist Approaches

Feminist theoreticians of the liberal school have advanced ideas that differ from the radical critique.[27] Contemporary writers (such as Sara Rudick and Carol Gilligan) who have associated the feminine experience and motherhood with such values as caring, antiviolence, or spirituality have laid the groundwork that has again made it possible to attribute agency to women who are infertile. They argue that radical feminism errs in denying the autonomy of motherhood and oversimplifies matters when it leaves no room for the complex and varied experiences of women. Women's desire for children is stronger and more fundamental than any supposed patriarchal mandate to procreate.[28] The liberals recommend applying a more critical eye toward reproductive choices and developing a comprehensive view that encompasses alternatives such as adoption. With respect to fertility therapies themselves, they call for better clinical standards and greater awareness of the differences among the various sorts of treatment. In their view, the key idea is freedom of choice.

Barbara Berg argues that the social forces that impel women to raise children (specifically biological ones) cannot themselves explain the desire of women to become biological mothers and to do so at a substantial cost.[29] Her clinical experience shows that most women who seek reproductive treatments are educated and accomplished women who have attained many other goals in their lives and still want to become biological mothers. The automatic reduction of that desire to pro-natalist cultural influences betokens a lack of sensitivity to the experience and feelings of infertile women.[30] It may well be possible that reproductive technologies diminish women's control and augment men's domination of them, but for women who cannot become pregnant naturally, these technological interventions may offer the sole hope for exercising any control at all over reproduction.

Nor, say liberal feminists, is the actual experience of women or their understanding of reality consistent with the radicals' assertion that patriarchal notions are responsible for the emphasis on genetic rather than sociological parental ties and that the desire for a biological child should be understood in that light. While the desire for genetic ties can be negatively associated with eugenics, narcissism, or a drive for immortality, it can also be viewed positively as the desire to create a new generation with recognized genealogical heritage. Moreover, the experience of raising an adopted child differs from that of raising a biological child, and it therefore should come as no surprise that women are interested specifically in biological motherhood. Adoptive parents have no automatic connection to the child, and they must be able to love a child who does not represent an extension of their own bodies. Berg believes that infertile women have given more thought to why they want to become biological mothers than have their fertile counterparts, for they are required to surmount greater obstacles to do so. One of the answers given by these women is that they are interested in the experience of pregnancy and birth no less than in that of parenthood itself, as well as in social recognition of their reproductive capability.

As noted, Overall and Rowland would deny the right of infertile women to reproductive therapies because recognizing that right might be harmful to women as a whole. Berg responds by asking whether "the good" of women as a social group can overcome the rights of individual women. Risky procedures, such as cesarean sections and amniocentesis, have not incurred sweeping demands that they be eliminated, nor has objection to abortion been expressed on the basis of the risk that female fetuses might be aborted because of their sex. That is so, Berg adds, even though it is harder, in her view, to show the potential harm to the community of women caused by reproductive therapies than to show the potential harm associated with undesired gynecological procedures.

Linda LeMoncheck believes[31] that if part of the role of the reproduction therapy provider is to enable the woman to define her reproductive life in her own terms, the provider must ensure that his or her counseling is based on a certain understanding of the patriarchal ideology under which provider and patient are operating, of the history of the exploitation of women through reproductive science, of the medical monopoly over female fertility and its near-total disregard for alternatives to technological intervention, and of the discriminatory manner in which IVF is offered (that is, only to people of economic means). Only then can a woman make responsible and effective reproductive decisions that strengthen both her and women in general.[32] As the subject of her reproductive experience, a woman must be equipped to express her reproductive identity and to determine whether and how identification as a mother has value for her. But she must also recognize that she might become an object subject to manipulation by patriarchal science. Accordingly, those caring for a woman would be well advised to examine their own attitude toward the issue of reproduction, unrelated to that of society or family. First, a greater amount of time should be dedicated to clarifying the needs and motivations of every woman and to present each patient with as many details as possible regarding the contemplated treatment, including the physical, psychic, and economic efforts that will be required of her. Second, because this ethics situates reproductive therapies in the wider social context of exploitation of women's procreative abilities, the providers must offer women the most up-to-date information available regarding the risks, prospects, and likely success of the procedure in the specific clinic in which she is being cared for. Additional information must be given regarding alternative or supportive treatments, the adoption option, and various sorts of birthing processes that are available; and meetings should be arranged with couples who have chosen to remain childless. In this way, the woman can truly be an active, conscious, and critical participant in all that takes place. It is self-evident that an ethics of this sort must treat all women equally—single women, lesbians, and lower-class women included—and not subject them to what others might regard as an "appropriate" standard of parenthood. A feminist ethics, accordingly, must be sensitive to the distress of infertile women and respect their choice and their desire for the greater control that fertility treatments can provide. At the same time, it must neutralize the influence of cultural constructs regarding the essential connection between women and procreation, constructs that, in their extreme form, can cause childless women to see themselves as lacking all value or purpose in life.

Surrogacy: Radical Feminist Views

SURROGACY AS COMMERCE IN BABIES AND EXPLOITATION OF WOMEN

The first and central argument of Katz-Rothman[33] is that surrogacy entails the purchase and sale of babies, both on the part of the surrogate, who sells the child that belongs to her (as its birth mother), and on the part of the sperm-donor father, who purchases his baby:

> We sell babies in "kit" form, purchasing the pieces and services separately: sperm here, an egg there, a rented uterus somewhere else. This is of course a "slippery slope" kind of situation—once you permit some people to buy some babies under some conditions, it is very hard to justify any given person not being allowed to purchase a baby under other circumstances.[34]

Her objection to surrogacy rests on values that treat human relationships and not genetic connections as central: motherhood is defined by the physical and emotional connection established during pregnancy and not by the mere biological donation. This is not to say that the motherly tie cannot be severed or that it is the most powerful of all relationships. A mother can give up her child and allow others to raise it; in so doing, she simply ends a relationship, as people often do. The tie that develops during pregnancy and birth may have greater weight than the genetic, the contractual, or the economic tie, but that does not contradict a woman's right to abort, for a woman who chooses to abort chooses not to enter into the relationships associated with motherhood. However, she can not sell her body for money.

An additional value, beyond the connection forged during pregnancy, involves physical autonomy, control of one's body. Katz-Rothman regards the fetus as part of the mother's body. The traditional patriarchal concept regards it as part of the father's body, a seed planted in the mother's body. From a feminist perspective, however, it belongs to the mother's body. It follows that the mother never carries someone else's fetus—not that of her husband, not that of the government, and not that of people who purchase a fetus through a surrogacy agreement. Every woman carries her fetus without regard to where the sperm or egg came from. Katz-Rothman recognizes that the new technologies allow for a surrogate to carry a fetus formed from the genetic sperm and egg of a couple, and she does not reject the possibility of a donated egg being fertilized in the body of another woman or of sperm donation. The problem, in her view, arises when these technologies are used for purposes of surrogacy—when the pregnant, birthing mother is recognized only as a "womb for hire" and the true mother is considered to be the woman who produced the egg.[35] She also rejects any resolution suggesting that though the pregnancy is, in fact, the surrogate's, the fetus belongs to the people who hired her, for the importance of the child who is so desired and precious will always overcome the value assigned to the cheap labor of the surrogate. That is the unavoidable outcome of a pregnancy that is understood not as a connection between mother and fetus but as a service that the mother provides to others, and of the idea that the woman herself is a mechanism to be used by other, more valued, persons. In that sense, surrogacy is a reductio ad absurdum of patriarchal, technological capitalism.[36]

Katz-Rothman appears, at first glance, to contradict herself. If a woman can sever the motherly bond by aborting a pregnancy and if she has autonomy over her body, she ought to have the sovereign right in a case of surrogacy to sever the motherly bond and give the child to others, just as in a case of adoption. To state it differently, her control over her body should allow her to use it for various purposes, including that of "a uterus for hire." It seems to me, therefore, that Katz-Rothman's objection to surrogacy is really an objection to the commercial aspect of surrogacy and to what she sees as the exploitation of women by others who are using her for cheap pregnancy labor. The woman's body is thereby reduced to a "vessel,"[37] that is, to a means for satisfying the interests of others. But given that she does not object to sperm or egg donation, I see no basis in her position for barring surrogacy where it is an entirely voluntary, altruistic act.

SURROGACY AS PROSTITUTION

The radical feminist arguments that compare surrogacy to prostitution warrant close attention. Is the comparison in fact a valid one?

If the primary reason for objecting to prostitution is that it entails selling access to intimate body parts not meant to be exchanged for money, it is unclear, indeed, why surrogacy should be seen differently. How does the uterus differ in essence from the genitals, given that it, too, is meant only for intimate, private use rather than for "mass" use? But if the primary objection to prostitution is its commercial aspect, usually associated with appalling exploitation of women on the part of a pimp who reaps most of the profits, the comparison to surrogacy is weakened. The thrust of the argument is no longer against the idea that women are entitled to engage in sexual relations whenever and with whomever they want in exchange for some form of compensation; rather, it is against the commercial exploitation of women. If surrogacy, then, has no commercial or class-related aspect, it can be seen as an altruistic act that actually strengthens women and respects their procreative abilities. Indeed Ruth Macklin argues that if one assumes the commercial and exploitive aspects are neutralized, it is inconsistent for feminists to claim that there is nothing wrong with maintaining nonmarital sex relations but nonetheless analogize surrogacy to prostitution.[38] The real question is whether these aspects of the matter can truly be "neutralized." In that context, Carole Pateman argues that women who are willing to serve as surrogates will inevitably fall victim to exploitation and degradation in a new sort of prostitution that will grow up against the background of commerce in women's reproductive services:

> The political implications of the surrogacy contract can only be appreciated when surrogacy is seen as another provision in the sexual contract, as a new form of access to and use of women's bodies by men.[39]

Surrogacy: Liberal Feminist Approaches

In contrast to the radical approaches, liberal feminists offer several arguments that, in principle, support the use of surrogacy contracts. Let me present the primary ones, on the basis of Lori Andrews's account.[40] In her view, the feminist heritage (especially with respect to procreation and motherhood) comprises the following principles:

1. Women must have the right to reproductive freedom and the right to control their own bodies. These include the rights to use birth control, to abort a pregnancy or initiate one, and to form nontraditional families, such as same-sex or single-parent families.
2. Biology is not destiny, and nonbiological parents can be just as good in that role as biological parents. That women carry children during pregnancy does not give them greater responsibility to raise them.
3. Surrogacy, to a substantial extent, is a foreseeable consequence of the feminist movement. Women who deferred childbearing or used birth control for many years while pursuing a career may find that their reproductive capacities have become impaired, in whole or in part, and turn to the solution offered by surrogacy. Feminism also allowed women wanting to use surrogacy to feel comfortable about that decision, for it

> taught that all women do not relate in the same ways to all pregnancies. Procreation pertains to a woman's body, and she has the right to control it. Intellectual developments of these sorts contributed to the freedom to be a surrogate.[41]

Against these arguments, there is a strain that would forbid surrogacy (at least commercial surrogacy, undertaken in exchange for payment) on the grounds that it causes symbolic harm to society, the woman, or the child. Andrews attempts to deal with these claims one by one.

Opponents of surrogacy contend, first, that the practice is tantamount to the sale of babies and that a society is demeaned when it is seen to be one that encourages that sort of commerce. But, Andrews says, that argument recalls the claim, rejected by feminists, that a society in which abortion is permitted is demeaned by being seen to be one that kills babies. In the abortion context, it is argued that abortion is not an act of baby killing as long as the fetus is in its mother's womb; and it can be argued just as well that surrogacy does not entail baby selling. The baby is not transferred, in exchange for money, to a stranger who can then treat it as merchandise. The payment is meant only to make it possible for the patron to bring his own biological child into existence. Does one purchase a child when one pays a physician for IVF or artificial insemination? In a surrogacy arrangement, one purchases, at most, the mother's pre-pregnancy waiver of parental rights—something analogous to a sperm donor's pre-pregnancy sale of paternal rights, which has been permitted for decades. According to Andrews, one of feminism's great contributions to the public debate over reproductive issues has been, and remains, its rejection of arguments based on traditions, symbolism, and an inflexible understanding of nature, and its concomitant openness to the influence of real life. Therefore, instead of considering the symbolic aspects of a supposed sale, or engaging in demeaning characterizations such as "reproductive prostitution," "reproductive servitude," or "womb for rent," it is better to focus on the propriety of waiving the rights of biological parenthood, whether by a man or by a woman. For example, if biological parenthood is important to parent or child, it may be proper to grant the biological parents the right to certain relationships with the child once it is born.

As we have seen, radical feminism argues that surrogacy has the potential to harm women. Andrews, however, believes that many aspects of these arguments themselves demean and debase women. For example, the claim that surrogacy entails a great potential for remorse, given that it is unnatural to expect a mother to give up her child, suggests that a woman must be protected against her own decisions. The opponents of surrogacy agreements contend that the model of informed consent does not apply here, inasmuch as a woman cannot imagine the intense emotions involved in giving up the child she has carried for so long in her womb. But Andrews sees that position as inconsistent with the legal doctrine of "informed consent." In what other context is the ability to give informed consent predicated on first having undergone the experience to which consent is given? Applying that condition would make it impossible for people to undergo sterilization, abortion, sex-change surgery, heart surgery, and all manner of other procedures. The legal doctrine of informed consent assumes that a person is able to anticipate in advance whether a given action will be useful to him or to her and to act accordingly. Macklin adds in this context that "informed consent," as a legal and moral concept, requires that a person understand the possible consequences of the action.[42] It is not realistic to maintain that the only way to achieve that understanding is to experience the action in question and the emotions that accompany it. And so, if surrogacy resembles other medical treatments, there should be no difference between the informed consent required for a surrogacy agreement and the informed consent required for, say, mastectomy or hysterectomy. If, on the other hand, surrogacy differs and requires a higher standard of informed consent, then only a woman who has experienced the birth and loss of a child can give that consent—a condition too bizarre, and almost certainly too cruel, to contemplate. Andrews therefore concludes that the argument lacks all merit.

A variation on the "informed consent" argument assumes that hormonal influences during the pregnancy will cause a woman to change her mind. To that, Andrews responds:

> Women are fully capable of entering into agreements in this area and of fulfilling the obligations of a contract. Women's hormonal changes have been utilized too frequently over the centuries to enable male dominated society to make decisions for them.[43]

Feminists, therefore, have good reason to be wary of "the argument from hormones."

In addition, the consent given by the surrogate has been regarded as involuntary. As we have seen, radical feminists question the real meaning of consent or choice in a society in which men as a group control not only the possibilities open to women but also the motivations that underlie their choices. Andrews believes such arguments are dangerous to feminism, for they can be interpreted as a reversion to the view that women are unequipped to make decisions. If a woman can decide to undergo an abortion, why can't she decide to become a surrogate?

Some feminists have argued that the financial incentive in surrogacy undermines the voluntariness of the decision; for a woman in need of money may enter into a surrogacy agreement out of necessity rather than free choice, and the economic compensation may lead to exploitation. Andrews certainly sees a need to ensure that all women have access to the labor market and that poor women not feel a need to enter into surrogacy agreements so they can feed their children.[44] But most women who become surrogates do so not to provide themselves with basic life necessities such as food or health care but to meet other, less basic needs. The premise that women planning to use funds for serious purposes are exploited impairs the legitimacy of women being in the workforce. The premise harks back to the idea that women work, and should work, only to earn "pin money." Also troublesome is the fact that when society suggests a particular activity should be altruistic and uncompensated, it is usually referring to women's activities.

Andrews completely rejects the argument that surrogacy entails potential harm to the children that result from it.[45] The analogy to the sale of children is invalid, for even if a sizable sum changes hands in exchange for the baby, it cannot be considered merchandise, since it is being placed under the protection of its biological parents[46] (as well as the relevant laws that protect it) and feels safe and secure. Nor is there any substance to the argument that the parents, having spent a sizable sum in connection with the child's birth, may be likely to expect more of it. Parents may also spend sizable amounts on fertility treatments, and there is no evidence that they expect more of the children that result from those therapies; such an argument is almost unheard of. The premise that extant children of surrogacy may be harmed by developing a fear of abandonment carries no weight, as long as the children are openly informed of their situation. It is odd, in Andrews's view, that feminists who favor amniocentesis and late-term abortions for children with genetic defects argue here that harm may result to children of surrogacy. What of the children of a woman who has chosen to undergo a late-term abortion? Might not her children, on learning of her decision, feel exposed to possible abandonment by their mother? If parents know how to direct and support their children's feelings, the children will feel safe and secure even where abortion or surrogacy is part of the picture.

Summing up her position, Andrews asserts that the arguments against surrogacy threaten to make all women into reproductive vessels, without their consent, by formulating a separate legal category for pregnancy. If pregnancy comes to be seen—even on the basis of a feminist argument—as something so distinct from other biological and sociological processes that it warrants separate legal standing and entitles a woman to reverse her decision to give up her child, it may come to be seen as unique in other areas as well, for special rights often entail special obligations. Andrews is concerned, for example, that a woman might to compelled, against her will, to undergo a cesarean section in order to save her child, although we would not compel elective surgery in other cases. She believes that the feminist arguments against surrogacy may well undermine the broader feminist agenda.

Macklin, meanwhile, would distinguish conceptually between the issue of commercialization and the practice of surrogacy per se;[47] as she sees it, only the former is ethically wrong. Accordingly, noncommercialized surrogacy—for example, on the part of women wanting to help their daughters or sisters—is not morally wrong and should not be prohibited, though even that sort of surrogacy might be considered morally wrong if it turned out to cause more harm than good.

In sum, we can say that radical feminism overwhelmingly objects to surrogacy arrangements for several reasons:

1. Surrogacy arrangements demean and degrade the concept of natural, unfragmented motherhood that encompasses all stages of childbearing.
2. Surrogacy arrangements exploit a woman's reproductive capacity for monetary compensation and are thereby substantially indistinguishable from prostitution.
3. Surrogacy arrangements cannot be compared to other contracts, for pregnancy by its very essence is something unique that defines the limits of gender equality. Accordingly, terms that are relevant to other sorts of

contractual agreements, such as informed consent, free choice, and individual responsibility, do not apply in this instance.

4. Surrogacy arrangements involve, in essence, the sale of babies, the sale of a woman's body, the commercialization of pregnancy and birth, and the exploitation of lower-class women.

In contrast, liberal feminists believe that almost all of the foregoing arguments can become a two-edged sword and that treating pregnancy and birth as so distinct allows for a reversion to the view that a woman is unable to escape her biological fate. Nor do liberal feminists see any essential flaw in surrogacy arrangements, and most would allow compensation for the surrogate's services. Macklin (and Katz-Rothman, according to my interpretation) appear to favor a middle ground: there is no essential moral flaw in surrogacy arrangements, but the commercial aspect, and the associated risk of exploitation, make it impossible to afford legal sanction to surrogacy, except where it is clearly noncommercial and done for purely altruistic reasons.

Despite the fundamental dispute between radical and liberal feminism regarding the gender significance of modern reproductive technology, both groups emphasize that gender is a critical lens for analyzing the moral issues that are likely to arise from widespread use of these technologies. Although liberal feminism tends to allow access to IVF and surrogacy more readily than the radical faction does, liberal feminists too are aware that uncritical acceptance of these technologies is bound to be problematic, especially with regard to women.

As noted, the next chapter will deal with halakhic positions on this topic. My primary claim is that the lenient approach favored by most of the halakhic decisors in the field embodies an essentialist attitude regarding women that still perceives motherhood as their primary—if not their exclusive—function in life. Thus, these decisors are not only blind to many of the issues that the use of reproductive technologies raise, but even were they made aware, it is likely that they would reject the concerns out of hand. The gap between the intense consideration of moral-gender issues in feminist bioethical discourse, on the one hand, and the absolute silence on these matters among contemporary halakhic decisors, on the other, highlights the extent to which gender concerns are absent from halakhic discourse.

CHAPTER SIX

Artificial Insemination, In Vitro Fertilization, and Surrogacy

HALAKHIC ANALYSIS

Artificial Insemination

Most halakhic analyses have considered artificial insemination with sperm from an outside donor (AID), for that poses the most significant halakhic challenges. But I want to consider as well artificial insemination with sperm from the husband (AIH), for I believe that analysis of using sperm from the husband is the necessary foundation for halakhic discussion of sperm from a donor and also for discussion of in vitro fertilization, which we will address later.[1]

The decisional literature on artificial insemination with sperm from the husband is focused primarily on whether it entails wasteful emission of seed and on whether conception through use of this technology fulfills the commandment to procreate. A minority of decisors forbid AIH on these grounds.[2] R. Benzion Meir Hai Uziel, one of the first decisors to forbid the practice,[3] reasons that the paternal link does not exist in a situation of artificial insemination, inasmuch as no actual sexual intercourse took place. Accordingly, the commandment to procreate is not fulfilled, and one who emits seed as part of the procedure is inherently engaging in wasteful emission. R. Uziel believes emission of semen is permitted only "in the usual way of the world," and that even if the commandment to procreate were fulfilled via AIH, there would still be concern about violating the prohibition, since "it is unavoidable that some drops will go to waste." In his book *Sha'arei 'Uzi'el*, he explains his determination regarding the absence of the paternal link, from which follows his moral judgment regarding AIH:

> In this way, we can limit this transgression, which is vile and disgusting in itself, and becomes more widespread under the camouflage of a syringe. But such should not be done in Israel, begetting children such as these who are created by [violating] the serious prohibition of wasting seed and creating flawed children such as these within Israel, a holy nation of well-defined paternal lineage.[4]

The author of *Divrei Malki'el*, in contrast, severs the link between ascription of paternity and the prohibition on wasteful emission of seed.[5] He rules, early in his responsum, that the offspring is not considered to be the son of the sperm provider and that the prohibition on wasteful emission therefore is violated. Later, however, he retracts the denial of paternity, though he maintains the view that the act entails wasteful emission of seed and therefore prohibits it. But his primary concern, repeatedly emphasized throughout the responsum, is the risk of the husband's semen becoming mixed up with someone else's, and that concern may be what leads him to ban the procedure outright.

R. Ovadia Hedaya believes it forbidden for the husband to emit semen for AIH, for the prohibition on wasteful emission of seed applies regardless of the purpose to which the seed is put.[6] According to R. Hedaya, the child is attributed to the sperm provider for paternity purposes, but the father is not considered to have fulfilled the commandment to procreate, for it has not been done through the pleasurable mechanism associated with the commandment: "There is not a scintilla of pleasure in this, not for the man and not for the woman, and this is certainly unrelated to the commandment; and even if he begets many sons and daughters through this mechanism, he has not thereby fulfilled the Torah's commandment to procreate."[7]

R. Waldenberg appears to adopt a middle ground on the issue.[8] His responsum is formulated as a summary of the positions taken by the various decisors, and while he does not clearly decide among them, his reservations about artificial insemination are quite evident. He does not close the door to the AIH, concluding the responsum with a reference to "a case in which a permissive ruling is issued," but he contemplates such a ruling only where it has become clear that conception by natural means is impossible and the couple has been married but childless for at least ten years. He also warns against any possibility of mixing up the husband's semen with someone else's.

To summarize the views of those who rule strictly and forbid the practice, most believe that the prohibition on wasteful emission of seed is violated in cases of AIH, but they differ on whether to attribute paternity to the donor-husband and on whether the commandment to procreate is fulfilled through artificial insemination. Some see a substantive link between the questions of paternity and of fulfillment of the commandment; others regard those issues as separate. It is possible to attribute paternity to the sperm donor even if he does not thereby fulfill the commandment to procreate.

This reliance on wasteful emission of seed as the basis for these decisions is surprising in a number of ways. First, R. Uziel himself, in another responsum, permits emitting semen for medical purposes, namely, to determine whether it is fertile.[9] There he writes that when the act is not done for promiscuous reasons, there is no prohibition: "But if one does this for medical reasons or to see if he is able to beget children, it would appear to be permitted."[10] Does it not follow a fortiori that it is permitted to emit seed for purposes of fulfilling the commandment to procreate? If the prohibition on wasteful emission of seed is related to the commandment to procreate—that is, it is the commandment to procreate that generates the prohibition on wasting seed—there should be no prohibition here, where the act is done for the sake of procreation. And if the prohibition is free-standing, unrelated to the commandment to procreate, one could still say that only wasteful emission is prohibited, but emission for a permissible purpose should be permitted, even if the commandment to procreate is not thereby fulfilled—precisely as in the case of examining the semen for medical purposes.[11]

Second, those who do not attribute paternity to the sperm provider appear to adopt an internally inconsistent position. One cannot say that in a case of AIH, the offspring is not considered the husband-provider's child (and he therefore has not fulfilled the commandment to procreate and has emitted semen wastefully) but say as well that AID should be prohibited lest the offspring unwittingly marry his half sister (from the same sperm donor). In other words, if the donor is not considered the father, then sperm donation even from a Jew should be legitimate, for there is no concern about the possibility of unwitting incest.[12] In view of the foregoing, it would appear that according to R. Uziel's approach, there is no reason to forbid sperm donation by a Jew (but for the concern about wasteful emission of seed). Sperm donation by a gentile should also be permitted, at least by the formal halakhic considerations of his approach. Nevertheless, he states in *Sha'arei 'Uzi'el* that he considers such procedures to be a great abomination, and that bearing such children of uncertain lineage impairs the sanctity of Israel. To put it differently, R. Uziel's formal halakhic position—that the paternity of children born through artificial insemination is not attributed to the sperm provider—could be used to warrant a lenient ruling regarding artificial insemination, but because his ethical position dictates his halakhic stance, the lack of lineage is treated as flawed lineage, and he therefore forbids all artificial insemination procedures.

According to those who permit AIH, the procedure entails no wasteful emission of seed, for it is undergone for the purpose of fulfilling a commandment. Some require that two physicians declare that the procedure will indeed be effective for the couple (that is, that the woman suffers no impediment to fertility and that there is a reasonable likelihood that a child will in fact be conceived).[13] On a technical level, there are preferred mechanisms for securing the semen; the couple should engage in sexual relations involving coitus interruptus or use of a condom, but the husband should not masturbate. According to R. Feinstein, emitting semen other than in the natural way violates the prohibition of adultery, even if the purpose is to bring about conception and birth.[14]

Despite the foregoing, the percentage of artificial insemination cases involving AIH is relatively low, and I will therefore focus on the halakhic rulings that consider AID, involving both married and unmarried women.

Artificial Insemination from a Jewish Donor

ADULTERY

The question posed with respect to AID is whether the Torah's prohibitions on sexual relations between certain partners (such as adulterers) are violated only when sexual contact takes place or whether the prohibitions extend to transfer of semen from a man to a woman even without bodily proximity. If AID is, in fact, considered adultery, the offspring would be a *mamzer*. This concern, of course, is pertinent only where the woman is married; if she is single, the issue does not arise.

Beyond that, even if AID does not entail adultery, it nevertheless is possible that several women will be inseminated with sperm from one donor; and all their offspring would be biologically related. That, in theory, could result in inadvertent incestuous marriages, and the offspring of those unions would likewise be *mamzers*. This concern is pertinent even if the woman being inseminated is not married.[15]

The plain meaning of the biblical verses provides little basis for reaching a decision: "None of you shall approach to any that is near of kin to him, to uncover their nakedness: I am the LORD. . . . And thou shalt not lie carnally with thy neighbor's wife, to defile thyself with her" (Lev. 18:6, 20; OJPS). Forbidden sexual relations generally are referred to as "approaching to uncover nakedness," suggesting a need for bodily contact. With respect to another's wife, however, the offense is described as "lying carnally" or, more literally translated, "placing your seed." Should this verse be understood to mean that where adultery is involved, the prohibition is violated even without bodily contact? Or should it be read as simply one example of forbidden relationships, all of which require "uncovering of nakedness," that is, physical contact? Nahmanides writes:

> *And thou shalt not lie carnally with thy neighbor's wife*—. . . . It is possible that he said *le-zara* in order to mention the reason for the prohibition, since it will not be known to whom "the child" belongs, and, as a result, great and wicked abominations might be done by both. . . . The correct interpretation appears to me to be that since another man's wife is completely forbidden to one, *whosoever toucheth her shall not go unpunished* [Prov. 6:29], therefore

> Scripture had to say here *le-zara*. For had it said only: "and thou shalt not lie with thy neighbor's wife," it would have appeared that it forbids [by punishment of excision] even lying with her just for embracing and kissing, since here [in this section] it speaks only of those forbidden relations that are punishable with excision. Therefore it was necessary to mention that the intimacy was *le-zara*, in order to explain that he is prohibiting here sexual intercourse. (Nahmanides, *Commentary on the Torah*, Lev. 18: 20; Chavel trans., pp. 257–258; footnotes omitted)

Nahmanides's comments are open to interpretation. One can read him as saying that scripture means to prohibit intercourse, but it can also be argued, as some decisors have done, that since the reason for the prohibition is that "it will not be known to whom the child belongs," AID is likewise included within this prohibition.[16]

The following talmudic passage constitutes the basic halakhic source on the question of whether AID constitutes adultery:

> Ben Zoma was asked: What is the status with regard to becoming married to the High Priest of a virgin who has been impregnated? Do we take account of the possibility raised by Samuel, for Samuel said: I can have intercourse [with a virgin] several times without producing blood; or do we say that Samuel is unusual [and should not be the basis for a decision]? He [Ben Zoma] said to them: Samuel is unusual, but we take account of the possibility that she was impregnated in the bath. But did not Samuel say: Semen that is not shot straight as an arrow does not impregnate? He was referring to semen initially shot straight as an arrow. (BT Ḥag. 14b–15a)

According to the Torah, the High Priest is forbidden to marry a woman who is not a virgin; he may marry only a woman who has never had sexual relations. The question is whether a pregnant virgin may marry a High Priest; that is, is she believed when she says that although she is pregnant, she has never had intercourse and her hymen is intact?

Two possible scenarios are suggested to account for her pregnancy: she may have had relations with a man in such a way that her hymen was left intact, or she may have been impregnated by semen from a man who had used a bath before she entered it. Logic suggests that, in the first scenario, she should be forbidden to the High Priest, for she has engaged in sexual relations even though, unusually, her hymen remained intact. In the second scenario, however, there would appear to be no reason for her not marry the High Priest, for she is still a virgin. But if we interpret Ben Zoma's assertion that "we take account of" (*ḥaishinan*) the possibility that she was impregnated in the bath as an indication to rule strictly and forbid her marriage to the High Priest, we may be warranted in inferring that the very fact of her pregnancy disqualifies her, even though we do not know whether intercourse actually took place. In other words, even impregnation in an unnatural manner renders the woman no longer a virgin. This conclusion has clear implications for the prohibition on adultery, for it suggests that the fact of pregnancy itself suffices to prove the sinful conduct associated with prohibited sexual relations and that sperm donation by an outsider (that is, AID) is tantamount to adultery.[17]

But it is also possible to construe the two references to "taking account of" as bases for a lenient ruling that would permit the impregnated woman's marriage to the High Priest. On that understanding, one may infer for our purposes that the fact of pregnancy does not, in itself, prove that the sin of adultery took place, and that adultery requires actual intercourse. Rashi elsewhere notes that the locution "we take account of" (*ḥaishinan*) sometimes indicates a basis for leniency (and gives the example from *Ḥagigah*),[18] and, on that understanding, the passage can indeed be understood to mean that a woman who became pregnant in the bath is permitted to the High Priest; that is, "we take account of that possibility" as a basis for the legal ruling. Given Rashi's silence in the first case, we may assume that he there understands "we take account of" as indicating a strict ruling; that is, where sexual relations took place, even if the hymen remains intact, she is forbidden to the High Priest. That interpretation may bolster the view that the factual predicate for all transgressions related to forbidden sexual relations is the existence of sexual contact and not simply impregnation; though it is possible to interpret Rashi as understanding "we take account of" to indicate leniency in both cases.

Tosafot treat the issue in three different places.[19] From their comments in *Ketubbot* and in *Niddah*, one may infer that a virgin becomes forbidden to the High Priest if she has engaged in sexual relations, and that the possibility of having become pregnant in the bath is adequate reason to permit her to the High Priest if she insists she is still a virgin. But their comments in

Ḥagigah are inconsistent with that conclusion. According to R. Isaac b. Samuel of Dampierre (Ri), cited in Tosafot, we should not accept Rashi's conclusion. Ri believes that in all instances, it is the physiological state of the hymen that determines a woman's virginity, not sexual contact itself. Accordingly, where there are many men such as Samuel who can engage in sexual relations without tearing the hymen, it is necessary to examine the woman physiologically. In the second case, where she became pregnant in the bath, she should be permitted to the High Priest, for there was no intercourse at all.[20]

Tosafot's comments in *Ḥagigah* have important implications for the question at hand: is the offense of engaging in forbidden sexual relations defined by sexual contact or by the presence of a man's semen in the woman's body? Rashi's comments suggest that the Talmud was speaking not solely of a woman's eligibility to marry the High Priest but, more generally, indicating that sexual contact constitutes the basis for the offense. But according to Ri's comments in *Ḥagigah*, we cannot infer a general rule regarding forbidden sexual relations, since the discussion is of a prohibition unique to priests.[21]

If we say that Rashi and Tosafot (at least in *Niddah* and *Ketubbot*) interpret the talmudic passage to mean that it is sexual conduct itself, and not impregnation, that renders a virgin ineligible to marry the High Priest, it follows that only sexual contact, and not impregnation alone, is the factual predicate for the transgressions related to forbidden sexual relations, such as adultery and incest. But even if we say that sexual contact is an essential element of adultery, the attribution of paternity to the sperm donor in cases of artificial insemination means that even if the woman is not married and there is no concern about adultery, the use of sperm from a Jewish donor entails a risk of inadvertent incestuous unions in the next generation and the consequent birth of *mamzers*:

> Rabbi Liezer says: Because he has relations with many women and it is not known which of them he had relations with, and she receives [semen] from many men and it is not known from whom she received, it follows that a man [inadvertently] marries his daughter or his sister and the whole world becomes *mamzers*. And that is why Scripture says "and the land [shall] become full of lewdness." (T Qid. 1:4)[22]

The concern expressed here is that uncertainties about lineage may lead to marriages between people who are unaware that they are relatives and forbidden to marry each other. When sperm is donated, the donor's identity is kept secret;[23] and despite the limits on the number of fertilizations that may be carried out with the sperm of a single donor, the concern raised in the Tosefta could become a real (albeit statistically unlikely) one, given that most opinions attribute the paternity of a child born through artificial insemination to the biological father, that is, the sperm source.

An illustration of a woman being impregnated by sperm other than her husband's is provided in a responsum by R. Perez b. Elijah of Corville, an important thirteenth-century Tosafist:

> I found in old annotations by our teacher R. Perez to *Sefer Miẓvot Qatan* that he had written that a menstrually impure woman could lie on her husband's sheets but must avoid sheets that some other man had lain on, lest she become pregnant from another man's semen. But why should she not similarly be concerned about becoming pregnant from her husband's semen while menstrually impure, thereby rendering the offspring a child of menstrual impurity? He answered that since there is no forbidden sexual intercourse here, even if she becomes pregnant from another man's semen, the offspring is entirely legitimate, as was Ben Sira;[24] but we are strict about distinguishing semen from another man, a measure taken lest he [the offspring] come to marry his half sister on his father's side.[25]

Two conclusions can be drawn from this.

1. In all matters related to prohibited sexual relations, the factual predicate for the commission of the sin is engaging in forbidden intercourse and not simply the placement of semen in the woman's uterus. This is consistent with the way in which Rashi and Tosafot understand (according to the annotations of *Baḥ*) the passage in *Ḥagigah*. In other words, AID does not entail adultery, and the offspring born through the procedure is not a *mamzer*.[26]
2. The distinction between the husband's sheets and those of another man is drawn "lest he [the offspring] come to marry his half sister on his father's side."[27] The premise implicit in that statement is that the paternity of a

> child born in this way is attributed to the source of the sperm;[28] accordingly, if the woman is impregnated by the other man's semen and the resulting child is erroneously attributed to her husband, or its paternity does not become known, the child may later, and unknowingly, come to marry his sister from his true father, the sperm source.[29] That conclusion may lead to a further conclusion, namely, that the sperm source has fulfilled the commandment to procreate, inasmuch as the offspring is considered his for all purposes.[30] It further follows, according to the line of thought of those decisors who forbid AIH, that the prohibition on wasteful emission of seed should not apply here, for the child born though the procedure is attributed to his father, the source of the sperm.

CERTAINTY OF LINEAGE

The attribution of the offspring to the sperm source is significant with regard not only to paternity but also to whether the use of artificial insemination allows the sperm provider to fulfill the commandment to procreate and whether, accordingly, it is permitted to emit semen for that purpose. To be sure, even those decisors who attribute paternity to the sperm source differ on whether the commandment is fulfilled, since the pregnancy does not result directly from the action of the sperm provider,[31] but the dominant view is that determination of paternity and fulfillment of the commandment are linked.

R. Perez's annotations to *Sefer Mizvot Qatan* make clear that, in his view, a child born of nonnatural impregnation is attributed to the provider of the sperm, but not everyone agrees with him.[32] The author of *Ḥelqat Meḥoqeq* has doubts about whether, in a case of impregnation through artificial means, the father has fulfilled the commandment to procreate and the child is considered his in all respects:

> *The child was a mamzer, etc.*—In the case of the woman who became pregnant in the bath, there is reason for uncertainty about whether the father has fulfilled the commandment to procreate and whether the offspring is considered his child for all purposes. And in *Liqqutei Maharil*, we find that Ben Sira was the son of Jeremiah, who had bathed in a bath. (Comment on *Shulḥan 'Arukh, 'Even Ha-'Ezer* 1:8)

But *Beit Shmu'el* (ibid., par. 10) writes "It appears it is his child for all purposes." R. Simeon b. Ẓemaḥ Duran (Tashbeẓ) had similarly ruled earlier that the son is attributed to the sperm source.[33] The *Taz* (ibid., par. 8) believes that the commandment to procreate is not fulfilled when the pregnancy is a matter of happenstance, as when it occurs in the bath, for the father has taken no action to bring it about, and he is considered the father only for purposes of ruling strictly. R. Ḥayyim Joseph David Azoulai (Ḥida), in contrast, severs the link between the sperm provider and the offspring. On the basis of a different manuscript that lacks the words "lest he come to marry his half sister on his father's side" and of a version "from a very old collection in a parchment manuscript," he concludes that R. Perez's argument is that "here, even though the rule of lest he marry his half sister on his father's side does not apply and *there is no father* [emphasis mine], it nevertheless is proper to be strict regarding the interposition of seed coming from somewhere else."[34]

The Mishnah's term for a child who does not know his father is a *shetuqi* (lit. "a silenced one");[35] such a child is thought to be a *mamzer*, on the premise that his mother may have become pregnant through a prohibited liaison. According to Ḥida, a child born of nonnatural insemination lacks a father by definition and may be a *shetuqi*, subject to other halakhic problems as well.[36]

In sum, we can say that there is no unanimity regarding the lineage of a child born of nonnatural insemination. Four views can be identified:

1. Paternity is attributed to the sperm provider, who is considered the child's father for all purposes.
2. Paternity is attributed to the sperm provider only where doing so imposes stringencies but not where it allows for leniencies.
3. The child is considered the provider's for all purposes, but the provider does not thereby fulfill the commandment to procreate.
4. Paternity is in no way attributed to the sperm provider.

In general, the identity of a sperm donor is kept strictly confidential, and the concern about possible incestuous relations in the succeeding generation, as well as psychological harm to the child who will be uncertain about his lineage, has led decisors to the conclusion that sperm donation by a Jew is halakhically forbidden.[37] But it is important to distinguish between those who forbid use of sperm from a Jewish donor on the grounds that it is genuinely tantamount to adultery, in which case revealing the donor's identity will not rectify the situation,[38] and those who do not believe adultery takes place in the absence of intercourse but are concerned about inadvertent incest and production of *mamzers* in the next generation, given the anonymity of the donor. On the latter approach, there is a theoretical possibility, and perhaps a practical one, that sperm donation by a Jew might be permitted on condition that the donor is identified and a precise record of the procedure is kept. Nevertheless, there are almost no lenient rulings of that sort.

To resolve the foregoing difficulties, decisors have considered sperm donation by a gentile, and that is the subject we next discuss.

Artificial Insemination from a Gentile Donor

The idea that the foregoing difficulties can be resolved by using sperm from a non-Jewish donor is premised on the halakhic rule that if a gentile man and a Jewish woman bear a child, paternity is not attributed to the father; the fact that he is the child's biological father is halakhically irrelevant. (The same rule applies in the case of a Jewish father and a gentile mother.) Accordingly, all concerns related to adultery, *mamzers*, and inadvertent incest are obviated, and it seems possible to resolve problems resulting from the husband's infertility.

That said, it is difficult to consider this procedure as legitimate, for it would appear to violate the Torah's prohibition on marriages between Jews and gentiles.[39] Moreover, the question of adultery, raised previously with regard to a Jewish donor, is pertinent here as well. Those who believe that the Torah's prohibitions on certain sexual relationships are violated only when there is actual sexual contact would argue here that since artificial insemination involves no sexual contact, sperm donation by a gentile poses no difficulty. They might also argue that sperm donation does not violate the prohibition on mixed marriages, because the Torah-stated rationale—"For they will turn your children away from Me to worship other gods" (Deut. 7:4)—is premised on cultural and religious influence being exercised by the gentile parent when the couple are living together (assuming, of course, that the reason for the prohibition is to be interpreted on the basis of environmental and cultural considerations). But for those who believe the Torah's forbidden-relations laws can be violated even without sexual contact, it is easy enough to interpret the prohibition on intermarriage as based not on cultural but on genetic or racial considerations. On that premise, intermarriage is prohibited because of a concern that a gentile's genetic makeup necessarily includes elements that will defile those who come in contact with it and entice them away from service of God. We shall see below that these themes, notwithstanding their racist basis, are present in contemporary decisors' deliberations.

Crystallization of the Halakhah in Recent Generations

RABBI M. FEINSTEIN

It is fair to say that the dispute over artificial insemination in general, and use of a gentile sperm donor in particular, was ignited by Rabbi Moses Feinstein's ruling, issued in 1959, permitting the procedure.[40] The issue had been dealt with earlier, but not with the degree of intensity that followed R. Feinstein's decision.[41]

R. Feinstein was asked about a couple "who are suffering greatly because of their yearning for a child," and the only way in which they could have a child was through AID. He responded:

> [The procedure] should be permitted with use of sperm from a gentile, for since the offspring will be a Jew because its mother is Jewish, there are no concerns of any sort. The offspring's paternity would not be attributed to the gentile father even had it been conceived though intercourse, and that is so a fortiori when it is conceived not through intercourse but in a bath . . . and the fact that the sperm is from a gentile also addresses the concerns of those who maintain that [a child born of] other semen [than that of the woman's husband] is a *mamzer* even [if conceived] without intercourse. . . . And so, in exigent circumstances when they are suffering greatly because of their yearning for a child, it is permitted to cast into the woman's innards semen coming specifically from a gentile. . . . As for the statement in *'Otsar Ha-Poseqim*, quoting *Sefer Menaḥem Meishiv*, that it would be terrible for a daughter of Israel to abandon herself to the artificial prostitution invented

> by the doctors—those are empty words, for this has nothing whatsoever in common with prostitution and the only prohibition is the possibility that the offspring might unknowingly come to marry his half sister on his father's side. Without the husband's consent, it would be forbidden on the grounds of her subservience to her husband . . . but with the husband's consent, and where they are suffering greatly, it should be permitted, but only with semen from a gentile. (*'Iggerot Mosheh*, *'Even Ha-'Ezer* 1:71)

The only halakhic problem that R. Feinstein sees in AID is the possibility of inadvertent incest in the next generation, given that paternity of the offspring is attributed to the sperm donor. He overcomes this problem by requiring the use of sperm from a gentile donor, a resolution premised on the halakhah's nonrecognition of a gentile father's paternity of a child he begets with a Jewish woman. That is the sole concern; in accordance with Rabbeinu Perez's determination, the procedure neither entails adultery nor produces a *mamzer*, both of which require actual intercourse.

R. Feinstein's permissive ruling received a stormy reception among his fellow decisors, who attacked it for all manner of reasons. In response, he wrote a letter in which he reemphasizes not only that his permissive ruling is meant to apply only in highly exigent circumstances but also that "a line must be drawn such that no rabbi, even the most eminent, will permit [the procedure]." Some saw the letter as a retreat in principle from the lenient ruling.[42]

The dispute with R. Feinstein was not always of a formal halakhic character. The participants' moral positions openly and expressly dictated their own opposing rulings and also led them to engage in personal attacks against R. Feinstein, some unprecedented in their ferocity. For the most part, it was revulsion at the very concept of insemination with gentile sperm that dictated a nonpermissive halakhic interpretation of the same sources that R. Feinstein had interpreted permissively. That is particularly prominent in the statements of R. Moshe Haim Ephraim Bloch, who refers to himself as a devoted student of the Maharsham (Rabbi Sholom Mordechai Schwadron), who, it will be recalled, permitted AIH.[43] R. Bloch believes that artificial insemination from a gentile donor is a vile and morally repellent act, prostitution, lust, adultery, filth, impurity, promiscuity, and a harsh blow to Judaism "from which we will never recover in all eternity."[44] He quotes

R. Jacob Moses Charlap, who wrote that "in the future redemption, the sanctity of the sons will be revealed. The sanctity of the sons is the sanctity of the seed, and it contains the loftiest sanctity in Israel." He goes on to speak in harsh personal terms of R. Feinstein: "all the tortured arguments raised by the Ga'on R. Moses Feinstein as a basis for permitting it are, in my eyes, fraudulent makeweights."[45] Only then does R. Bloch turn to the halakhic question itself. His principal argument is with the determination that actual intercourse is an essential element of adultery. Were that so,

> It would be a wonderful ruse to circumvent all the forbidden sexual relationships written in the Torah. A woman could become pregnant and give birth, by means of a pipette, from other seed [than her husband's]—from seed of a gentile, or seed of her father, her father-in-law, her brother, all her relatives; and she has no need for her principal partner.[46]

One of the longest and most exhaustive responsa on the subject was written by R. Jacob Breish. Though he presents a wealth of arguments, it appears that his dispute with R. Feinstein turns on two central considerations—the question of *ḥaliẓah* (the procedure for avoiding levirate marriage, explained further below) and the prospect of "desecrating God's name." Halakhah provides that if a man dies without (biological) children, his widow must receive *ḥaliẓah* from the deceased's brother, if there is one, before remarrying.[47] R. Breish is concerned that if the husband of a woman who has borne a child through AID should die, his widow might be ashamed to reveal that the child was not her late husband's and remarry without undergoing the *ḥaliẓah* that is required because her husband died without biological children.[48] The second claim, regarding desecration of God's name, may be the more interesting and is unique to R. Breish:

> Is it possible that a renowned decisor would permit something so revolting and disgusting? It is something that even the Catholics and their leaders have forcefully attacked, forbidding such vile actions, which resemble the ways of Egypt and Canaan with their abominations. Should we, the precious and chosen people, permit something as revolting and disgusting as this? Is it not the greatest desecration of God's name? (*Ḥelqat Ya'aqov, 'Even Ha-'Ezer* 14:1)

As noted, the claim of "desecration of God's name" was voiced in connection with abortion as well, and I have suggested that it appears, albeit implicitly, in the strict rulings on birth control issued by early-nineteenth-century rabbis in Hungary and Germany; here we see it reiterated in connection with artificial insemination. The argument regarding "desecration of God's name" entails a degree of circularity, for the decisor assumes in advance the ethical stance he wants to adopt and then goes on to find support for that stance in non-Jewish circles. R. Breish's moral position regarding AID with a gentile donor is clear and explicit—in addition to calling the procedure "vile and disgusting," reminiscent of the abominations of Canaan (see previous quote), he writes:

> We should not increase the number of flawed and polluted [offspring] in Israel. . . . That means it is forbidden to mingle and damage Israel with unfit seed, of people with corrupt qualities. (Ibid., *'Even Ha-'Ezer* 13, summary of the responsum, par. 5).

R. Breish is caught in a thicket of contradiction. On the one hand, he is very interested in increasing the Jewish birthrate, especially after the Holocaust, as is evident in his positions on birth control. On the other hand, it is precisely in the generation that suffered the Holocaust that he is unable to conceive of the nation of Israel "becoming mingled" with gentile seed, the unfit seed of corrupt people, as he puts it, who are capable of carrying out such acts. In view of that concept, he believes that allowing AID from gentile sperm is a "desecration of God's name," since even the Roman Catholic Church forbids it. But it appears that citing the position of the Church as support for the premise that AID from gentile sperm constitutes moral degradation and impairs the sanctity of Jewish seed is itself a moral paradox of the highest order. The moral justification for forbidding the procedure relies on the position of those whose seed is considered totally unfit! Isn't this a logical failing as well as a moral one?

The journal *Ha-ma'or*, primarily through its editor, R. Meir Amsel, was also enlisted in the war against R. Feinstein's legal rulings. The articles that appeared there, directed at other writings on the subject as well,[49] are strikingly harsh, to the point that the editor was compelled to publish a clarification disavowing any personal attack on R. Feinstein or any insult to him and explaining that the opposition was only to his halakhic position on this subject.[50]

Though aware of the sweeping prohibitions and powerful opposition aroused by his permissive ruling, R. Feinstein did not retract it. He emphasized his rejection of the criticisms and reiterated that everything he said remains valid:

> Everything I wrote in my responsum is true and clear as a matter of law, and there is no reason to regret my words and no concern related to injection of gentile seed. As a practical matter, however, I did not teach that this should be done, for it is ineffective in fulfilling the husband's obligation to procreate, and the woman has no such obligation; and it may result in great jealousy on the part of her husband, so it is ill-advised. . . . Certainly one should not advise doing this, for the reasons I have set out, but if one did so, the offspring is fit even for the priesthood. . . . As for what his Torah Excellency [an honorific applied to the correspondent] wrote regarding the main concern being that of [the offspring] marrying his [half] sister, that does not apply with respect to [seed from] gentiles, as I wrote in my responsum. (*'Iggerot Mosheh, 'Even Ha-'Ezer* 4:32)[51]

Despite his forceful rejection of his critics, and even though his permissive ruling stands, at least in principle, some believe that R. Feinstein changed his mind about the matter, noting that he does not recommend applying the ruling in practice lest household harmony be disrupted.[52] In any case, it appears from everything said above that even if the permissive course is ill-advised for a married woman, that should not be the case for a single woman. According to R. Feinstein's logic, there should be no basis (at least on this ground) to forbid the use of AID by a single woman, since there is no formal halakhic prohibition that pertains to it.[53]

RABBI E. WALDENBERG

Among decisors who deal extensively with issues of medical halakhah, R. Waldenberg is prominent in his sharp and forceful objection to AID. Regarding AIH, meanwhile, his position is rather ambiguous. After reviewing the positions of decisors in the generation preceding his own, he goes on to convey reservations about the procedure along with a willingness to permit it in exigent circumstances in which there is clear proof that the couple will be unable to bear children naturally. He appears to be less concerned about wasteful emission of seed[54] or about the procedure's inability to fulfill the husband's obligation to procreate than about eliminating any possibility of insemination with sperm other than the husband's.

There is no ambivalence in R. Waldenberg's position on AID, however; his opposition to the procedure, whether for a married woman or a single woman, is firm and unambiguous. His halakhic analysis and the resulting prohibition revolve around several points. First, he believes the commandments related to forbidden sexual relations are violated by placement of semen in the woman even without sexual contact and that the passage in BT *Ḥagigah* pertains only to the special case of a High Priest and a virgin, allowing for no inferences regarding the law of adultery. Beyond that, he believes there is an express prohibition against bringing into the world children of unknown paternity. He offers two reasons: first, that the divine presence dwells only on those whose lineage is known; and, second, the risk of inadvertent incest and of problems related to *ḥaliẓah* and *yibbum* (levirate marriage). As for AID with sperm from a gentile, his position does not appear to be driven by clearly halakhic considerations. Indeed, I think one can go further and say that his concerns about AID with gentile sperm are what dictate the interpretive moves that he makes regarding AID with sperm from a Jew and even his reservations about AIH. AID with sperm from a gentile represents the bottom of the "slippery slope" and is so serious a matter, in his view, that it shapes his position on the entire subject.

R. Waldenberg expresses his moral reservations about AID with sperm from a Jew in clear and explicit terms:

> This entire business of introducing into a married woman's womb semen from another man is a great abomination within the tents of Jacob and there is no greater family desecration within the dwelling places of Israel. It destroys all the lofty concepts of the purity and sanctity of Jewish family life at which our nation has excelled from its beginnings, and it severs the chains of lineage running from sons to fathers. Instead of the fathers being the glory of their sons, we will come, God forbid, to have dust instead of glory,[55] as we see a generation that says to wood, "you are my father." The result of bearing these children of confusion . . . is that many Jewish households will come, God protect us, to be involved with seed not their own to the point of

exchanging wives with one another, as a breach invites a thief . . . whether they know it or not. And after that breach, who will set them straight? (*Ẓiẓ 'Eli'ezer* 9:51, *Qunteres Refu'ah Ba-Mishpaḥah, sha'ar* 4, chap. 4, par. 1)

He is speaking here not only of the slippery slope that will lead to use of sperm from a non-Jew but also of coming to treat the prohibition of adultery lightly. For if semen from an outsider is not forbidden, there is reason for concern that the revulsion at adultery will be attenuated.[56] R. Waldenberg speaks even more harshly about sperm donation by a gentile:

> And what shall we say from this perspective when the issue is accepting semen from a gentile? . . . Words cannot describe the ugliness and filth inherent in such an act, or the terrible destruction and frightening spiritual devastation that such measures will bring to the House of Israel in general and to the individual households engaging in them in particular. And how terrible to think it possible to permit assimilation to the nations of the world through penetration of their semen into the womb of a Jewess. (Ibid., par. 2)

Gender Concepts

It has been suggested that the sharp divergence between R. Waldenberg's stringent position and R. Feinstein's permissive one can be understood as a disagreement between the two decisors regarding the extent of a husband's control over his wife's reproductive ability.[57] That is, R. Waldenberg believes the husband to have the exclusive right to activate his wife's reproductive powers, and AID therefore impairs the very essence of the marital relationship, whereas R. Feinstein limits the wife's subservience to her husband to the sphere of sexual activity alone.

In my judgment, this explanation does not satisfactorily account for the differences between them, if only because it does not account for R. Waldenberg's reservations about AIH. If the issue were really about the husband's exclusive rights, there would be no reason to limit AIH—which fully preserves the husband's exclusive status with respect to his wife's reproductive capabilities—to an after-the-fact, last-resort remedy that can be used only after ten years of childless marriage or after other medical possibilities are ruled out.[58] A fuller understanding of the dispute between decisors requires consideration of the broader picture with regard to procreation, and that broader picture suggests other conclusions.

As we saw in the earlier chapters, R. Waldenberg rules very permissively on matters of abortion, while R. Feinstein is extremely strict and sees every abortion—including those during the first forty days following conception—as a violation of the biblical prohibition of murder. Their views on birth control are not such polar opposites, but it still appears that R. Waldenberg has fewer reservations about use of the pill than does R. Feinstein. When it comes to artificial insemination, however, their positions are very much reversed—R. Feinstein is more permissive and R. Waldenberg far less so—and I believe this is no coincidence.

It may well be that R. Waldenberg is very strict with regard to artificial insemination (and even more so with regard to in vitro fertilization and surrogacy) but quite permissive with regard to abortion because *he recognizes the existence of values more important than the commandment to procreate*. To put it differently, he is not prepared to adopt the "procreation at any cost" position that came to dominate the world of halakhic rulings during the past generation. In the case of abortion, he assigns importance to the quality-of-life concerns of parents called upon to raise a child with birth defects or a short lifespan and to the situation of a mother required to endure a pregnancy that will be harmful to her physical and psychological health. His rulings, as we have seen, are not entirely free of gender biases; still, his leniencies can foster a willingness to see women as subjects, not merely objects, in matters related to procreation. And so, too, with respect to artificial insemination. His strict rulings appear, at first glance, to ill serve women who yearn for children of their own. In the long term, however, his position is likely to promote a more equal balance between "woman" and "Eve" and strengthen the tendency to view a woman as a subject, not an object meant primarily to procreate.

R. Feinstein's positions, meanwhile, point in the opposite direction. To say that a woman cannot abort a defective fetus or a fetus that endangers her physical well-being (short of actual mortal danger) but may nevertheless use artificial insemination even with sperm not from her husband is to paint a troubling picture of her position in life. A woman is meant as a receptacle for a man's (any man's) seed and is obligated, at almost any price, to bring that seed to "fruition," forgoing in that process any concern about her bodily well-being or other human needs. In none of R. Feinstein's writings on abortion or on artificial insemination have I been able to find expression of even a single reservation from the woman's perspective, but he is quite sensitive to the effects of these technologies on the husband. In the case of AID, for example, he considers the psychological state of a man called upon to act as father to a child who is not genetically his—a situation likely to affect the tranquility of the household and the relationship between husband and wife. That concern for the husband's situation led R. Feinstein to retreat from his own permissive ruling, as he says:

> As a practical matter, however, I did not teach that this should be done, for it is ineffective in fulfilling the husband's obligation to procreate, and the woman has no such obligation; and it may result in great jealousy on the part of her husband, so it is ill-advised. (*'Iggerot Mosheh, 'Even Ha-'Ezer* 4:32)

R. Feinstein did not have the opportunity to deal with questions of in vitro fertilization, egg donation, and surrogacy, but it is worth noting that in other halakhic discussions, I found no consideration of such matters as the psychological state of the surrogate mother who is not destined to retain the child she bears. It appears that every scientific innovation that may enhance fertility is accepted without taking account of the woman's perspective, which is entirely absent from the halakhic discussion. R. Waldenberg's reservations, to be sure, are not driven specifically by a concern for the interests of women; but whatever their motivation, they have the effect of establishing a more cautious stance regarding new fertility-enhancing technologies and thereby limiting the extent to which "woman" is equated with "procreation."

To sum up the positions of contemporary decisors, we may say that AIH is permitted by most and AID with a Jewish sperm donor is forbidden by all.[59] AID with sperm donated by a non-Jew is becoming more widely accepted in the wake of the positions taken by important decisors such as R. Feinstein and R. Auerbach.[60]

In Vitro Fertilization and Surrogacy: The Problems in Principle

Most of the halakhic problems associated with artificial insemination become even more severe when the discussion turns to in vitro fertilization, for IVF entails total severance of the fertilization process from its natural course.

Moreover, IVF technology opens the door to surrogate pregnancy and the difficult questions it poses: should the practice be permitted altogether and, if so, who should be considered the offspring's mother?

There are several different scenarios in which these questions must be answered:

1. IVF using sperm and egg provided by the couple and placement of the fertilized egg in a surrogate's uterus
2. IVF using the wife's egg and donated sperm, and placement of the fertilized egg either in the wife's uterus or that of a surrogate
3. IVF using the husband's sperm and a donated egg and placement of the fertilized egg in the wife's uterus, in the donor's uterus, or in the uterus of a third-party surrogate

Resolving the issue of IVF is no simple matter, for there are no clear precedents from which guidance may be drawn; indeed, this appears to be a classic instance of a legal lacuna. In such instances, in which pertinent legal norms are lacking, a judge enjoys wide discretion. That is the case as well with respect to surrogacy, for there is no clear halakhic rule on how to decide whether the procedure is permitted and, if so, who should be considered the mother. But that lacuna may actually render the moral and gender-based considerations that guide rulings in these areas clearer and more easily identifiable. Moreover, we can compare the principles that guide the rulings on artificial insemination (where it is most often the husband whose infertility necessitates the procedure) and on IVF and surrogacy (where the fertility problem is most often the wife's) and examine whether they treat the issues equally. For example, does the principle that paternity is ascribed to the genetic father apply as well to assign maternity to the genetic mother in a case of surrogacy, where the genetic mother does not bear the fetus? If not, what accounts for the difference?

ATTRIBUTING THE OFFSPRING TO THE GENETIC FATHER AND MOTHER

Before the advent of artificial insemination and IVF, the question of whether a child's lineage should be attributed to the parents who raised that child did not arise, for the rule was "the preponderance of sexual unions are with the husband."[61] That presumption meant that "a child born to a married woman is presumed to be that of its mother's husband,"[62] even if rumors of the wife's unfaithfulness were in circulation. Of course, if the facts show that the husband could not possibly be the father, the presumption is rebutted. The halakhic effect of artificial insemination and IVF is to narrow the applicability of the presumption that "the preponderance of sexual unions are with the husband." The fact that the "meeting" between the sperm cell and the ovum (that is, fertilization) takes place outside the womb rather than within it in the aftermath of intercourse raises concerns about the severance of the halakhic link between the child and the sources of the gametes that provide its genes. In the case of IVF, given that the presumption noted above can no longer be relied on, there is uncertainty regarding the child's lineage—especially, though not solely, when the donor of the sperm or the egg is unknown.

We have seen that some approaches to artificial insemination rest on the premise that the offspring's paternity is not attributed to the sperm provider. The analogous question arises with respect to the genetic mother, given that the fertilization of her ovum is accomplished by artificial means, outside its natural location in the uterus. It is fair to assume that those who believe the paternity tie is severed in the case of artificial insemination will reach the same conclusion in cases of IVF, with respect both to the man and the woman who provide the genetic material. Conversely, the majority who believe paternity is not negated by the "artificiality" of the insemination, and that the sperm source is the child's biological father, can be expected to reach the same conclusion regarding the ascription of maternity to the woman who has provided the ovum and to whose uterus the ovum will be returned after its extrauterine fertilization. Surrogacy is an additional, complicating variable.

THE MAN'S FULFILLMENT OF THE COMMANDMENT TO PROCREATE

In cases of artificial insemination, one might argue that the natural fertilization process is preserved to a considerable degree, but IVF is quite different in that regard. In some instances, indeed, micromanipulation[63] may be used to compel a sperm cell to penetrate an ovum after both have undergone a process of enhancement. According to those who say that fulfillment of the commandment to procreate is conditioned on preserving the natural processes and on fertilization taking place "in the usual way and with the usual pleasure,"[64] the absence of those conditions precludes saying that a man who begets children through IVF has fulfilled the commandment to procreate.

THE PROHIBITION ON WASTING SEED

The foregoing question, as we have seen, has a direct bearing on whether emitting seed for use in these procedures entails forbidden waste. In contrast, once again, to artificial insemination—where all the semen is injected into the woman's body and it may be said that there is no waste—IVF presents a situation in which most of the semen is not needed, especially since the ongoing refinement of the procedure diminishes the number of healthy cells needed to achieve fertilization. Meanwhile, the relatively low (albeit increasing) success rate for IVF means that several attempts will likely be made before pregnancy is achieved, requiring repeated emissions of seed, most of which may be considered "wasted."

OVERSIGHT DIFFICULTIES

When artificial insemination is performed, it is relatively easy to oversee the procedure and be certain that the woman receives her partner's semen and not the semen of some more fertile man. IVF, however, takes place entirely within the laboratory, continues for a lengthy time, and by its nature is not subject to the same sorts of oversight as is artificial insemination. Accordingly, some decisors see that concern as reason enough to forbid the procedure outright.[65]

LEGITIMACY OF THE OFFSPRING

The offspring's legitimacy—that is, its not being a *mamzer*—was considered in connection with artificial insemination, and the same halakhic question seems to be posed here: is forbidden intercourse itself a prerequisite to the offspring being considered a *mamzer*, or is it enough that genetic materials from two individuals forbidden to have intercourse are mingled? To answer the question, it is necessary to consider whether the same basic premises apply with regard to the sperm and egg donation. As noted, the use of sperm from a Jewish donor is totally forbidden because of the concern about inadvertent incest in the next generation. It would be fair to assume that the same reasoning precludes the use of ova donated by a Jewish woman, though the likelihood of a problem arising is much lower in the case of egg donation, since sperm from one donor can easily fertilize many women whereas the use of eggs is more limited. While there are many disagreements concerning use of sperm from a gentile, a fair number of decisors follow R. Feinstein's position and permit it. One therefore may ask whether use of an egg donated by a non-Jewish woman would be permitted even if use of one donated by a Jewish woman would be forbidden.

DETERMINATION OF MATERNITY IN CASES OF SURROGACY

Biological paternity is invariably the same as genetic paternity; there is no difference between them. Maternity, in contrast, encompasses two functions that, in the natural course, take place in the same woman: the genetic function of providing the egg to be fertilized, and the physiological function of carrying the fetus to birth. IVF allows for the functions to be divided between two women, one providing the egg and the other carrying the resulting fetus. If the birth mother lacks working ovaries or is elderly, she will need egg donation; on the other hand, a woman lacking a healthy uterus or unable to become pregnant owing to other health problems can have her fertilized egg carried to term by a surrogate.

Halakhic paternity and halakhic maternity differ significantly in how they are determined. Paternity, according to most views, is attributed to the sperm provider, but views differ with respect maternity. At least four approaches can be identified: (1) maternity is attributed to the birth mother; (2) maternity is attributed to the egg provider; (3) maternity is attributed to both the egg provider and the birth mother, so the offspring has two mothers; (4) maternity is attributed to neither, so the offspring lacks a halakhic mother.

In Vitro Fertilization without Outside Donation: Halakhic Approaches

PROHIBITORY APPROACHES

The most prominent of the decisors who prohibit all forms of IVF is R. Waldenberg.[66] We have already seen the main elements of his position in the discussion of artificial insemination, but his objections are even more pronounced when it comes to IVF and surrogacy, where the "slippery slope" becomes, to his thinking, even more worrisome. What lies at the bottom of the slope here is cloning along with disruption of the entire natural order as created by God and the possibility that this will lead to rampant apostasy:

> Particularly since we already read that the culmination of this process of test-tube fertilization will likely bring about, sooner or later, the formation of a child in a test tube, that is, the entire pregnancy will begin and end outside the woman's body, in the test tube itself, with the formation within it of womb-like conditions. Thereafter, one can envision the frightening process of duplicating a human being without the pairing of two gametes. . . . This distortion of creatures, the bringing of them into the world in this manner, will destroy the image of the human being, and chaos will prevail over all childbirth as it becomes a laboratory with no human character. . . . It will also lead indirectly to the intrusion of apostasy among the simple masses in various ways, may God help us, that I have no desire to detail here, and who can tell where it will end[?] (*Ẓiẓ 'Eli'ezer* 15, 45, par. 4)

R. Waldenberg's concerns are clear: he fears that increased "technologization" will eliminate the human dimension in procreation; beyond that, he has a theological concern that the ever-increasing human intervention in the natural process of creating life, something that touches on the divine creative powers, will lead to the undermining of faith in God and to increased apostasy. R. Waldenberg thus derives his halakhic position from his theological position and is led to the conclusion that the greater the human intervention in the act of procreation, the more severely it is prohibited.

The halakhic rationales that applied with respect to artificial insemination apply, in his view, much more forcefully with respect to IVF. Adequate oversight is impossible, since IVF takes place over a period of time and is performed in a laboratory, out of the couple's sight. The prohibition on wasteful emission of seed is even more severe in the context of this technology, for reasons explained earlier, and neither the commandment to procreate nor even the commandment to "settle the earth" is fulfilled, because it is the test tube, as a "third party," and not the couple that brings about the fertilization. Moreover, the test tube is a place "without lineage"; that is, it cannot provide a basis for attributing parenthood. Because the ovum is separated from its natural place of growth and its relationship with the woman is thereby severed, R. Waldenberg determines, in an unprecedented ruling, that a child born through in vitro fertilization has no father and no mother for halakhic purposes.

In view of all this, it seems clear that egg donation and surrogacy would be absolutely forbidden. And yet, in a 1993 responsum on impregnation of a woman with a donated egg fertilized by her husband's sperm, such that the fertilized egg would be implanted in her own uterus, R. Waldenberg says it is preferable that both the donor and the physician performing the procedure be non-Jews.[67] His rhetoric in that responsum clearly suggests a lack of symmetry between the intense moral revulsion he expresses over fertilization of a Jewish woman with sperm from a gentile donor and fertilization of an egg from a gentile donor with sperm from a Jewish man. The asymmetry may be explained by formal halakhic considerations. R. Waldenberg does not permit IVF at all, even where sperm and egg are provided by the husband and wife, and the entire discussion in this responsum is after the fact. If the egg donor is Jewish, the possible impairment of her reproductive organs that may be caused by the donation process may run afoul of the rabbinic prohibition against sterilizing a woman. Accordingly, it is preferable that the donor be a non-Jew.

Similar considerations are raised by R. Moshe Sternbuch,[68] though he makes it clear that his principal concerns relate not to wasteful emission of semen or to the offspring's uncertain parentage but to the harm to Israel's sanctity that results from confused and impaired lineage.[69] R. Sternbuch adds that he heard a reliable account that R. Ḥayyim Kanievsky likewise forbade IVF.

R. Meir Amsel presents a more balanced view. He, too, believes all the prohibitions and concerns raised in connection with artificial insemination apply with full force here as well, but he suggests that if the woman is certain that the sperm is her husband's, it may be possible to permit the procedure.[70]

PERMISSIVE APPROACHES

For the same reasons described in connection with artificial insemination, most decisors permit IVF using the couple's own sperm and egg.[71] Even though the natural process is barely preserved in IVF, they do not believe that factor outweighs the considerations that led them to permit artificial insemination, and they allow IVF as well.

R. Ovadia Yosef takes the view that the offspring is attributed to its biological parents; the prohibition against wasting seed does not apply, because the seed here is not wasted but used; the offspring is not a *mamzer*, since no forbidden sexual relations take place; and the husband fulfills his obligation to procreate. He therefore finds it possible to permit the procedure, but with the following reservations:

> The practical conclusion regarding a test-tube baby is that he has the same legal status as a child produced through artificial insemination, which recent authorities have permitted when it is impossible for the wife to become pregnant in any other way, in the usual manner. But great care must be taken that the husband's sperm not be replaced by that of some other man; and it would be best if it were done by two religious physicians providing full supervision from the emission of the semen until its introduction into the uterus. (*Yabi'a 'Omer*, part 8, *'Even Ha-'Ezer* 21)[72]

R. Shlomo Goren offers similar reasons for permitting IVF using the couple's own sperm and egg,[73] and he also discusses the maternity of a child born through IVF of an egg provided by the woman into whose uterus the embryo is then reintroduced.[74] He believes that since most decisors attribute the child in a case of artificial insemination to the source of the seed, that should be the case a fortiori with respect to the status of the provider of the egg used in an IVF situation where the genetic mother also carries the fetus to term.[75]

R. Judah Gershuni believes a test-tube baby derived from a couple's own sperm and egg is attributed neither to its father nor to its mother and that the father therefore does not discharge his obligation to procreate.[76] Unlike R. Waldenberg, however, he believes the father does not violate the prohibition on wasteful emission of seed, since the seed is used to fulfill the commandment "to populate the earth."[77]

R. Jacob Ariel takes a similar position.[78] While he does not believe IVF fulfills the commandment to procreate, he nevertheless finds the emission of seed permissible for the purpose of bringing children into the world, inasmuch as the commandment "to populate the earth" is discharged through the use of IVF. In other words, he does not draw a necessary connection between the obligation to procreate and the prohibition on wasteful emission of seed.

The other decisors who permit the procedure treat IVF according to the same criteria they apply to artificial insemination. They see no difference in principle between the two procedures, and no reason to forbid IVF simply because it takes place outside the woman's body.[79]

In Vitro Fertilization Using a Donated Egg: Halakhic Approaches

The principal questions to be asked with regard to use of a donated egg are as follows:

1. *Is egg donation permissible?* In theory, this should be a simpler matter than sperm donation, since there is no prohibition on removing an ovum that parallels the prohibition on wasteful emission of semen.
2. *Is it permissible to use an egg from a Jewish donor?* Even if one gives a positive answer to the previous question, it must be recalled that the principal objection to use of sperm from a Jewish donor was the concern about inadvertent incest in the ensuing generations. The same concern ought to apply with respect to ova from a Jewish donor, notwithstanding the smaller likelihood that the problem would actually arise.[80] But sperm donation involves only the sperm itself, and biological paternity is based solely on the contribution of genetic material. In a case of egg donation, however, there are two biological inputs: the genetic input of the donor and the physiological input of the woman who carries the fetus. Accordingly, halakhic maternity is more complicated to define. If the genetic mother (the egg provider) is considered to be the halakhic mother, the concern about a Jewish sperm donor would apply to a Jewish egg donor as well, and it would be reasonable to assume that the procedure would similarly be forbidden. (We will

consider the question below and find that some responsa are not consistent in that way.) If, however, it is the mother carrying the fetus who is the halakhic mother, the genetic source of the ovum becomes irrelevant; it has nothing to do with the determination of maternity, and there is no longer any concern about inadvertent incest in the next generation.

3. *Is it permissible to use an egg from a gentile donor?* Problems might arise here given that Jewish status is a matter of matrilineal descent.[81] In addition, it is necessary to determine whether the revulsion voiced by the decisors over the prospect of using sperm donated by a gentile man applies with equal force to using an egg donated by a gentile woman. And what of a case in which the woman carrying the fetus is Jewish but the fetus was formed by from an ovum donated by a gentile? Is there a difference between penetration of a Jewish woman's body by sperm from a gentile and fertilization of a gentile woman's egg by a Jewish man's sperm?

Most if not all of these questions are clarified in the context of a discussion regarding determination of motherhood in cases of surrogacy, and that is the issue to which we now turn.

MATERNITY IN SURROGACY CASES

A small number of decisors permit IVF using the couple's own gametes but absolutely forbid surrogacy in both its forms: gametes from the husband and wife forming a fetus carried to term by another woman, or sperm from the husband fertilizing an egg from an outside donor, with the resulting fetus carried to term by the wife. R. Samuel Ha-Levi Wosner, for example, believes that as a matter of Torah law, such activities are forbidden for the reason that AID is likewise forbidden, namely, that the biblical directive "a man . . . shall cleave unto his wife, and they shall be one flesh" (Gen. 2:24) is understood to refer to the offspring formed from the two of them:

> In case you should think this reprehensible act is permitted by the Torah and that it is possible to cleave to his wife but to form one flesh with his fellow's wife through the offspring formed by them, the Torah here sets the first condition of marital relations as a matter of biblical law, that their

> marriage and cleaving to each other be what produces offspring coming from the two of them, the father and mother becoming one in the offspring formed by the one for whom the Torah determined the rule that he shall cleave to his wife and not to his fellow's wife. (*Shevet Ha-Levi*, part 3, 175:2)

In the responsum at issue, R. Wosner does not deal directly with surrogacy, but, as the author of *Nishmat 'Avraham* reports, he directly ties the prohibition on surrogacy to the rationales set forth in that responsum.[82] R. Yosef Shalom Elyashiv and R. Shlomo Zalman Auerbach likewise object to surrogacy. R. Elyashiv cites the confusion it could cause and is concerned that people might think that just as it is permitted to bring about pregnancy and birth through two women, so, too, is it permitted to use sperm from a donor other than the husband. R. Auerbach also bans the procedure because of the (unspecified) confusion and disorder it will cause; and after the fact, in view of the doubt about the child's maternity, he requires the child to undergo conversion to Judaism if the surrogate was a gentile.[83]

The decisors who permit IVF do not forbid surrogacy[84] or even egg donation if necessary. The primary question that concerns them is who should be considered the child's halakhic mother. A minority of the decisors believe that the genetic criterion should be assigned greater weight than carrying the fetus and that the provider of the egg therefore should be considered the halakhic mother for all purposes. Treating the genetic criterion as determinative is helpful where the provider of the egg wants a child but cannot carry the pregnancy. Where, however, the would-be mother is able to carry the pregnancy but lacks fertile eggs of her own, it is more helpful to make the opposite determination and find the birth mother to be the halakhic mother.

Pinchas Schiffman, meanwhile, suggests an entirely different criterion (applicable to both members of the couple), and would determine parentage on the basis of intention rather than biology,[85] though the halakhah would appear to reject that as a matter of principle. According to Schiffman's criterion, "the parent is the person who took an active part in bringing the child into the world."[86] Just as an anonymous sperm donor should not be seen as the father of the child, so, too, should an anonymous egg donor not be seen as its mother. Use of an outside surrogate, however, sharpens the issue, since two women both play an active part in the birth of the child. The genetic mother is not an anonymous donor; on the contrary, it is she who initiates the process of bringing the child into the world. At the same time, it is the birth mother who forms a physical connection with the child during the course of the pregnancy. According to Schiffman, the parties' original intentions and expectations should be enforced. Accordingly, in a case of anonymous egg donation, the birth mother who wanted to bring about the child's birth should be considered its mother; but where the genetic mother provides the egg to initiate the process and retains a surrogate, the former should be considered the mother since the outside surrogate agreed at the outset to serve only as host for the growth of the fetus. Schiffman's approach is foreign to halakhic thinking, however,[87] and in the following paragraphs I will consider the various halakhic positions that have been advanced.

The Child Is Attributed to the Provider of the Egg

R. Goren is among the few to take the position that the genetic mother is the halakhic mother. In his view, the axis around which the question revolves is whether maternity is determined by the woman's participation in the process of establishing the fetus's potential or by her role in bringing about the realization of that potential, of the fetus's essence. In the former case, maternity, like paternity, would be assigned to the provider of the gamete; in the latter case, maternity would be assigned not to the egg provider but to the woman who carried the fetus to term in her womb.[88]

R. Goren finds support for his view that the genetic mother is the halakhic mother in the following *baraita*:

> Our rabbis taught: Three partners share in the formation of a person: the Holy One, blessed be He, his father, and his mother. His father's seed provides the white substance, from which are formed bones, tendons, and fingernails, the brain in his head, and the white of the eye. His mother's seed provides the red substance, from which are formed skin, flesh, hair and the dark of the eye. And the Holy One, blessed be He endows him with spirit and soul and facial appearance, with vision, hearing, and speech, with the capacity to walk, and with understanding and reason. (BT Nid. 31a)

In R. Goren's view,[89] one can infer from this source that just as the father's sperm caries the genetic material from which the fetus develops in the mother's womb, so, too, does the mother's egg. Maternity is determined on the basis of the genetic link that is potential in the egg and becomes actualized only during the course of the pregnancy. Although the father plays no part in the process of actualizing the characteristics embedded in his sperm, paternity is nevertheless determined solely by virtue of the potential genetic link embedded in his sperm. Maternity likewise should be determined solely on the basis of the genetic potential embedded in the egg, and not on the basis of actualization of that potential in the womb.

Decisive proof that maternity is determined by the woman's potential partnership with her mate in the genetic material they jointly contribute can be found, in R. Goren's view, in the debate between Rabbi Judah the Prince and Antoninus (BT Sanh. 91b). As additional support, he cites a source in the Zohar, which interprets the verse "Honor your father and your mother" in a way that bolsters the view of the child as obligated to honor both parents because he is formed from both of them as one.[90] He ultimately concludes that because it is clear that the true mother is the provider of the egg and not the birth mother, "who will know that the child belongs not to the woman who bore him but to another woman, and who will disclose who the woman was who donated her egg for implantation?"[91] In such circumstances, there is a real risk of marriage between siblings on their mother's side (that of the woman who provided the egg), and for that reason widespread surrogacy-on-demand should be forbidden. But in isolated cases, in which the purpose is to resolve difficult issues and surrogacy will help preserve family life that is at risk of being destroyed, "perhaps it is possible to find some way to permit it in order to save the peace of the household; and great is peace."[92]

I find R. Goren's ultimate ruling quite surprising. Once it is decided that the genetic mother is the halakhic mother, consistency would seem to call for him to prohibit egg donation by a Jewish woman, given the concern over inadvertent incest, just as he forbade all sperm donation by a Jewish man for the same reason. Why his turnabout with respect to egg donation? R. Shlomo Aviner indeed challenged him on that point,[93] suggesting that because one could reasonably argue as well that the halakhic mother is the pregnancy carrier rather than the egg donor, one can rely on that view—which obviates concern about inadvertent incest, given the certain identity of the birth mother—in exigent circumstances where a couple's childlessness is especially harsh.

But R. Goren does not stop there and raises a second, even more surprising, rationale for the asymmetry between egg and sperm donation by a Jew. He argues that in cases of egg donation, the couple can always clarify who donated the egg and can even demand the information from the physicians. In cases of sperm donation, however, the source of the sperm cannot be ascertained, since the donor would never divulge the information to others[94] nor will the physician divulge the information to the woman inseminated by the donation, and the concern about widespread inadvertent incest is therefore quite serious. But while R. Goren's first rationale can be explained from the perspective of halakhic logic, the underlying assumptions of the second rationale are not at all clear. Why should a woman agree to remove the veil of anonymity and identify herself as an egg donor while a man "would never divulge that to the world"? Is egg donation psychologically easier for a woman than sperm donation is for a man? Is a woman more willing to acknowledge her maternity than a man is to acknowledge his paternity? Is a woman more easily persuaded than a man? If all that is the case, it becomes clear that these judgments rely on gender concepts that are not at all certain.[95]

R. Jacob Ariel takes a position similar to R. Goren's and likewise argues that maternity follows the genetic source, not the carrying of the pregnancy.[96] Because he believes it preferable to use an egg donated by a gentile and then convert the child to Judaism, and because the fertilization in any event is artificial, he believes it preferable to bear a boy rather than a girl, to avoid the question of whether the girl could marry a *kohen*.[97] On the other hand, if the husband is a *kohen* and he begets a child in this manner, he must change his family name and inform his son that he is not a *kohen*. Here, too, I find both determinations problematic from a gender perspective. If the husband is a *kohen* and the son born to him is a convert with no paternal lineage, the problem is less severe as a matter of formal halakhah—though no less severe from a psychological and emotional perspective—than it would be in the case of a girl infant who would have to be converted and therefore be unable to marry a *kohen*. Why does R. Ariel believe it simpler to inform a son that he is not a *kohen*, thereby revealing the story of how he came into the world (a fact that the parents may be uninterested in), than to take care that a daughter not marry a *kohen*? Perhaps he means to avoid the problem from the outset, but would he, for the same reason, tell a prospective woman convert not to pursue her conversion plans? Is he unaware of the powerful effects of what he says—namely, that it would encourage the use of IVF technology to determine the sex of a fetus in a patriarchal society and culture that already tends to favor sons over daughters?[98]

Like R. Goren before him, R. Ariel is prepared to favor egg donation from a close relative, for then the concerns about future inadvertent incest are obviated inasmuch as everything takes place within the narrow family circle and everything is known to all participants. Why are similar suggestions not offered with respect to sperm donation (in consequence of which it becomes necessary to permit sperm donations from a gentile)? Why should one permit egg donation within the narrow family, in connection with which there would be no doubt about the fetus's genetic identity, but regard sperm donation in the same situation as impossible? Would R. Ariel allow sperm donation by a Jew on condition that the donor's identity be divulged? In other words, why is a sperm donor's anonymity so strictly protected, while that of an egg donor is not?

The Child Is Attributed to the Birth Mother

Although using the genetic criterion to determine parenthood may be consistent with scientific developments that emphasize the centrality of genetics in human biology, most decisors believe it is the birth mother who is the halakhic mother. The attempts to prove that proposition are ambiguous, convoluted, rely in part on precedents from the world of animals and plants, and are open to refutation. Nevertheless, I believe the proposition rests on sound halakhic logic, which I will address at the end of the section. First, let me discuss the ways in which advocates of this position have sought to prove it.

"TWO TWIN BROTHERS" One of the talmudic sources most frequently cited in this context deals with two twin brothers who converted to Judaism; on the basis of that passage, R. Zalman Neḥemiah Goldberg and R. Abraham Iẓḥak Ha-Levi Kilav[99] conclude that the birth mother is the halakhic mother. The passage follows:

> Come and hear: If two twin brothers convert, or, similarly, [if two twin Canaanite slaves] are emancipated, [and one dies childless, the other] is not required to perform *ḥaliẓah* or engage in levirate marriage [with the deceased's widow], and they are not bound by [the law forbidding marriage to] one's brother's [former] wife [after death of the brother or divorce]. If

> they were conceived outside of sanctity [that is, while the mother was still a gentile] but born within sanctity [after the mother's conversion], they are not required to perform *ḥaliẓah* or engage in levirate marriage, but they are bound by [the law forbidding marriage to] one's brother's [former] wife. (BT Yev. 97b)

The rationale for the passage's rulings is that a new convert is considered to have the status of a newborn child, and all his (or, in this case, the twins') preconversion genetic ties are annulled. If, however, the twins are Jewish because their mother converted during the course of the pregnancy, they are still exempt from levirate marriage and *ḥaliẓah* (because being subject to levirate marriage depends on paternal ancestry, and they have no father, since the seed of a gentile is treated as the seed of an animal, as is established later in the passage). But they are considered to be brothers for purposes of the prohibition on marrying one's brother's widow (except for levirate marriage) or divorcée, inasmuch as their mother gave birth to them when she was already a Jew in all respects. On that basis, R. Goldberg tries to prove that giving birth suffices to establish halakhic maternity, since the brothers were conceived while their mother was still a gentile and, as noted, her conversion annuls their past genetic ties to her. To put it differently, before the mother converted, the twins were considered brothers for all purposes. With her conversion during the course of her pregnancy, the fraternal bond between them was canceled, for "a new convert is like a newborn child" and all his genetic ties are annulled. Accordingly, one can say that at the moment of the mother's conversion during her pregnancy, they cease being considered her children, yet the passage goes on to determine that there exist fraternal ties between them, established at the time of birth.

This proof has been much discussed in the halakhic literature, and various reservations about it have been expressed. R. Ariel and R. Mordechai Halperin reject the proof, arguing it can be shown that the principle of "a new convert is like a newborn child" does not apply to an unborn fetus. Conversion confers newborn status on one already born but not on one still unborn, consistent with Rashi's approach to the passage in *Yevamot*.[100] R. Ezra Bick likewise rejects the proof; he believes that while the birth establishes that the convert is the twins' mother—because they were formed in her body and from her ovum—the rule of "a new convert is like a newborn child" applies only with respect to lineage and not with respect to biological fact.[101] Accordingly, one could reason that while the birth is indeed the cause for assigning maternity to the woman, the genetic tie is the precondition to doing so (and the conversion does not alter the biological fact). R. Bick believes that the usual halakhic method of using analogy to determine the applicable halakhic rule does not lend itself to application here, for there is no source that can be said to supply the precise analogue needed.[102] Z. Lev similarly rejects any effort at proof from the case described in the Talmud, arguing that the case at hand does not resemble it.[103] The case in the Talmud speaks of one body, one woman, whose halakhic status underwent a change during the course of the pregnancy. She did not become another woman, and a new convert is not considered to be an actual newborn; the statement that the convert is such pertains only to lineage. In contrast to all that, the case of surrogacy involves two real women, two different bodies. A pertinent precedent would have to deal with two separate bodies and a single offspring.

"A FETUS IS A LIMB OF ITS MOTHER" R. Joseph Engel, in his book *Beit Ha-'Ozar*, attempts to prove from a passage in BT *Megillah* that paternity is determined at the beginning of the pregnancy but maternity is determined only after birth.[104] The passage in question (BT Meg. 13a) relates to the seemingly superfluous repetition in Esther 2:7; the verse states: "He was foster-father to Hadassah—that is, Esther—his uncle's daughter, for she had neither father nor mother . . . and when her father and mother died, Mordecai adopted her as his own daughter." The Talmud comments: "*For she had neither father nor mother*—[Given that statement,] what need have I for *when her father and mother died*? Said Rav Aḥa: After impregnating her [mother], her father died; after giving birth to her, her mother died." Rashi, based on close reading of "she had neither father nor mother," adds that not even for one day of her life did she have a father or a mother: "when her mother became pregnant, her father died, meaning that from the time one might be called a father, she had no father; and when her mother bore her, her mother died, meaning she was never called 'mother.'" On that basis, it is clear to Engel that paternity is determined at the time of conception and maternity at the time of birth, and he connects that to the fact that "a fetus is a limb of its mother":

> The mother of a fetus is not called a mother, and the reason should be that because the fetus is a limb of its mother, it is considered part of her body and it makes no sense to call her its mother, for it is as one of her limbs.[105]

Still, as Halperin properly notes, this does not necessarily prove anything with regard to maternity in a case of egg donation.[106] Even if the time for determining maternity is at birth, there remains a need for a genetic link that gives the determination force. In other words, deciding that maternity is determined at birth does not necessarily obviate genetic maternity.

"A YOUNG SHOOT GRAFTED ONTO AN OLD TREE" As early as the start of the twentieth century, R. Benjamin Aryeh Weiss was asked about a case in which infertility had been successfully dealt with by transplanting another woman's ovary into the infertile woman.[107] The case closely resembles that of surrogacy, in that the eggs formed in the ovary are not those of the woman carrying the pregnancy, who is to be the birth mother.

Weiss begins his responsum by arguing that ovary transplantation is forbidden because it constitutes sterilization of a woman; he so rules even though the prohibition is only rabbinic and a lenient ruling could be imagined. As for the question itself, he holds that the offspring is the child of the birth mother in all respects. His source is a statement in BT *Sotah* 43b: "Now, Rabbi Abahu said: If a young shoot [lit. "a girl"] is grafted onto an old tree [lit. "an elderly woman"], the [legal status of the] young shoot is annulled by [that of] the old tree, and it is not subject to the rules of *'orlah*."[108] In the case described, the young shoot is taken from a tree that is already able to bear fruit and is subject to the restrictions of *'orlah*, and is grafted onto the trunk of a tree that is already past the period of *'orlah*, and the question relates to status of the fruit produced on the grafted shoot. Genetically, the fruit is the produce of the young shoot subject to *'orlah*, but it is grafted onto a trunk that is already past that point. Rabbi Abahu's comment implies that, for halakhic purposes, the fruit is ascribed to the old trunk, the body that receives the graft, and not to the shoot or the limb that is engrafted. On that basis, Rabbi Abahu would infer that a woman's ova implanted into the body of another woman are assimilated into the second woman's body and lose their connection to the woman who provided them.[109]

R. Waldenberg—who, as already noted, objects to artificial fertilization and, accordingly, to surrogacy—likewise believes that if the process has nevertheless taken place, the birth mother should be regarded as the halakhic mother. His ruling relies on R. Weiss's comments on the issue and on the proof adduced from the discussion of *'orlah*.[110] R. Ariel, in contrast, belies that the analogy drawn by the proof does not withstand analysis, given the differences between grafting and surrogacy. The former is an irreversible implantation of a shoot; that is, the shoot becomes permanently part of tree, and it stands to reason that it is legally subsumed within it—that is, annulled as a separate entity. The latter, meanwhile produces a fetus that is destined to emerge from the womb in which it is implanted, and it therefore is not annulled by being considered part of the woman carrying it, and its maternity certainly could be ascribed to the egg provider. Moreover, the young shoot is annulled and considered part of the tree only with respect to the rules of *'orlah*. With regard to its status for purposes of the prohibitions on interspecies grafting, it is the shoot that is determinative.

RECOGNIZING THE UNCERTAINTY AND ATTRIBUTING THE OFFSPRING TO BOTH WOMEN: "A STALK THAT PRODUCED A SHOOT" According to Lev, a talmudic passage regarding "new grain"[111] is a good analogue for surrogacy, for it involves two separate entities. He acknowledges that the analogy "is a bit audacious, for the proof is brought from plants, which have no vital soul and spirit,"[112] but he nevertheless tries to draw conclusions from it:

> Rabbi Simeon ben Pazi asked: if a stalk produced one-third of full growth before the time for the *'omer*, and [the farmer] plucked it and planted after the *'omer* and it grew taller, what is its status? Do we look to the original shoot, so that the passage of the *'omer* permits it to be used, or do we look to the additional growth, in which case it cannot be used until after the ensuing *'omer*? The question stands unresolved. (BT Men. 69b)

The passage considers a case in which a stalk is replanted in other soil after having grown to about one-third of its full size.[113] The initial growth took place before the *'omer*, and the replanting took place after the *'omer*.[114] The question is whether the principal growth took place during the first stage, in which case the passage of the *'omer* allowed for use of the wheat, or whether it took place later, in which case it would be necessary to await the ensuing *'omer*. In other words, if the first plot of soil is analogous to the genetic mother, whose egg was fertilized, and the second plot of soil is analogous to the surrogate mother, "do we look to the original shoot" and attribute the fetus's growth in the surrogate's womb to the natural mother's egg that was fertilized, given that the potential offspring resided entirely in the fertilized egg, as modern genetics shows? Or "do we look to the additional growth," in which case the fetus's continued growth in the surrogate's womb is determinative? Inasmuch as the Talmud leaves the question unresolved (as does Maimonides), Lev believes the status of the fetus carried by a surrogate mother is likewise unresolved, and one must acknowledge, from a halakhic perspective, the maternity of both women.[115]

Halakhic Discourse and Feminist Discourse

An overview of feminist theory regarding fertility treatments and surrogacy was presented earlier, and for good reason. These are sensitive issues, bearing on the most personal and intimate feelings, aspirations, and emotions a human being, and especially a woman, can have. At the same time, we are dealing with morally complex issues, and we have not yet exhausted the thicket of considerations and arguments that might be raised in connection with them.

In stark contrast to the wide range of concepts and opinions held by feminists and ethicists on these issues, the contemporary halakhic discussion of in vitro fertilization and (especially) of surrogacy is striking in its disregard of the ethical element. Did the decisors here sense "the ethical poverty of their halakhic sources," as R. Lichtenstein put it in another context,[116] or might there be some other explanation for their silence with regard to the ethics of these practices?[117] To put it differently, how can so morally complex an issue as surrogacy become entirely a question of "who is the mother," however important a halakhic question that may be (and it is important)? How can it be that all the energy and wisdom of halakhic authorities is devoted solely to searching for the proper halakhic analogy that will "prove" whether it is birth or provision of genetic material that defines motherhood, when other morally weighty matters are on the agenda as well? Alternatively, how is it that scarcely any of the decisors express discomfort regarding the analogies that are offered, some of which are taken from the botanical world and have absolutely nothing to do with real life, with motherly sentiments, or with human bonds?

The halakhic questions that are raised in discussions of in vitro fertilization and surrogacy are also striking in that they have nothing to do with the gender aspect of the subject. And that is so even though the technologies at issue directly affect not only a woman's body but also, perhaps primarily, her sense of self as a person and as a potential mother. For example: Is it proper to permit egg donation, which, unlike the relatively simple process of sperm donation, entails a medical procedure requiring total anesthesia and a degree of risk to the donor? What are the psychological and emotional aspects of "dividing" motherhood, and are they not likely to have a bearing on the halakhic determination regarding the offspring's maternity? What are the halakhic aspects of commerce in a woman's reproductive organs? What are the likely effects of surrogacy on the family life of the couple employing it and on the surrogate and her partner? Do any of the decisors consider the objectification of women and their transformation into receptacles for almost anything designed to increase fertility and birth, be it sperm from an outside donor or a fertilized egg that is not in any way hers and her partner's and that will not belong to her after it is born? Doesn't fertility therapy, under prevailing patriarchal notions, construe the primary role of women to be that of bearing and raising children? Doesn't it entail excessive control of women's procreative abilities? When an infertile woman chooses to undergo fertility therapy, is her choice truly voluntary? Does surrogacy entail elements of commerce in babies and exploitation of lower-class women? What is the difference between sale of sexual services and sale of reproductive services, and might there be some substance to the comparison of surrogacy to prostitution?

Despite the wide range of relevant ethical considerations, the entire halakhic analysis is centered on the question of who should be regarded as the fetus's halakhic mother. Moreover, some of the halakhic precedents invoked in that analysis make one uncomfortable at best; at worst, they convey a sense of moral and emotional apathy. Can so difficult a question really be decided on the basis of cases dealing with shoots from a young tree grafted onto a mature tree? Can plant life provide answers to questions of human motherhood?[118] The premise that doing so is possible necessarily implies unstated assumptions about the nature of motherhood as an institution and the relation of women to it. To compare motherhood to a shoot from a young tree implanted in a mature tree is to imply that the woman onto whom the shoot is "grafted" becomes the fetus's mother involuntarily, whether she has invited the "grafting" or not. Surprisingly, the determination by most decisors that the birth mother is the halakhic mother means, in practice, that she is required to give up a child who, halakhically, is hers.

If pregnancy is the significant link between mother and child, then the tendency evident in the halakhic rulings—that is, to regard the birth mother as the mother of the child—would appear to be consistent with Katz-Rothman's feminist approach. At odds with her theory, however, is the decisors' willingness to allow the birth mother to give up the child who is hers or even to sell it.

At this point, we should broaden the inquiry and ask whether assigning priority to the birthing criterion rather than the genetic one has implications beyond the formal halakhic analysis and whether it is possible to identify interests transcending those posed by the specific question under discussion. I would answer that such interests are indeed at stake and that the halakhic assignment of maternity to the birth mother indirectly advances the pro-birth discourse that we saw in the earlier sections of the book. That discourse provides the theoretical and ideological underpinning for the specific decisions that are issued, including those permitting the use of all the aforementioned technologies.

The ruling (of most decisors) that the birth mother is the halakhic mother parallels, I believe, the authorization of artificial insemination with sperm from a gentile. Just as use of sperm from a gentile provides an escape from the concerns about inadvertent incest that arise in the context of artificial insemination with donated sperm, so, too, does denying the genetic mother's maternity provide an escape from the same concerns that might arise in the context of egg donation. Once it is determined that the birth mother is the halakhic mother, the identity of the mother becomes certain, and concerns about inadvertent incest in the next generation fade away, which would not necessarily be the case if the genetic mother—the egg donor—were assigned maternal status. In other words, these rulings remove all impediments to permitting use of these procedures, for they obviate what remains a serious concern even according to the lenient view that requires actual intercourse for transgression of the law against improper sexual unions. We have seen that even R. Goren, who believes the genetic mother is the halakhic mother, is willing to permit, in exigent circumstances, egg donation from a family member,[119] although he assumes that widespread use of the procedure on demand will not be allowed under such conditions. Treating the birth mother as the halakhic mother, in contrast, removes concern about inadvertent incest and opens the door to mass usage of the permissive ruling.

It is important, however, to note that the picture I have painted, whereby halakhah treats the birth mother as the halakhic mother, reflects the tendency in mainstream halakhic discourse up until 2006, when I completed the primary research for this study. Since the field of reproductive technology is itself constantly developing and changing, the halakhic discourse, which responds to these changes, is also in constant flux. Therefore, it is possible that the picture may have already shifted slightly, in the direction of assigning greater weight to the genetic factors.

Of course, one cannot prove with certainty that the decisors have acted with full awareness of the considerations I have enumerated. Still, I think the data show that a less-than-fully conscious desire to take advantage of scientific developments related to fertility has exercised a tacit influence on the halakhic analyses and decisions. Even those who ascribe maternity to the egg donor assume that the practice of surrogacy is permitted and say, in their rulings, that procreation is important enough that it can displace weighty moral considerations; but it is the majority view ascribing maternity to the birth mother that allows broader access to surrogacy by obviating concerns about inadvertent incest. One could argue, to be sure, that if the halakhah were really interested in promoting procreation at almost any cost, it would allow sperm donation even by a Jew, on condition that his identity be disclosed. To this I would respond that, indeed, it seems that the decisors discount this possibility simply because they do not believe that sperm donors will agree to disclose their identities. This assumption, which is not raised with regard to egg donors (as I have demonstrated), is in itself gender-biased.[120] In any case, that counterargument does not detract from the fact that when all is said and done, a way has been found to permit the use of all forms of modern reproductive technology. The authorization to inseminate a woman with sperm from a gentile and the determination that the birth mother is the halakhic mother serve alike to advance that goal.[121]

Some would argue that the foregoing presentation misreads the reality and that it could be argued just as well that all these lenient rulings stem from the decisors' concern for the distress felt by individuals, men and women alike, who want nothing more than a child that is genetically theirs and are willing to submit to difficult or painful fertility therapies in order to attain that. The argument is not without merit, but I believe it falls short of fully accounting for the situation. People's desires are influenced by their cultural surroundings, and one cannot draw a line between, on the one hand, the express and tacit messages in the halakhic rulings and the atmosphere generated by that discourse and, on the other, the uncompromising desire for a biological child. If the halakhic decisors had greater reservations about these technologies, other channels to parenthood—such as adoption, which is not yet considered with adequate seriousness—would gain legitimacy and social support of the kind that affects a couple's decision-making.[122] In that way, it might be possible to ease the suffering of many women who undergo repeated (and progressively riskier) cycles of treatment with no results.

My principal argument in this chapter—beyond uncovering the halakhic tendency to permit all reproductive technologies—is that halakhic decisors take little account of weighty moral and gender considerations when they come to rule on these sorts of issues and, in that sense, they consider the end to justify almost all the means. It is possible that because procreation is considered an important commandment incumbent only on men, while most of the moral considerations related to in vitro fertilization and, even more so, to surrogacy pertain to the lives and status of women, the decisors, themselves being men, may simply have been unaware of them. But the gap between the extensive treatment of those considerations from an ethical-feminist perspective and the decisors' silence only heightens the sense that if the establishment entrusted with formulating and interpreting the halakhah had not been exclusively male, the picture we see today might have been significantly different.

AFTERWORD

The Gender Project in the Philosophy of Halakhah as an Exercise in Criticism

In the seventh of his "Theses on the Philosophy of History," the philosopher and culture critic Walter Benjamin writes that the role of the historical materialist is to "brush history against the grain."[1] He uses this image to emphasize that there is more to history than the "official" version that is written by the "victors" who control the historical narrative. The task of the historian is to tell the "other" story, that of the history that has been withheld, and the historian's critical approach can reveal new directions in thought.

"Brushing against the grain" serves a dual purpose. First, it demonstrates the extent to which history should be seen as the story of the powerful, of those who exercise control. But it also attempts to uncover who it is that pays the price for "the history of the victors." That sort of exposure can call into doubt the desires and interests of the powerful, who controlled the shaping of history, as well as their goals and their values. Moreover, "brushing against the grain" can produce an alternative historical story, thereby showing that the "official" story is not the inevitable one. Revealing this element of contingency in the official story can open the door to new readings not previously encompassed within the range seen as reasonable. It can thereby liberate the "oppressed classes" by offering them new horizons.

The recasting of history as a contingent rather than necessary narrative appears most prominently in the philosophy of Michel Foucault. His historical studies, devoted primarily to fact-based description (albeit from a new perspective), proved influential mainly in the normative sphere. The principal method used by Foucault to accomplish the move from necessity to contingency was that of genealogy.[2] Simply understood, genealogy is the study of descent, of origins. The genealogy proposed by Foucault in *Madness and Civilization* and in *History of Sexuality* adopts a critical stance that is meant to liberate—in the one case, from the dichotomy between madness and reason; in the other, from a particular perspective on sex and sexuality. Genealogy in its critical sense is explained as follows:

> First and foremost, the genealogical method seeks out the variances between the links in the chain. In a seemingly somewhat paradoxical matter, it looks for linkages that are not inevitable, not essential, not substantive. One may even say that it attempts to show the absence of any linkage. It displays a chain in order to demonstrate that it is not a chain; that there is nothing at all here that is continuous over time, no fixed essence.[3]

The genealogical method's principal value lies in its presentation of the historical development of the object of study. If something has a history, it may not be an inevitable part of present reality; it may be, rather, the product of a particular time and place, one alternative among many that might have developed. In that sense, genealogy has a therapeutic value, for it liberates us from notions of imagined necessity:

> It is this change in perspective that makes it possible for us to reexamine our positions and maintain them responsibly. The more solidly rooted the idea of necessity and the more powerful the mythologization of the present, the more significant the change in perspective with regard to the reflective-therapeutic process.[4]

The move from a perspective of necessity to one of contingency was central to the Critical Legal Studies (CLS) movement. That movement sought to divest law of its mantle of neutrality and objectivity and to demonstrate that a legal decision is not necessarily the product of formal deductive deliberation and, therefore, not necessarily derived from earlier legal precedents. Judges, CLS proponents would argue, are not "bound" by the law in a sense that precludes a broad exercise of discretion, and the adjudicatory act is not as absolute as it is said to be.

I would argue that what CLS has done for the field of law, a gender critique can do for halakhah.[5] My study is essentially a work of criticism, and to give it a solid grounding, I made use of the tools developed by the CLS movement and, primarily, by feminist legal thinkers. To put it in Walter Benjamin's terms, the study seeks to "brush against the grain of halakhic rulings," that is, against the explicit and perceptible assumption that halakhic truth can be objectively attained, without invoking gender prejudices and other preconceived sociological biases.

Brushing halakhic rulings against the grain reveals that interpretive moves and halakhic decisions that ultimately determine the official and binding narrative of the halakhah can be perceived as the "history of the victors." The decisors enjoy a monopoly of power, and it is they who determine the content and authenticity of the "story"—what is considered fit to be included in the halakhic corpus and what is to be denied legitimacy and therefore forgotten and left to disappear. Brushing against the official grain has demonstrated that the story of the "victors" has occasionally failed, consciously or unconsciously, and has, at points, silenced the voices and vital interests of anyone who does not occupy a position of power and is not entrusted with the interpretation and shaping of "halakhic truth."

In Foucault's terms, the genealogical method—displaying the historical development of the halakhic sources—can demythologize the regnant concepts as it shows us that halakhic rulings are not the inevitable outcome of a necessary chain of events. In so doing, it can contribute to the establishment of different halakhic rulings. In our case, those other rulings could have great therapeutic value, especially for women.

Accordingly, in this study I adopted a two-tiered approach of inquiry. First, I set about to uncover the historicity of halakhic rulings. By "historicity" I do not mean historical development in the sense typically used by historians; I have not examined halakhic rulings in the context of their times, their places, and the cultural influence on their formulation. The historical development I am referring to is primarily diachronic, but it is internal to the world of halakhah; that is, I have attempted to locate, within the halakhah's own process of development, the modes of thought and alternative interpretations that were relegated to the margins. Having done so, I believe a historical study of the conventional sort would round out the picture in an interesting and important way, but such a study is beyond the scope of this project.

My second area of inquiry was the rhetoric used by the halakhic establishment to justify its interpretations and rulings. Rhetoric, which appears in the selection of the sources and in the explanations provided for rulings, both shapes social consciousness and reveals, sometimes through inadvertence, the rationale for a decision; hence the importance I ascribe to it. We have seen that even when the halakhic conclusion of a given responsum could be considered respectful of women and properly sensitive to their interests, the rhetoric of that responsum sometimes points in the opposite direction. One can identify with R. Lichtenstein's rulings on abortion, for example, yet still reject his declaration that "from the perspective of the fetus and those concerned with its welfare, liberality in this direction comes at the expense of humanity," which implies that the interests of women are at odds with a humane stance. One might agree with the position of R. Isaac Weiss, who permitted temporary use of the pill by a woman who was too weak to endure a pregnancy, yet find that his unwarranted construction and interpretation of the sources attest to his gender-based position and his belief that the primary purpose of a woman is procreation.

The methods I have used in this study are drawn, for the most part, from critical feminist theory. I might therefore be subject to challenge on the grounds that those methods themselves are not without a gender bias. At a minimum, it might be said that they are "political" in the sense that they are not neutral; they are, instead, directed toward uncovering the gender-based values and concepts that I believe to be present in a corpus that, by definition, is clearly masculine. That claim may have merit, but, as Bartlett notes, the political nature of the method arises only because it seeks information whose very existence is denied. The argument that the information in fact exists, and that the "woman's question" must be considered, is political only to the extent that the contrary argument—that the information does not exist—itself is political. The method's bias (that is, its prejudice) is simply a partiality for revealing a different type of bias. The method uncovers biases whose gender consequences are concealed, and if that is a "bias," feminists must insist it is a salutary or correct one.[6]

In this study, I have examined the place of gender considerations in halakhic determinations related to procreation. Among my conclusions is that halakhic decisions in this realm manifest a clear tendency to promote childbearing. On the one hand, the decisors amass obstacles to allowing birth control and family planning and to permitting abortions except in cases of actual mortal danger to the mother. On the other hand, they permit, almost without reservation, the use of all the new fertility technologies, including some practices—such as surrogacy—that are a matter of debate among philosophers, ethicists, and feminists.

But my principal criticism of halakhic rulings in this area is directed not at their promotion of childbearing but at the negative conception of women that they necessarily imply—a view of women that fails to acknowledge their worth as full-fledged human beings. While those who exhibit a pro-natalist tendency may be quite likely to understand the role of women in functional terms, that outcome is not inevitable. Moreover, I have shown that a substantial number of contemporary halakhic rulings in fact fail to treat the women in question as subjects, as ends in their own right; instead, they define women's value as people primarily through their reproductive function. Not only are these concepts wrong in principle, but their effects can be destructive to women's lives, for they maintain, almost irredeemably, this image of women. In the chapter on birth control, I argued that if the decisors recognized the absolute value of a woman as a person, beyond the procreative context, there would be no justification to forbid her use of effective birth control mechanisms in cases where her health was in jeopardy—particularly since mainstream interpretive possibilities allow for that conclusion. Nor would there be any justification to forbid planning for reasonable intervals between births, consistent with a woman's abilities, needs, and interests.

This critique gains additional force when it comes to abortion. I showed that framing the question solely from the perspective of the fetus does more than simply reflect a blatantly male perspective; it also construes a woman's value in material, biological terms, as if she is nothing more than a vessel for the formation of new life. A review of various feminist theories helped clarify these conclusions. While I reject the liberal notions that justify abortion on demand in all circumstances, I believe that the feminist critique raises a whole series of considerations related to the prohibition on abortion and the way it affects the day-to-day life of women—considerations that are totally absent from the decisors' deliberations over whether to permit or forbid an abortion.

With regard to the reproductive technologies considered in chapters 5 and 6, meanwhile, I showed a reverse trend, for the corpus of halakhic rulings on those issues tends to be extremely lenient. Of course, the stringencies highlighted in the first four chapters and the leniencies highlighted in the fifth and sixth draw on a common source. The inclination to promote childbearing, which I inferred from the data presented in the first four chapters, is confirmed by the data in the fifth and sixth chapters, which complete the picture. The response to sex without procreation is a tendency to rule strictly, but procreation without sex generates a tendency to rule leniently, on the premise that procreation is the goal, at almost any cost. And so we found that a woman, who serves as a vessel for procreation (as long as she is married), can be inseminated with almost any semen and can carry any pregnancy, without any serious inquiry into the pertinent moral questions.

I recognize that I may be misunderstood as calling for the rejection of all artificial fertilization technologies on the grounds that they emphasize a woman's procreative function, but that is not my intention. I certainly recognize both the difficulties and intense suffering experienced by infertile women and men and the capacity of these technologies to offer them a way out of their straits. My principal quarrel is with the lack of balance and proportion within the corpus of halakhic rulings. On the one hand, for example, no recognition is granted to the desire of mature, unmarried women to bring children into the world. On the other hand, married women are subjected to norms of "procreation at any cost," which themselves impose suffering on infertile women who feel obligated to undergo painful and risky treatments in order to achieve that goal. The almost unquestioning acceptance of all available reproductive technologies indirectly promotes the idea that a woman's primary purpose is procreative, and it thereby can obscure her value as a person who is an end in her own right, not merely a means for creating new life.

Studies of halakhah rarely if ever note the place of gender considerations in halakhic decision-making. Examining these studies closely can provide an instructive example of the state of halakhic research from a gender perspective. Scholars appear uninterested in the issue for a number of reasons. First, there is the basic belief that halakhic decisors are, in fact, treating women as fairly as they can, given a halakhic corpus marked by hierarchal or patriarchal preconceptions. If we find a lack of gender fairness, it can be attributed to sociological circumstances or, alternatively, to a moral understanding that the differences between men and women justify halakhic rulings that differentiate between them in certain circumstances. Second, the research itself on halakhic topics was and remains predominantly male. It is entirely possible that the male scholars in this field have simply been unaware of gender issues.[7]

As a matter of methodology, I believe that examining the ways in which gender considerations figure in halakhic decisions can shed new light on the decision-making process, highlighting its characteristically patriarchal and hierarchical approach. The method I have adopted thus opens many new lines of study that themselves may illuminate the purposes, values, and decisional factors in halakhic decision-making and, where needed, call for critiques of them.

In a classic essay on legal theory, Robert Cover distinguishes between "*nomos*" and "narrative."[8] Nomos represents the realm of law within which we live and which determines what is lawful and what is unlawful, what is in force and what has been annulled. But that realm is but a small part of the normative world that commands our attention. The conventional legal framework cannot exist without a narrative that determines its meaning and transforms the law from a system of rules to a complete world. Every directive entails context and discourse, historical background and purpose; conversely, every narrative entails a directive and moral significance. The narratives are models through which we experience change; they point to the horizon toward which the community is moving.[9] Following Cover, Thomas Ross wrote that feminist legal theories create a new narrative that makes possible the creation of a different "nomic" world—that is, the formation of a different legal constitution in the spirit of an egalitarian ethics.[10]

The importance of this work, I believe, lies in its forming another stratum in the new narrative that has been generated in recent years. This is the narrative of women who feel committed to halakhic discourse but also to the values of equality. The new "halakhic story" they are creating affords the women of this generation the possibility of a considerable degree of liberation and opens the door to future change as well.

Notes

Abbreviations

The following abbreviations are used throughout this book's endnotes.

BOOKS OF THE BIBLE

Deut. Deuteronomy
Esther Esther
Gen. Genesis
Isa. Isaiah
Job Job
Lev. Leviticus
Prov. Proverbs

RABBINIC TEXTS

BT Babylonian Talmud
JT Jerusalem Talmud
M Mishnah
T Tosefta
'Arak. *'Arakhin*
BB *Bava Batra*
'Eduy. 'Eduyot
Git. *Gittin*
Ḥag. *Ḥagigah*
Ḥul. *Ḥulin*
Ket. *Ketubbot*
Meg. *Megillah*
Nid. *Niddah*
'Ohal. *'Ohalot*
Pes. *Pesaḥim*
Sanh. *Sanhedrin*
Shab. *Shabbat*
Sot. *Sotah*
Ta'an. *Ta'anit*
Yev. *Yevamot*
Yoma *Yoma*

Introduction. Epistemology, Jurisprudence, and Halakhah

1. For a thorough analysis of subjectivity in halakhah, see Kirschenbaum (1992), pp. 61–91; Lichtenstein (2002); and Irshai (in press).

2. In this context, Nelson's comments are striking: "At a recent symposium on feminism and science, several participants discussed feminist criticism of androcentric bias in developmental psychology. Granting that many of the criticisms were warranted, a psychologist balked at the relationships others found between them

and feminism. In reference to one of the issues under discussion, he maintained, '*Anyone* can see that you can't build a theory about psychological development from studies limited to males. There is no need to assume there's a relationship between feminism and the ability to see that.' I waited for someone on the podium to ask the obvious question: if the problem with an empirical base limited to males—a common limitation in developmental psychology—was obvious, then *why*, prior to the advent of feminist science criticism, had developmental psychologists *not* recognized it?" (Nelson [1996], p. 286).

3. The arguments are grounded in articles by Dalima and Alcoff (1993), pp. 217–244; Lloyd (1996), pp. 149–165; Jaggar (1996), pp. 166–190.

4. Positivism continues to structure the practice of many social scientific disciplines, but systematic changes have taken place in the field over the past thirty years, and today the positivist approaches are being challenged by historians and sociologists of science as well as by feminist scholars. See Hawkesworth (1998), pp. 204–212; Code (1998), pp. 173–184.

5. Harding (1996), pp. 235–248.

6. Rakover (1992), pp. 5–12.

7. See, e.g., Yannai (1992), pp. 13–20.

8. For a selective listing of feminist legal writings, see Ross (1993), n. 3; Bartlett and Kennedy (1991).

9. In the context of this study I will not consider post-1990 feminist criticism concerned primarily with presenting the differences among women themselves and with criticizing earlier waves of feminist writing on this point. That is not because I consider these theories to be unimportant; it is, rather, because those theories are unable, at least at this stage of critical writing about the halakhah, to serve as useful theoretical tools for productive comparative analysis.

10. See Gilligan (1982).

11. For the further development of this approach into what has been called "feminist ethics," see primarily Held (1995).

12. See Menkel Meadow (1985); Friedell (1992), and the citations in his article regarding the application of Gilligan's ideas to feminist legal theory, especially note 8.

13. Posner (1998), p. 125.

14. See MacKinnon (1987); MacKinnon (1990–91).

15. MacKinnon (1987), p. 37.

16. For her critique of the decision's right-to-privacy rationale, see MacKinnon (1989), pp. 181–194; MacKinnon (1990–91).

17. Dworkin disagrees here with MacKinnon, contending that she confounds several different concepts of privacy. See Dworkin (1995).

18. According to MacKinnon, even normal sexual relations bear certain similarities to rape; she suggests that society and culture regard sexuality itself as domination of women by men. For her criticism of the concept of "consent" and the laws of rape, see MacKinnon (1989), pp. 171–183. MacKinnon's approach has been widely criticized, primarily for its absolute nature and its premise that the experience of all women is the same, regardless of race, class, or sexual orientation. See Harris (1990).

19. West (1988).

20. In this connection, see also West (1993).

21. West (1988), p. 58 et seq.

22. Ibid., pp. 41–42, 59–60.

23. Bartlett (1990). Other methods discussed by Bartlett include "a practical mode of thinking" and "raising consciousness."

24. The renowned examples in rabbinic literature are Beruriah and Yalta. See BT Eruv. 53b–54a; BT Pes. 62b; Rashi on BT AZ 18b, s.v. *ve-'ikka de-'amerei mi-shum ma'aseh de-beruria*; BT Ber. 51b; BT Nid. 20b.

25. On halakhic rulings by women, see Ariel (2003–4). Although he writes that, in principle, he can envision women issuing halakhic rulings, the tone of his comments makes it clear that he would not view such a development positively. See also Bin-Nun (2004).

26. On the characteristics of legal formalism, see Schauer (1988); Weinrib (1988). For a broader analysis of halakhic formalism, see Irshai (in press).

27. See, especially, Soloveitchik J. B. (1983); Soloveitchik J. B. (1986).

28. Soloveitchik J. B. (1982), pp. 76–78.

29. Thus, for example, some of Rabbi Soloveitchik's students maintain that any religious experience not shaped by the halakhah resembles paganism. Women's prayer groups do not constitute a halakhic category; accordingly, not only are they illegitimate, but women seeking to participate in them are marked as placing personal experience above faithfulness to halakhah. See Ross (2004), pp. 75–77.

30. See, e.g., Halbertal (1997); Sagi (1998).

31. For a broader discussion of this subject, see Irshai (in press).

32. See Irshai (2010).

33. Shagar (2006), p. 81.

34. Under Jewish law, a woman whose marriage has ended can remarry only if there is legally acceptable proof of her first husband's death or if he has given her a bill of divorce. An *'agunah* (lit. "one who is anchored"; pl. *'agunot*) is a woman unable to remarry because she remains "anchored" to her first husband, who has abandoned her or has otherwise disappeared or who refuses, perhaps out of spite or to gain leverage in negotiating the terms of divorce, to grant a bill of divorce.

35. Even in a book that tends to be well disposed to the feminist revolution, Rabbi Yair Dreyfuss notes that "this cordiality [toward feminism] is accompanied by an awareness of the dangers posed by this revolution to the traditional family structure" (Dreyfuss [2006], p. 7).

36. See Hartman (2007), pp. 45–61.

37. See Ross (2011).

38. See, e.g., Adler (1983); Ozick (1983); Berman (1973).

39. See Wahrhaftig (1979–80); Elon (1994), vol. 2, pp. 978–986.

40. Wahrhaftig (1979–80), pp. 121–130.

41. Elon (1994), p. 984 (emphasis mine).

42. See Irshai (forthcoming).

Chapter 1. "Be Fruitful and Multiply"

1. See United Nations (1975), p. 8.

2. Ibid., pp. 15 et seq.

3. See United Nations (1975); Chaudhury (1978); Jensen (1995); Jordan (1976). The journal *Studies in Family Planning* is devoted almost entirely to these issues and to the application and effectiveness of projects related to family planning.

4. Fullam (1975), p. 6.

5. Chaudhury (1978).

6. United Nations (1975), p. 27.

7. See Jensen (1995), p. 63. Jordan's study (1976) particularly emphasizes women's low educational levels as a significant contributor to high birthrates.

8. Firestone (1970); Oakley (1974); Polatnick (1983); O'Brien (1981); Ruddick (1989); Rich (1976).

9. M Yev. 6:6.

10. See the collection of rabbinic statements in BT Yev. 61–64 and BT Shab. 34a. On the importance in rabbinic thought of the commandment to procreate, see Satlow (2001); Daube (1977); Gafni (1989), pp.13–30; Cohen (1989); Safrai (1983), pp. 69–81; Cohen (1998), pp. 83–96; Boyarin (1993); Schremer (2003); Lorberbaum (2004).

11. BT Git. 41b.

12. BT Ber. 10a.

13. Tosafot on BT Git. 41b, s.v. "*lo tohu bera'ah lashevet yeẓarah*." See also Tosafot on BT Shab. 4a, s.v. "*ve-khi 'omerim lo*"; and Tosafot on BT Git. 38a, s.v. "*kol ha-meshaḥrer 'avdo*."

14. *Sefer Ha-Ḥinukh*, commandment 1.

15. *Shulḥan 'Arukh, 'Even Ha-'Ezer* 1:2: "A Torah scroll may not be sold except [to enable one] to study Torah or take a wife."

16. Lorberbaum (2004), pp. 386–435.

17. The term "theurgy" has a bivalent meaning, referring both to divine activation of man and human activation of the divine. Historians of late antiquity applied the term to rituals having the purpose of purifying the soul and thereby allowing it to free itself of the body and unite with the divine. See Lorberbaum (2004), pp. 156–169.

18. See note 10.

19. On the tension between the duty to procreate and the duty to study Torah, see Boyarin, Satlow, and Schremer, above, note 10.

20. "Biblical law" (*de-'orayeta*) and "rabbinic law" (*de-rabbanan*) refer to two very broad categories of norms within Jewish law. Their precise meaning and relationship is a highly complex matter; for present purposes it should be understood that a rule binding as a matter of biblical law has greater normative force and is less subject to countervailing considerations than is a rule binding as a matter of rabbinic law—*translator's note.*

21. R. Simhah Meir of Dvinsk, author of *Meshekh Ḥokhmah*, commenting on Gen. 9:7, writes that the Torah exempts women from the commandment to procreate because "its ways are ways of pleasantness," and it therefore does not impose on women a duty that entails danger and pain. See also Millen (2004), who enumerates five possible reasons for exempting women from the commandment.

22. M Qid. 1:10; BT Qid. 29a–35b.

23. For example, women are obligated to observe some commandments that are time-determined, such as eating matzah on Passover, rejoicing on festivals, and gathering for the septennial reading from the Torah; meanwhile, they are exempt from some commandments that are not time-determined, such as Torah study and redemption of the firstborn.

24. See, e.g., the statements attributed to Rabbi Eleazar ben Azaryah at JT Sot. 3:4: "A woman's only wisdom pertains to the loom"; see Meiri, *Beit Ha-Beḥirah* on *Sotah*, chap. 3 (p. 46), who understands this statement as confirmation of the assumption that a woman has only limited cognitive abilities.

25. See the discussion at BT Sot. 21 and Rashi ad loc. s.v. "*ke-'ilu*," suggesting that women understand deviousness and act in secrecy. So, too, Bartenura on M Sot. 3:4.

26. Safrai (1995).

27. Zohar (1988).

28. See, e.g., Ozick (1983); Adler (1983, 1998). Compare the differing view of

Aiken (1992), who does not see women's exemption from certain commandments as expressing disdain for their worth or standing before God. Instead, she adopts the view that men need more external reminders than do women in order to attain spiritual goals.

29. Berman (1973).

30. Daube (1981).

31. Ibid., p. 57.

32. Wegner (1988), p. 171.

33. Ibid., p. 42.

34. Even if it could be argued that to attain this goal, it would have sufficed to exempt only those whose "souls craved only Torah" (on the model of Ben-Azai), the fact is that the blessing of fertility was reformulated as a commandment in the context of a struggle against tendencies to cast off the burden of child rearing. It could be argued, therefore, that the sages were not interested in various exemptions that might erode the commandment's importance. At the same time, however, they did not disregard men's intellectual needs, channeled through the commandment to study Torah. In a patriarchal world, exempting women from the commandment while treating men as fully bound by it indirectly benefits men: on the one hand, it achieves the goal of reinforcing the commandment's ability to withstand the forces tending to challenge it; on the other hand, the woman's exemption allows her to used various birth control mechanisms to free the man from total subservience to the commandment.

35. See the discussion below of sterilization of men and women.

36. See T Yev. 8:4.

37. See JT Yev. 6:6. Schremer (2003), pp. 38–39, reaches a similar conclusion; see also Ellinson (1977b), pp. 13–16.

38. M 'Eduy, chap. 4.

39. It should be made clear, however, that the commandment to procreate has another aspect, referred to in the halakhic literature as "[God] formed it for habitation." Its significance pertains to the question of whether the commandment to procreate is fulfilled even if one or both of the children do not survive. To state it differently, is the biblical-law obligation to beget two children, or is it to populate the world? And are we speaking here of a broadening of the commandment to procreate, or are these two separate commandments? If so, it may be that women are bound by "for habitation"; that is, they must bear at least one child who survives, even though they are not bound by the commandment to procreate. See Tosafot, s.v. "*she-ne'emar lo tohu bera'ah*"; BT BB 13a. See also Tosafot on Git. 41b, s.v. "*lo tohu*

bera'ah," which takes the view that a woman, as well as a slave, is subject to the commandment of "for habitation." Later scholars, too, are divided on the issue.

40. See Ellinson (1977b), p. 14, and Feldman (1995), pp. 48–49, regarding this issue.

41. See *Hilkhot Rav Alfas*, Yev. 62b, 19b.

42. See *Ha-ma'or Ha-Gadol* on Rif, ibid.

43. Rosh on Yev. 62b, chap. 6, sec. 9.

44. *The Code of Maimonides*, book 4, "The Book of Women," trans. from the Hebrew by Isaac Klein (New Haven and London: Yale University Press, 1972).

45. In his commentary on *Hilkhot 'Ishut*, R. Jonathan Eibeschutz likewise understands Maimonides in this way. See *Benei 'Ahuvah* 1, *'Ishut* 15:1.

46. *Maggid Mishneh* on *Hilkhot 'Ishut* 15:7.

47. See *Leḥem Mishneh*, ibid., s.v. "*lo yissa 'adam 'aqarah.*"

48. Nahmanides, *Novellae on Yevamot* 62b.

49. See *Tur*, *'Even Ha-'Ezer* 1.

50. M Yev. 6:6.

51. For a broad and systematic treatment of the disinclination to compel performance of the commandment to procreate, see Cohen (1989), chap. 4; Westreich (2002), esp. pp. 50–53, 106–127.

52. See Westreich (2002), p. 173.

53. Maharam Minẓ 1:42.

54. Albeit not with an explicitly permissive ruling to that effect.

55. An exception is R. Solomon Luria, a contemporary of Rama, who disagrees with him and takes the view that a Torah scroll must be sold if necessary to marry a woman who has had children, even if the husband has already fulfilled the commandment to procreate. See *Yam Shel Shelomoh* on *Yevamot*, chap. 6, sec. 27.

56. Taz, *'Even Ha-'Ezer* 1:1; *Beit Shmu'el, 'Even Ha-'Ezer* 1:1; *Birkei Yosef, 'Even Ha-'Ezer* 1:2.

57. Cf. Gen. Rabbah 31:18.

58. See Ran's commentary on Rif, BT Ta'an. 11a.

59. Maimonides, *Mishneh Torah*, *Hilkhot Ta'aniyot* 3:5; *Shulḥan 'Arukh*, *'Oraḥ Ḥayyim* 240:12. In sec. 574, the *Shulḥan 'Arukh* limits the prohibition, requiring a man to engage in intercourse with his wife on the night of her immersion even during times of famine.

60. Annotation to *Shulḥan 'Arukh*, *'Oraḥ Ḥayyim* 240:12: "And that is the rule with regard to other troubles that are like famine." Rama is consistent in his view that the commandment of "in the evening" lacks absolute halakhic force, and he therefore expands the conditions under which one refrains from it, as I showed

earlier in connection with his reference to "family well-being." See Rama on *'Even Ha-'Ezer* 1:8.

61. *Qorban Ha-'Edah* on JT Ta'an. 1:6 (Vilna, 1922).

Chapter 2. Birth Control and Family Planning

1. The Hebrew term here, *sirus*, is often translated "castration." As will be seen, however, it refers to a procedure that may be performed on women as well as on men, so the term "neutering" will be used except where the reference is more specific.

2. See Steinberg (2003), vol. 1, pp. 123–140.

3. See also T [Zuckermandel] Mak. 5:6.

4. The term "drinking roots" or "a cup of roots," here usually translated as "a sterilizing potion," evidently refers to a beverage that was known to prevent pregnancy or induce early abortion because of its poisonous quality. Some believe it caused permanent sterilization. The term appears at M Shab. 14:3, and the composition of the beverage is mentioned at BT Shab. 110a. See also Rashi and Malbim on Gen. 4:19. The Hebrew term itself (*'iqqarin*) is variously associated with the sterilization (*'iqqur*) caused by the plant root (*'iqqar* in Aramaic) from which it is made; the roots are able to prevent ovulation (see Steinberg [2003], vol. 1, pp. 248–249). See also Jakobovits (1975), p. 162, n. 64.

5. *Tosefta Ki-Feshuta, Yevamot*, pp. 67–70. That reading of the Tosefta also appears in the *Maggid Mishneh* commentary on Maimonides's *Mishneh Torah, Hilkhot 'Issurei Bi'ah* 16:2, and in the *Beit Yosef* on the *Tur, 'Even Ha-'Ezer* 5:12.

6. See BT Shab. 111a in the Schottenstein edition and Naḥmanides's novellae on BT Shab. 110b.

7. BT Yev. 65b.

8. Tosafot on BT Shab. 110b, s.v. "*ve-ha Tanya.*" This conclusion is reiterated by Tosafot later in the passage; see ibid., s.v. "*Bi-zeqeinah u-ve-'aqarah.*"

9. See., e.g., *Yabi'a 'Omer* 8, *'Even Ha-'Ezer* 14, and sources cited there.

10. Maimonides, *Mishneh Torah, Hilkhot 'Issurei Bi'ah* 16:11.

11. Maggid Mishneh, ibid., s.v. "ha-mashqeh 'iqqarin."

12. *Sefer Miẓvot Gadol*, neg. comm. 120; *Tur, 'Even Ha-'Ezer* 5.

13. *Shulḥan 'Arukh, 'Even Ha-'Ezer* 5:11–12.

14. *Sefer Miẓvot Gadol*, neg. comm. 120.

15. Commentary of the Gra on *Shulḥan 'Arukh, 'Even Ha-'Ezer* 5:28.

16. See, for example, the comments of Rabbi Breisch, who questions that ruling: *Ḥelqat Ya'aqov, 'Even Ha-'Ezer* 61:5.

17. That is the case at least over the last two centuries. See *Ḥatam Sofer*, part 6, *Liqqutim* 40; *Torat Ḥesed, 'Even Ha-'Ezer* 44.

18. For discussion of just what a *mokh* is, see *Tur*, *'Oraḥ Ḥayyim*, sec. 264. R. Isaac b. Moses, author of *'Or Zaru'a*, writes as follows: "The people of Lombardy state that cotton wool is a form of grass, having nothing in common with flax or hemp; it is a sort of fruit that grows from the grass as a sort of nut, within which is the cotton wool; its roots and leaves are entirely grass. And the *'Arukh* states that a *mokh* is "cotton wool" (*Hilkhot 'Erev Shabbat* 40). Following the lead of several decisors, Rosner (2000), p. 84, identifies the *mokh* with the modern diaphragm.

19. The prohibition on wasting seed is a highly complex issue with implications for male birth control mechanisms as well. I cannot deal with it in detail here, though it will come up marginally because it has been inextricably linked, since the medieval authorities, to discussions regarding use of a *mokh*.

20. In BT Yev. 34b, in a discussion of Onan's actions (Gen. 38), the opinion regarding "treads inside and sows outside" is attributed to Rabbi Eliezer.

21. That is, the new fetus that results from intercourse may impair the development of the existing one. See Rashi on BT Yev. 12b: "*Sandal*—a fetus whose face is not formed."

22. Parallel passages appear at BT Ket. 39a; BT Yev. 100a; BT Nid. 45a; BT Ned. 35b (this passage considers only the case of a minor).

23. Thus the version in ms. Munich (95) (Leiden, 1912) and in the first printing.

24. Albeit not great danger: in the case of the pregnant woman, the danger is only to the fetus; in the case of the minor, it might be argued that her ability to conceive indicates she is mature enough to bear the pregnancy safely; and in the case of the nursing mother, pregnancy is usually prevented by nursing (though not in all cases). The three situations are alike in that none involves unambiguous mortal danger. On mortal danger with connection to this *baraita* see Meacham (2009b).

25. See BT Nid. 3a, from which we can draw at least one clear inference: a *mokh* is mentioned as an everyday item, without any reference to particular categories of women who use it, as mentioned by Feldman (1995). See also BT Yev. 42a; BT Yev. 34b.

26. Tosafot on BT Meg. 13b note that Esther used a *mokh* in her relations with Ahasuerus.

27. Quoted in Harkavy (1887), p. 169.

28. See Rashi "Use a *mokh* in intercourse" on BT Yev. 12b; BT Ket. 37a, 39a: BT Nid. 3a, 45a.

29. Many responsa by later authorities discuss Rashi's surprising attribution to the sages of the view that one is permitted to expose oneself to a not-insignificant degree of danger. See, for example, *Divrei Yissakhar*, *'Even Ha-'Eezer* 138; Radbaz, part 3, no. 596; *Penei Yehoshu'a* on BT Ket. 39a; *'Aḥi'ezer*, *'Even Ha-'Ezer* 23.

30. *'Avnei Nezer* infers that all decisors who follow Rashi believe he forbade a

postcoital *mokh* as well. See *'Avnei Nezer, 'Even Ha-'Ezer* 81. According to the *Ḥatam Sofer* (*Yoreh De'ah*, 172), Rashi referred specifically to a precoital *mokh* because a postcoital *mokh*'s "medical efficacy is not confirmed."

31. See Urbach (1980), pp. 625–629, who determines that while R. Eliezer of Touques edited the Tosafot on *Ketubbot*, his original source was the Tosafot of Sens. I am grateful to Dr. Rami Reiner for this reference.

32. Tosafot on BT Meg. 13b supports the view that Rabbeinu Tam held the view that all women are permitted to use a *mokh*.

33. Urbach (1980), pp. 620–621.

34. This exegetical intuition is shared by some of the later authorities; see *Torat Ḥesed, 'Even Ha-'Ezer* 44, par. 15–20, and *Mishpetei 'Uzi'el, 'Even Ha-'Ezer* 43.

35. See Feldman (1995), pp. 194–198. See *Torat Ḥesed, 'Even Ha-'Ezer* 44; *Mishpetei 'Uzi'el, 'Even Ha-'Ezer* 2:16. These authorities largely harmonized Rashi's view and Rabbeinu Tam's but declined to rule decisively because of their different understanding of the medievals.

36. See *Ḥiddushei Ha-Ramban Ha-Shalem* [Complete novellae of Naḥmanides], *Ketubbot* 39a, s.v. "*ve-zeh leshon Ha-Ramban zal shalosh nashim meshameshot be-mokh*"; novellae of Naḥmanides on BT Nid. 13a, s.v. "*nashim de-lav benot hargashah ninhu meshubaḥat*"; novellae of Rashba on BT Yev. 12b and Nid. 13a; novellae of Ritva on BT Yev. 12b, s.v. "*shalosh nashim meshameshot be-mokh*" and Ket. 39a; *Beit Ha-Beḥirah* on BT Yev. 12b; novellae of Ran on BT Ket. 39a; *Tosafot Ha-Rosh* on BT Yev. 12b, s.v. "*shalosh nashim meshameshot be-mokh*"; Rosh on BT Ned. 35b, s.v. "*shalosh nashim meshameshot be-mokh*"; *Tosafot Ha-Rosh* on BT Nid. 3b, s.v. "*meshameshot be-mokh*"; *Teshuvot Ha-Rosh, kelal* 33, 3, s.v. "*ve-she-sha'alta.*" Rosh, too, rejects Rashi's interpretation, but he is inconsistent with respect to whether use of the *mokh* is precoital or postcoital. His comments on *Nedarim* and his responsum allow the inference (though not requiring it) that he permits precoital use, but his addenda to *Yevamot* and his interpretation of *Niddah* suggest that he permits only postcoital use.

37. The claim that many of the medieval authorities prohibit postcoital use of a *mokh* is rejected by many of the later authorities. See, for example, *Divrei Malki'el, 'Even Ha-'Ezer* 70; *Zikhron Yonatan, 'Even Ha-'Ezer* 3.

38. See the analysis in Feldman (1995) of Maimonides's omission, pp. 203–208.

39. See note 36.

40. See *Damaseq 'Eli'ezer, 'Even Ha-'Ezer* 92, disagreeing with him on this point, and *Divrei Malki'el, 'Even Ha-'Ezer* 70, agreeing with him.

41. Some entirely ignore him (I consider that phenomenon below); some disagree with him (such as R. Waldenberg; see below); and some interpret him as referring

only to someone who has already fulfilled the commandment to procreate (*Heikhal Yiẓḥaq*, *'Even Ha-'Ezer* 2:16) or as ruling leniently only in situations where danger is present (Jakobovits [1975], p. 169).

42. Responsa *Ḥatam Sofer*, *Yoreh De'ah* 172. The responsum is undated.

43. Ibid.

44. Part 6 (*Ḥoshen Mishpat, Liqqutim*), 40.

45. *'Even Ha-'Ezer* 20.

46. Rappeld notes that Rama prevailed in his competition with his contemporary, the author of *Yam Shel Shelomo*, and that the latter's ruling remained marginalized. See Rappeld (1990), pp. 217–223. Among other things, he finds (but ultimately rejects) suggestions that Luria's rulings were not accepted because of his forcefully held opinions and eccentric personality.

47. See Feldman (1995), p. 219.

48. See, for example, R. Akiva Eger's *Teshuvot Ḥadashot*, *'Oraḥ Ḥayyim* 5, s.v. "*gam mah*," referring to *Yam Shel Shelomoh* on *Bava Qamma*; *Yoreh De'ah* 12, s.v. "*'akh 'adayyin*," referring to *Yam Shel Shelomoh* on *Yevamot*. It is evident, then, that though the commentary on that tractate was not as widely disseminated as were R. Luria's novellae on other tractates, it was well know to Eger. *Yam Shel Shelomoh* on *Yevamot* was printed twice, in Altona (1740) and again in Statin (1862). Between 1861 and 1862, the entire *Yam Shel Shelomoh* was reprinted. The *Ḥatam Sofer* likewise mentions the *Yam Shel Shelomoh*. See *Ḥatam Sofer*, *Qoveẓ Teshuvot*, sec. 21, s.v. "*'aval ha-kesef meshaneh*" (referring to *Yam Shel Shelomoh* on the chapter known as *Gid Ha-Nasheh*); ibid., sec. 67, s.v. "*ma'alat kevod torato ramaz li*" (referring to *Yam Shel Shelomoh* on *Yevamot*). In the latter context, R. Sofer even notes that "I searched in the *Yam Shel Shelomoh* [on *Yevamot*] and did not find it." See also *Ḥatam Sofer*, part 3 (*'Even Ha-'Ezer* 1), sec. 43: "And the *Yam Shel Shelomoh* at the end of *Yevamot*, sec. 25, expressed surprise at the position of Rosh on this point but did not presume to disagree with him." See also *'Even Ha-'Ezer* 2, sec. 127.

49. See *'Even Ha-'Ezer* 2, sec. 127.

50. That was in 1796. See Katz (1968), p. 129.

51. See Kunstlicher (1993), 314.

52. Part 3, *'Even Ha-'Ezer* 1:20.

53. Part 6, *Liqqutim*, sec. 40.

54. *Yoreh De'ah* 172.

55. See Noonan (1965), chap. 13.

56. On those concerned about the *Ḥatam Sofer*'s ruling, see especially *Maharam Schick*, *Ḥoshen Mishpat* 54 (expressly stating that since the *Ḥatam Sofer* , R. Akiva Eger, and the *Minḥat 'Eliyahu* all forbade use of the *mokh*, "what can we say

after them, and how could we rule contrary to their words?"); *Minḥat 'Eliyahu, 'Even Ha-'Ezer* 2; *Naharei 'Afarsemon, 'Even Ha-'Ezer* 29; *'Avnei Nezer, 'Even Ha-'Ezer* 81. See also Goldstein (1981), in his collected comments on the *Ḥatam Sofer*'s responsa.

57. See *Hit'orerut Teshuvah, 'Even Ha-'Ezer* 17.

58. *Torat Ḥesed, 'Even Ha-'Ezer* 44. For additional responsa adopting similar interpretive options, and permitting precoital use of a *mokh* in instances of danger, see especially *'Or Gadol* 31; *Ḥemdat Shelomoh, 'Even Ha-'Ezer* 46; Maharsham 1:58; *'Aḥi'ezer* 1, *'Even Ha-'Ezer* 23; and *Zikhron Yehonatan, 'Even Ha-'Ezer* 3.

59. The *Zemaḥ Ẓedeq, 'Even Ha-'Ezer* 1:89, follows a similar course, as do *Ḥemdat Shelomoh* (*'Even Ha-'Ezer* 46) and *Minḥat Yeḥi'el* (2:22), who believe that the prohibition against endangering oneself is of biblical authority, based on the verse "Take good care of yourselves" (Deut. 4:15). Accordingly, they say, the intention was to allow sexual relations without a *mokh* where the risk is remote, but where there is genuine danger, miracles are not to be relied on.

60. Rabbi Steinberg is the author of the *Encyclopedia of Jewish Medical Ethics* (Jerusalem and New York: Feldheim, 2003).

61. Steinberg (2003), vol. 1, p. 243.

62. Steinberg (1983), p. 143.

63. Steinberg (2003), vol. 1, p. 247.

64. Steinberg (1983).

65. Ibid., p. 147.

66. Aviner (1984), pp. 35–36.

67. Ibid., p. 35.

68. See, e.g., Kahn (2002), pp. 283–287.

69. See *Ẓiẓ 'Eli'ezer* 9:51; *Sha'ar* 2, chap. 4, sec. 11. Recently, however, controversy has arisen within the medical community regarding the pill's safety.

70. At least not for married women after the commandment to procreate has been fulfilled as a matter of biblical law. I consider below, under the heading "Family Planning," the implications of using the pill before or after fulfillment of the commandment.

71. See *Yehudah Ya'aleh, Yoreh De'ah* 222.

72. Even the *Ḥatam Sofer* believes that only before fulfilling the commandment of "to inhabit" is use of a sterilizing potion restricted to cases of difficult birth; once the commandment has been fulfilled, it may be used even in the absence of difficult birth (*Ḥatam Sofer, 'Even Ha-'Ezer* 1:20). See also *Ḥelqat Ya'aqov, 'Even Ha-'Ezer* 61:5.

73. *'Iggerot Mosheh, 'Even Ha-'Ezer* 1:13.

74. In an article published in 1978, R. Feinstein explained his ruling and noted explicitly that many disagreed with R. Elijah of Vilna. He recognized that he had been strict in his 1955 ruling because "she had been advised to use a *mokh*" (Feinstein [1980], pp. 328–331). He believed that even if most authorities believe the prohibition to be rabbinic only, "not all rabbinic prohibitions are equally subject to waiver in cases of hardship or great need." In other words, because he assigns great importance to a woman's procreative capacity, he is unwilling to forgo it even if the prohibition on doing so is only rabbinic. I believe that to be the idea that underlies his strict ruling.

75. In chronological order: *'Iggerot Mosheh, 'Even Ha-'Ezer* 1:63 (1935); *'Even Ha-'Ezer* 4:70 (1936); *'Even Ha-'Ezer* 1:67 (1951); *'Even Ha-'Ezer* 1:62 (1952); *'Even Ha-'Ezer* 1:13 (1956); *'Even Ha-'Ezer* 1:64 (1958); *'Even Ha-'Ezer* 4:74 (1960); *'Even Ha-'Ezer* 1:65 (1961); *'Even Ha-'Ezer* 1:66 (1961); *'Even Ha-'Ezer* 4:67 (1961); *'Even Ha-'Ezer* 2:17 (1962); *'Even Ha-'Ezer* 3:15 (1965); *'Even Ha-'Ezer* 3:21 (1965); *'Even Ha-'Ezer* 3:22 (1966); *'Even Ha-'Ezer* 3:13 (1972); *'Even Ha-'Ezer* 3:24 (undated); *'Even Ha-'Ezer* 4:72 (1972); *'Even Ha-'Ezer* 4:68 (1978); *'Even Ha-'Ezer* 4:69 (1978); *'Even Ha-'Ezer* 4:71 (1978); *'Even Ha-'Ezer* 4:73 (1981).

76. *'Iggerot Mosheh, 'Even Ha-'Ezer* 4:74.

77. *'Iggerot Mosheh, 'Even Ha-'Ezer* 1:63.

78. In this responsum, R. Feinstein attacks the discussion of birth control mechanisms that had appeared in certain (Torah-oriented) journals and had expressed the view that a *mokh* could be used where danger existed. He determines that a discussion of this sort should not take place before an audience of ordinary people who simply want lenient rulings and who therefore are not debating the issue for the sake of Heaven (that is, in an exalted effort to identify the truth). Interestingly, Rabbi Amsel, editor of *Ha-Ma'or*, identifies his own journal as the target of R. Feinstein's attack. See *Ha-Ma'or*, Tammuz 5722 [1972], p. 7.

79. *'Iggerot Mosheh, 'Even Ha-'Ezer* 4:74.

80. *'Iggerot Mosheh, 'Even Ha-'Ezer* 1:67.

81. *'Iggerot Mosheh, 'Even Ha-'Ezer* 4:68.

82. *'Iggerot Mosheh, 'Even Ha-'Ezer* 4:67.

83. *'Iggerot Mosheh, 'Even Ha-'Ezer* 4:73.

84. *'Iggerot Mosheh, 'Even Ha-'Ezer* 2:17.

85. *'Iggerot Mosheh, 'Even Ha-'Ezer* 4:74.

86. *'Iggerot Mosheh, 'Even Ha-'Ezer* 4:32.

87. *'Iggerot Mosheh, 'Even Ha-'Ezer* 4:72.

88. See, e.g., Ellinson (1977b); Aviner (1984).

89. *Shevet Ha-Levi* 3, 177.

90. *Shevet Ha-Levi* 3, 179.

91. *Divrei Yaẓiv, 'Even Ha-'Ezer* 31.

92. Landau (1979), pp. 23–25.

93. Neubart (2002), p. 135.

94. A detailed discussion of types of Orthodoxy is beyond the scope of this work. The term "National-Ḥaredi," perhaps less familiar than either Ḥaredi or Modern Orthodox, refers to a segment of the Orthodox world that shares the Ḥaredi outlook overall but takes a positive view of the state of Israel and is more actively involved in its society.

95. Aviner (1984), p. 37.

96. See also his later book *'Aḥoti Kallah* (Aviner [2002]), in which he characterizes his decisions as tending to be lenient.

97. Published on the NRG website (offering Hebrew-language daily news), www.nrg.co.il, 22 June 2006.

98. *Benei Banim*, part 1, 30.

99. Ibid., p. 95.

100. *Ẓohar* is a journal published by rabbis associated with Religious Zionism.

101. Levy (2002), pp. 205–216.

102. BT Nid. 9a.

103. Levy (2002), p. 209.

104. In his opinion, most physicians, even the most senior, are unfamiliar with the findings of the studies he cites in his article (ibid., p. 212).

105. Katan (2003), p. 28.

106. Ariel (2002).

107. Ibid., p. 224. The title of R. Kahana's work, *Tahorat Bat Yisra'el*, may be translated "The Purity of the Daughter of Israel."

108. Ibid.

109. Ibid., p. 234.

110. Ibid.

111. Wolfson (2002), pp. 137–140.

112. Ibid., p. 138.

113. Ibid., p. 140.

114. Ellinson (1977b), p. 18. That same year, Ellinson also published an article in the journal *No'am* in which he wrote that the commandment to procreate could not be deferred (Ellinson [1977a]). Asked by Rabbi Henkin about this inconsistency, he said he had changed his mind about what he had written in *No'am*. See Henkin (2003), pp. 149–150.

115. Ellinson (1977b), p. 23.

116. Lichtenstein (1988), p. 29.

117. Among them, a widower with children taking a second wife who is unlikely to be quarrelsome even though she is known to be infertile. See *Terumat Ha-Deshen*, 263.

118. Introduction to Ellinson (1977b).

119. Thereby at least fulfilling the commandment of "to inhabit." See *Be-'Ohalah Shel Torah* 1, *'Even Ha-'Ezer* 66–67.

120. Ibid., p. 338.

121. Ariel (2002), pp. 223–236.

122. Lau (2003), pp. 135–148.

123. Ibid., p. 138.

124. Ibid., p. 143 (emphasis mine).

125. Maharit, part 2, *Yoreh De'ah* 47.

126. See R. Henkin's critical comment on this point in Henkin (2003). Henkin himself permits deferral of the commandment for six months after the wedding (reasoning that the husband is free to choose a career as a sailor, and a sailor is required to engage in conjugal relations with his wife only once every six months) but finds no basis for permitting a longer deferral. I discussed R. Henkin's gender-based ideas earlier, and they are evident here as well.

127. See Knohl (2005), pp. 287 et seq. In a similar vein, see also Y. Sharlo, http://www.kolech.org.il/show.asp?id=32738.

128. Tong (1989), p. 121.

129. Gordin (2005), pp. 102–103 (emphasis mine).

130. Zoloth (2003), pp. 21–53; Kahn (2000).

131. Polatnick observes that one of the reasons men do not want to raise children is that they favor the status, prestige, and power afforded by professional activity in the public sphere—factors that make their way into the power structure within the family as well. See Polatnick (1983).

132. See Foucault (1984).

133. Ibid., pp. 57–58.

Chapter 3. Halakhic Rulings on Abortion: A Historical Survey from the Rabbinic to the Modern Period

1. See, for example, Rudy (1996), p. 110; Dworkin (1995), p. 51. Of course, positions such as these must be seen as exceptions that say nothing about the rule. As a practical matter, their proponents appear not to have remained part of the feminist movement.

2. Singer (1993); Tooley (1989), pp. 45–60; Warren (1989), pp. 75–92.

3. See Singer (1993), pp. 138–143, who refutes every effort to identify definitively the point in a pregnancy that should be used to determine the legitimacy of an abortion. For the contrary view, see Robertson (1994).

4. Dworkin (1995).

5. Ibid., p. 81.

6. Ibid., p. 93.

7. Thomson (1971), pp. 29–44.

8. On abortion from the perspective of gender power relationships in which unwanted pregnancies ensue, see primarily MacKinnon (1989), pp. 184–194.

9. West (1990–91), pp. 43–106.

10. Sherwin (1992).

11. The contemporary dilemmas regarding mercy killing suggest that such equivalence may, in fact, be possible. That brings us back to Dworkin's discussion of the value and sanctity of life as flowing from the very fact that it was given (in the biological sense) or from the human investment embodied within it.

12. Halbertal (1997) has noted that many halakhic midrashim follow a schema in which two interpretive possibilities are presented and the Midrash decides in favor of one of them. This overall model suggests that the Midrash most often does not offer an automatic, unselfconscious reading of the biblical text. Instead, it exercises choice, usually between two possible interpretations, and moral considerations are taken consciously into account.

13. See *Mekhilta De-Rashbi*, pp. 168–169. *Mekhilta De-Ri* likewise understands the word *ason* to refer to the woman, not the fetuses; see *Mekhilta De-Ri, Mishpatim, Masekhta De-Neziqin, Parashah* 8, pp. 275–276.

14. For detailed discussion of Hellenistic exegesis see Irshai (2006).

15. Other versions of the text refer to its head or most of its head emerging. See M 'Ohal. 7:6, "once most of it has emerged"; thus ms. Kaufman (1978), vol. 2, and ms. Parma (De Rossi 138) (1979); M Nid. 3:5, "if it emerged cut or torn, once most of it has emerged, it is as if born; if it emerged normally, once most of [its head; what is most of] its head? Once its forehead has emerged" (per ms. Kaufman, ibid., p. 542); per ms. Parma: "if it emerged normally, once most of its head emerged. What is most of its head? Once its forehead has emerged" (vol. 2, p. 371); JT Sanh. 8:9: "once its head and most it has emerged, it is not touched" (per ms. Leiden [1961], p. 1310; BT Sanh. 72b: "Once its head has emerged, it is not touched" (so, too, ms. Munich [1971], p. 696, and the Venice printing [1920]).

16. See *Ḥasdei David* on T Git. 3:13.

17. T [Zuckermandel] 'Arak. 1:4. The Tosefta requires that the fetus extend its hand as a condition to delaying execution. *Ḥasdei David* on the Tosefta ('Arak. 1:2)

explains that the Tosefta thereby disagrees with the Mishnah, holding that if the mother is simply in labor (but the fetus has not yet extended a hand) the sentence is carried out without delay. The Tosefta thus becomes concerned about the status of the fetus only at an even later stage than does the Mishnah, seeing the fetus as a life only once it has extended a hand but not at the onset of labor.

18. The case is one of adultery, in which both the man and the woman are to be put to death. The seemingly redundant "both of them" (*gam sheneihem*) is understood to include the fetus as well if the adulterous woman is pregnant; her execution need not await delivery of the child.

19. The sources that refer to the fetus as "its mother's limb" include BT Git. 23b; BT Tem. 30b; BT Naz. 51a; BT Ḥul. 58a; BT Sanh. 80b and Tosafot ad loc., s.v. " *'ubar*"; and BT BQ 46b. Urbach notes in this regard that no *tanna* believes the fetus to be a body in its own right or considers it a "life"; the reference in the Babylonian Talmud to a *tanna* who believes the fetus is not its mother's limb is merely a suggestion. As a matter of halakhah, the opinion does not predate the time of the *'amora* R. Yoḥanan. The early view of the *tanna'im* thus was that "a fetus is its mother's limb," though that formulation appears neither in tannaitic sources nor in the Jerusalem Talmud and is not attributed to any of the earlier *'amora'im* in the Babylonian Talmud. See Urbach (1976), pp. 214–218.

20. The source for the rule is M Yoma 8:7—"If a building collapsed on someone [on the Sabbath], and it is uncertain whether or not he is there, the pile of rubble is combed through [in order to rescue him]." The Talmud (BT Yoma 85a–b) cites the views of various *tanna'im* regarding the basis for the rule; among them is that of Rabbi Simeon ben Menasya: "Desecrate one Sabbath on his behalf so he will [survive to] observe many Sabbaths." The *'amora* Samuel explains it on the basis of "*by . . . which man shall live* [Lev. 18:5]—and not by which he shall die" and maintains his explanation is superior to those of the *tanna'im*. In the ensuing discussion, the *gemara* explains, in the name of Rabba, that all the explanations except Samuel's can be refuted. See also T Shab. 15:16.

21. As Urbach says, "there is no indication that the 'mind' of the fetus is taken into account." Urbach (1976), p. 216.

22. See how *Ha-Noda Bi-Yehudah* (*Mahadura Tenina, Ḥoshen Mishpat* 60) understands their dispute as pertaining to the essence of the law of *rodef*. Zohar (1998) argues that the moral basis for the law of *rodef* lies primarily in the attacker's guilt. Accordingly, a minor, a small child, and certainly a fetus that unknowingly endangers another cannot be regarded as a *rodef*.

23. One could understand the *gemara* to be applying the rubric of *rodef* to the *mishnah* in *'Ohalot* and arguing that only at the time of birth itself would the fetus

not be considered a *rodef*, for it is only natural that a fetus endanger the mother as it emerges from the womb. That interpretive option seems a bit farfetched, however, for why, in that case, would it be forbidden to kill the fetus once its head or most of its body has emerged—something the *mishnah* expressly attributes to its at that point being considered a "life"?

24. The text of the printed version is identical to that of ms. Leiden (ed. Zusman).

25. The commentaries have difficulty understanding this turn of phrase and explain that it refers to a minor who was being pursued but gathered his strength and turned the tables, becoming the *rodef* with respect to the person who had initially pursued him. It appears, however, that the text is corrupt and should read "if an adult becomes [pursued by] a minor." See Aptowitzer (1942–43), p. 16, end of note 23. Still, as already noted, the printed edition of the text is identical to that of ms. Leiden, and we have no other manuscript versions that might support the alternative reading. The structure of the sentence, however, suggests that it is dealing with cases in which the tables are turned—the *rodef* becomes the one pursued; the minor pursues the adult. The question posed later in the passage also supports that view—is it permitted to save the adult at the cost of the minor's life? That is, the minor is the *rodef*.

26. For a comprehensive treatment of the status and obligations of Noahides, see, among others, Rakover (1989), pp. 19–57; Broyde (1997); Lichtenstein (1986).

27. The Hebrew *ba-'adam*, translated above as "by man," could also mean "in a man." Rabbi Ishmael appears to understand it that way, as do some versions of the Septuagint: "One who sheds the blood of man in a man, his blood shall be shed."

28. That would not necessarily imply the absence of a biblical prohibition against feticide. Those who posit such a prohibition all concur that one who commits feticide is not subject to capital punishment by a court even though he has violated the prohibition against murder. (One who kills a person who has already been mortally wounded likewise violates the prohibition against murder but is not executed by the court.)

29. Weiss (1904) argues that the prohibition of feticide by Noahides is directed at the Roman practice of killing fetuses with a potion that induces abortion. Aptowitzer (1942–43) disagrees, taking the view that the sages interpreted the verse in an effort to ascertain how to judge Noahides when Israel had the power to do so (p. 28, n. 59).

30. As the talmudic passage unfolds, it becomes clear that that maxim is not without exceptions.

31. The talmudic discussion suggests that for a Jew as well, a trivial taking would

be theft, though the victim would absolve the perpetrator. The distinction strikes me as semantic, for absolution means the act is not considered to be actual theft.

32. Rosh on BT Yoma 8:13. Elsewhere, Rosh defines the fetus as "possibly a life"; see *Shittah Mequbbeẓet* on BT 'Arak. 7a, s.v. "*yashevah 'al ha-mashber.*" A careful analysis of his words, however, shows that the status of "possibly a life" is attributed only to a fetus that has begun to emerge from the womb; otherwise, it would be necessary to defer execution even where the fetus had not begun to emerge, contrary to the Mishnah's ruling. See Soloveitchik A. H. (1998), who understands Rosh in this manner.

33. Ran on Rif, BT Yoma chap. 8, 3b.

34. "Doubt about whether it is alive or dead," according to the *Meqitẓei Nirdamim* edition (Berlin, 1892).

35. *Torat Ha-'Adam, 'Inyan Ha-Sakkanah*, pp. 28–29.

36. See Rosh on BT Yoma 8:13 and his understanding of Naḥmanides.

37. Rosh, ibid., quotes Naḥmanides's comments about the author of *Halakhot Gedolot* almost in their entirety, omitting only his conclusion that *Halakhot Gedolot* allows for the inference that the Sabbath may be desecrated even for a fetus less than forty days after conception, and some have taken this to indicate Rosh's disagreement with Naḥmanides on the point. But Naḥmanides is simply conveying his understanding of the view taken by the author of *Halakhot Gedolot* (who does not expressly make the point himself), and it does not necessarily follow that Naḥmanides himself adopts that view, as some of the later authorities have concluded. Their positions are discussed below.

38. Ritva, in novellae to BT Nid. 44b, agrees with the author of *Halakhot Gedolot* that the Sabbath is desecrated on behalf of the fetus alone but says he does not understand the *Halakhot Gedolot*'s view, as interpreted by Naḥmanides, that the ruling applies as well to a fetus less than forty days from conception (see Ritva, s.v. "*di-khetiv ve-'ish ki yakkeh kol nefesh 'adam,*" especially notes 325 and 326). The authorization to desecrate the Sabbath on account of the fetus's future human potential might be said to have implications for its status in the present, but in his novellae to *Niddah* (see below), Naḥmanides seems to reject that possibility.

39. Naḥmanides, novellae on BT Nid. 44b. This understanding of Naḥmanides's comments is adopted as well by R. Weinberg, *Seridei 'Eish* 3:127, and by Stern (1980). R. Feinstein rejects it outright (*'Iggerot Mosheh, Ḥoshen Mishpat* 2, sec. 69).

40. *Minḥat Ḥinukh, miẓvah* 296, par. 8.

41. *Magen 'Avraham, 'Oraḥ Ḥayyim* 330:15.

42. See Ta-Shma (2000), p. 47.

43. *Semag,* neg. comm. 164.

44. Rabbeinu Beḥye, commentary on the Torah, Deut. 22:26.

45. *Beit Ha-Beḥirah*, BT Yev. 69b.

46. See discussion earlier in this chapter regarding desecration of the Sabbath to save a fetus.

47. Maharit, part 1, nos. 97 and 99.

48. *'Iggerot Mosheh, Ḥoshen Mishpat* 2, 69:3. See also *'Aryeh De-Vei 'Ila'ai, Yoreh De'ah* 19, who does not argue that the second responsum is a forgery but nevertheless believes Maharit maintained the view in the first responsum that feticide is forbidden.

49. For R. Waldenberg's full reconstruction of Maharit's responsum, see *Ziẓ 'Eli'ezer* 9:51, *sha'ar* 3, chap. 3, 1.

50. Ben-Ḥaim (1994). See also Hibner (1969), p. 33, who senses the problematic nature of the second responsum's text but does not treat the contradiction between the two responsa.

51. *Ha-Kenesset Ha-Gedolah, Yoreh De'ah* 280 (on the *Beit Yosef*). The author of *Ha-Kenesset Ha-Gedolah* writes of a scribal error in his teacher's words, but I did not find him to have written of "confusion in the responsa of Maharit." But that does not affect the conclusion that there appears to have been a single responsum whose text became corrupted in printing.

52. *Ẓiẓ 'Eli'ezer, Yoreh De'ah* 100, par. 5.

53. Maharit, part 1, no. 99.

54. *'Emunat Shemu'el* 14.

55. Sometimes translated "bastard," *mamzer* has a much more limited connotation than the English legal term. It refers not to any out-of-wedlock child but specifically to the child of a forbidden (that is, incestuous or adulterous) union. Such a child, according to halakhah, is permitted to marry only another *mamzer*.

56. *Ḥavvot Ya'ir* 31.

57. Ibid.

58. *She'eilat Ya'avez*, 1:43.

59. Ibid.

60. Ibid.

61. A *tereifah* is generally defined as a person who is going to die. See Steinberg (2003), vol. 2, p. 743.

62. *Ha-Noda Bi-Yehudah, Mahadura Tenina, Ḥoshen Mishpat*, sec. 59.

63. Ibid.

64. In other words, these women want to abort a pregnancy not because of concerns about life and limb but for the same reasons that lead many women today

to seek abortions—the difficult burdens of bearing another child or the inappropriateness of a pregnancy at a particular point in their lives. This historical account demonstrates that it is not feminists who "invented" or promoted the need for abortion. The formulation of the question also shows that those women did not make an effort to ask rabbis about the permissibility of the practice at issue, for R. Ayyash writes that "my heart moved me to investigate and look into what I have heard about some women." It also suggests that abortion was a clearly female matter, for which women possessed the needed folk information even without medical intervention.

65. R. Waldenberg notes here that if R. Ayyash did not take the view that the prohibition on feticide was rabbinic only, he would not have been able to permit it in the case of the nursing mother. See *Ẓiẓ 'Eli'ezer* 9, 51, *sha'ar* 3, chap. 3, par. 11. R. Ovadia Yosef, however, takes a different view and understands the *Beit Yehudah* to permit only the drinking of a drug to abort the fetus (under the halakhic rubric of "indirect causation"); but if the feticide is committed directly, the *Beit Yehudah* would regard the violation as biblical. See *Yabi'a 'Omer* 4, *'Even Ha-'Ezer* 1.

66. For listings of those who ruled leniently and those who ruled strictly, see *Sedei Ḥemed, Pe'at Ha-Sadeh, Ma'arekhet Ha-'Alef, Klal 52*; *Ẓiẓ 'Eli'ezer* 9, 51, *sha'ar* 3, chap. 3, par. 11; Steinberg (2003), vol. 1, pp. 4–15. For a comprehensive analysis of the responsa of the later authorities, see Schiff (2002), chap. 4 et seq.

67. See *Sefer Ha-Ḥinukh*, commandment 600; *Shulḥan 'Arukh*, *Ḥoshen Mishpat* 425:2. *'Arukh Ha-Shulḥan, Ḥoshen Mishpat* 425:7, notes the clear contradiction between Maimonides and the *mishnah* in *'Ohalot* and even questions the significance assigned to the emergence of the fetus's head, but he leaves the issues as "requiring inquiry."

68. For a comprehensive review of attitudes toward Maimonides's ideas about the *rodef*, see Stern (1980), pp. 24–51; Feldman (1995), pp. 275–284.

69. See *Koaḥ Shor*, part 1, 20.

70. The work is a collection of seventeenth- and eighteenth-century responsa by a number of sages, including the authors of *Tosafot Yom Tov*, *Bayit Ḥadash*, *Turei Zahav*, and *Maginei Shelomoh*. Each responsum bears the name of its author.

71. The discussion appears at *'Even Ha-'Ezer* 42:17.

72. *'Aḥi'ezer* 3:72.

73. *'Ohel Mosheh* 3, 15:16.

74. Similar positions are taken by Maharam Schick (*Yoreh De'ah* 155) and the author of *Ḥavvot Ya'ir* (31).

75. R. 'Aaron Ha-Levi Soloveitchik (the grandson of R. Ḥayyim of Brisk) sees Maimonides as taking the position that feticide while the woman is in labor would

constitute murder and therefore may be permitted only if the fetus is a *rodef*. He believes his grandfather says nothing contrary to that conclusion, but Rabbis Unterman and Feinstein infer from the comments of R. Ḥayyim of Brisk, as we shall see below, that the fetus is a life even before it begins to move toward emergence. I believe their view is a more straightforward reading of what R. Ḥayyim says. See Soloveitchik A. H. (1998).

76. Soloveitchik Ḥ. H. (1986), *Hilkhot Roẓeiaḥ U-Shemirat Nefesh*, p. 95.

Chapter 4. Abortion in Contemporary Halakhic Rulings

1. See Rafael (1976), p. 5.

2. Unterman (1963).

3. Ibid., p. 1.

4. In *Shevet Mi-Yehudah*, R. Unterman broadly considers issues related to preserving life, including that of desecrating the Sabbath for the sake of a fetus. He concludes, in sum, that it is permissible to desecrate the Sabbath for a fetus, even though it is not considered a life and one who kills it is not subject to capital punishment. He reasons that we consider the future, when the fetus will have become a person; accordingly, the rationale of "so he may observe many Sabbaths" applies in the case of a fetus as well. See ibid., pp. 3–12.

5. Unterman (1963), pp. 5–6.

6. R. Unterman emphasizes that most decisors are of the opinion that the law of saving a life applies to a fetus and it follows that the prohibition of murder bars cutting off its life. Citing Naḥmanides, he asserts that the those who permit desecration of the Sabbath for the sake of a fetus permit it even during the first forty days, "and we find no one who disagrees on this point" (ibid., p. 360). These comments are surprising, for there is disagreement even among the medieval authorities, as we have shown, and some later authorities take the view that Naḥmanides believes the Sabbath is not to be desecrated for the sake of a fetus that has not yet begun to emerge (see *Magen 'Avraham*, *'Orah Ḥayyim* 330:15, and *Ha'ameq She'eilah*'s understanding of Tosafot on BT Nid.). Accordingly, it is not clear how he can say so decisively that there is "no one who disagrees."

7. *Shevet Mi-Yehudah*, p. 357.

8. The only exception is R. Unterman's questioning of R. Emden's opinion regarding a fetus that is a *mamzer*, where he refers to the passage in *'Arakhin* but dismisses it as pertaining to a situation in which the woman's fate has been finally adjudicated; at earlier stages, he believes, the interpreters take the view that the legal proceeding is suspended until she gives birth. Here, too, it is unclear why in principle

the status of the fetus should be affected by whether or not the final verdict against the mother has been issued.

9. Unterman (1963), p. 94.

10. See *'Iggerot Mosheh, Ḥoshen Mishpat* 2:69.

11. See discussion earlier in this chapter regarding the Tosafot's position on the Noahides.

12. This responsum was issued during Sukkot 5737 (that is, in 1976), but the basic decision on the matter is much earlier, going back to 1935. See *'Iggerot Mosheh, Yoreh De'ah*, part 2, 60:2.

13. See *Tif'eret Yisra'el* on M 'Ohal.

14. As I have shown, however, Naḥmanides's wording does not establish that the status of the fetus depends on whether the Sabbath is to be desecrated in order to save it. Moreover, there is no need to understand Naḥmanides himself to believe there is a duty to desecrate the Sabbath for the sake of a fetus.

15. BT 'Arak. 4a.

16. R. Uziel (*Mishpetei 'Uzi'el* 46) offers an interesting refutation of the claim of "scriptural decree." He argues that if it were, in fact, forbidden to kill the fetus, there would be an imbalance between the rule forbidding delaying the mother's execution and the rule forbidding the feticide: transgression of the former involves sitting passively by and not executing her, while transgression of the latter involves the action of killing and is consequently more serious. Those who maintain the existence of the "scriptural decree" would have to say "the prohibition of feticide comes and displaces the prohibition against delaying execution"; but the Talmud in fact reaches the opposite conclusion.

17. See discussion earlier in this chapter regarding the Maharit.

18. Ibid.

19. See 'Iggerot Mosheh Ḥoshen Mishpat 2:69.

20. As I have shown, it may be impossible to infer from the Sabbath desecration discussion anything at all about the status of the fetus, for most of the medieval authorities, with the exception of Naḥmanides's reading of the author of *Halakhot Gedolot*, see no way to isolate danger to the fetus.

21. See, in this regard, R. Waldenberg's penetrating criticism (*Ẓiẓ 'Eli'ezer* 14, 100, par. 2).

22. *Yabi'a 'Omer* 4, *'Even Ha-'Ezer* 1.

23. See Steinberg (2003), vol. 1, p. 10, n. 153.

24. *Shevet Ha-Levi* 9, 266–267.

25. Cited in R. Elyashiv's name by Zilberstein and Rothschild (1987), pp. 408–

409, par. 3. The paragraph begins with a reference to the *Ḥazon 'Ish*, who forbade abortion in a case of danger to the mother's limb (as distinct from her life).

26. Lichtenstein (1974).

27. Ibid.

28. I consider R. Lichtenstein's position further below.

29. *Mishpetei 'Uzi'el, Ḥoshen Mishpat* 46–47.

30. M Nid. 5:3—"If one kills a one-day-old infant, he is liable."

31. *Mishpetei 'Uzi'el, Ḥoshen Mishpat* 46–47.

32. Ibid.

33. It is forbidden to kill another to save one's own life on the premise that no one's "blood is redder" than anyone else's. See BT Pes. 25b. Accordingly, actively taking the life of another to save one's own life is forbidden.

34. *Mishpetei 'Uzi'el, Ḥoshen Mishpat* 46–47.

35. BT Nid. 44a.

36. *Mishpetei 'Uzi'el, Ḥoshen Mishpat* 46–47.

37. *Ẓiz 'Eli'ezer* 7:48—*Quntres 'Orḥot Ha-Mishpatim*, chap. 1, par. 8 (1963); 8:36 (1964); 9:51—*Quntres Refu'ah Ba-Mishpaḥah* (1967). This is the central and most detailed responsum, and I will deal primarily with it. See also 13:102 (1975) (dealing directly with Tay-Sachs disease); 14:100 (1978) (responding to R. Feinstein with respect to Tay-Sachs); 14:101–102 (1978–79) (dealing with amniocentesis and abortion where there is a finding of Down's syndrome).

38. That is how he interprets *Ha-Noda Bi-Yehudah*, the *Ḥavvot Ya'ir*, and *Ge'onei Batra'i*. He sees Maharam Schick, who considers feticide to violate the prohibition on appurtenances of bloodshed, as breaking new ground with that unprecedented opinion (*Ẓiẓ 'Eli'ezer* 9:51, *sha'ar* 3, chap. 1, 14).

39. *'Arukh La-Ner* on BT Sanh. 59a, s.v. "*leika mide'am. ha-kuti she-shavat ḥayyav*."

40. As we saw earlier, he believes Maharit wrote a single responsum (not two seemingly conflicting responsa) and ruled in it that the prohibition on abortion is rabbinic only.

41. See *Ẓiẓ 'Eli'ezer* 9, 51, *sha'ar* 3, chap. 3, the summary of the responsum, par. 15.

42. The absence of any reference to the position or needs of the adulterous man—the father of the fetus—is irrelevant, for there is no need to assume that his adultery, which has no physiological manifestations, will ever be made public. It should be noted as well that in addition to the woman—whether married and adulterous or single, but certainly in a case of rape—there will always be a man who is jointly or solely responsible for the sin. In contrast to the woman, he will not bear the consequences of his sin throughout his life, but that fact, too, is disregarded by the decisors who rule strictly.

43. *She'eilat Ya'avez* 1:43.

44. *Ẓiẓ 'Eli'ezer* 9, 51, *sha'ar* 3, chap. 3, par. 8.

45. R. Waldenberg argues that following R. Emden's reasoning to its logical conclusion would require forbidding abortion even if the woman had been raped—something that made no sense at all to him. He therefore believed that in both cases—the fetus that is a *mamzer* and the woman who was raped—the reason for permitting the abortion is "for great need." See *Ẓiẓ 'Eli'ezer*, ibid.

46. See *Mishpetei 'Uzi'el*, part 3, *Ḥoshen Mishpat* 47.

47. R. Joseph Ḥayyim (author of the *Ben 'Ish Ḥai*) was asked a similar question about aborting a fetus that was a *mamzer*. Though he did not render a decision, his comments suggest he was inclined to rule leniently because the case can be considered one of "great need" (*Rav Pe'alim* 1, *'Even Ha-'Ezer* 4).

48. Zweig (1964), p. 54.

49. Lichtenstein (1977).

50. Published in English as Lichtenstein (1991); originally published in Hebrew as Lichtenstein (1974).

51. "Who among us has not sometimes felt, and been pained by, the ethical poverty of his halakhic sources?" See Lichtenstein (1977), p. 10.

52. I refer here specifically to the modern decisors who are witnesses to advances in embryological medicine and their effects on how fetuses are seen as human beings. It seems to me that stringent rulings in earlier generations were motivated more by a desire to discourage forbidden sexual liaisons than by concern for the fetus's status as an independent being. This is evident, for example, in the *Ḥavvot Ya'ir*, whose author recants his lenient interpretation because of his desire to close "the breaches caused by licentious conduct and those who follow it" (*Ḥavvot Ya'ir* 31).

53. See Noonan (1970), p. 39.

54. For more on the influence of the Church's stand, see Sinclair (2003 English), p. 50.

55. Zweig (1964), pp. 55–56.

56. See *'Iggerot Mosheh*, *Ḥoshen Mishpat* 2:69. R. Feinstein's strict position on abortion predates the women's movement, going back to 1935, but the emphasis on placing a boundary around the Torah in an environment in which legalization of abortion is on the rise suggests that his extreme view, under which abortion is permitted only in cases of certain mortal danger to the mother, should be seen against that background as well. It should be recalled, too, that the family planning movement goes back to the late nineteenth century, and one may assume that the early-twentieth-century feminist activists did not escape R. Feinstein's notice.

57. Chaves (1997), pp. 158–192.

58. His argument supports the feminist contention about the dominant male concept that sees every effort to work for change as a challenge to male hegemony or a diminution in the worth of men.

59. Tzuriel (2005).

60. Ibid., p. 64.

61. Ibid.

62. He enumerates at least twelve decisors who believe the prohibition is rabbinic. See ibid., n. 15.

63. Jakobovits (2000).

64. Ibid., p. 147.

65. In a conversation with R. Prof. Abraham Steinberg (editor of the *Encyclopedia of Jewish Medical Ethics*), I learned that R. Waldenberg attended the hospital's synagogue because of its proximity to his home. People there naturally enough posed to him their halakhic questions with respect to medicine, physicians, and patients, but he was never officially appointed rabbi of the hospital.

66. That is the implication of his responsum on amniocentesis. See *Ẓiẓ 'Eli'ezer* 14, 101.

67. On active euthanasia, see *Ẓiẓ 'Eli'ezer* 8, *Ramat Raḥel*, chap. 29. On passive euthanasia, see *Ziẓ 'Eli'ezer* 14, 80.

68. On chemotherapy during pregnancy, see the exchange of letters between R. Bakshi-Doron and Silberstein (2004). Here, the situation is reversed: the woman wanted to be treated, but the physician objected because of the mortal danger to the fetus and the small likelihood that the therapy would effect a cure. R. Bakshi-Doron justified the physician's refusal to treat, and the stringency reflected in his comments appears consistent with the idea that the woman's life is not regarded as an end in itself. See Bakshi-Doron and Silberstein (2004).

69. According to John Locke, an important shaper of the modern liberal idea, ownership rights over one's body are the paradigm for ownership rights in general. It follows that subjecting an ill person to treatment against his will, even to save his life, partakes of violence. He puts it this way in his *Second Treatise on Government*: "Every man has a property in his own person. This nobody has any right to but himself. The *Labour* of his body, and the *Work* of his hands, we may say, are properly his." See Locke (1988), chap. 5, pp. 287–288.

70. Maimonides, *Mishneh Torah, Hilkhot Roẓeiaḥ* 1:4.

71. See Raziel (1981); Rafael (1992); Sinclair (1999).

72. See Radbaz, *Hilkhot Sanhedrin* 18:6—"For a man's life is not his own property

but that of the Holy One blessed be He, as it is said, 'All lives are mine' (Ezek. 18)." For criticism of the idea, see Zohar (1994).

73. See Zohar (2008).

74. Robertson (1994), p. 48.

75. I assume, for example, that even a sweepingly permissive position would not allow abortion during the eighth month for purposes of research.

76. Sherwin (1992).

77. *'Aqedat Yizḥaq, Bereshit, sha'ar* 9.

78. MacKinnon (1989), p. 186.

79. Greenberg (1976), p. 201.

Chapter 5. Artificial Insemination, In Vitro Fertilization, and Surrogacy in Liberal and Radical Feminist Approaches

1. Tong (1997), pp. 160–162.

2. See the positions of Rosemary and Kass and other theologians and bioethicists in Sherwin (1987), pp. 267–273.

3. Heyd (1992), pp. 221–222.

4. See Stanworth (1987), pp. 1–3.

5. Stanworth (1987); LeMoncheck (1996); Sherwin (1987).

6. See Thompson (2002), p. 52.

7. De Beauvoir (1953).

8. Firestone (1970).

9. See Rowland (1992); Thompson (2002); Oakley (1987); Katz-Rothman (2000); Corea (1985); Corea (1987); Dworkin (1983). This understanding of things implies a very clear agenda: rejection of male technology and advocacy of "natural" birth by and for women.

10. See Rowland (1992), p. 14.

11. Stanworth (1987).

12. Ibid.

13. Dworkin (1983).

14. Ibid., p. 181.

15. Ibid., p. 188.

16. See Corea (1985); Corea (1987); Corea (1988).

17. That is an overstatement with respect to Jewish culture, notwithstanding the contention by Wegner (1988) that the Mishnah treats women more as objects than as persons. For example, even in the past women could own property and could not be compelled to engage in sexual relations against their will.

18. Something similar goes on to this day in India. Low-caste women acting as surrogates primarily for Western couples are housed in special hostels so they may be supervised during their pregnancies. See the film *Google Baby* at http://www.docaviv.co.il.

19. Overall (1987), pp. 137–165.

20. Sherwin (1987), p. 277.

21. Rowland (1992).

22. Katz-Rothman (1984).

23. Rowland (1992), p. 283.

24. Ibid., p. 5.

25. Rowland (1987), p. 84.

26. Ibid., p. 27.

27. For a partial summary of these positions, see Tong (1997), pp. 162–186; Thompson (2002), pp. 61–78.

28. See Sandlowsky in Thompson (2002), p. 62; Berg (1995); Sawicki (1991); LeMoncheck (1996).

29. Berg (1995).

30. Ibid., pp. 84–85.

31. LeMoncheck (1996).

32. Ibid., p. 170.

33. Katz-Rothman (2000).

34. Ibid., p. 161.

35. Ibid., p. 171.

36. Ibid., p. 172.

37. Ibid.

38. Macklin (1988).

39. Pateman (1988), p. 210.

40. Andrews (1988); see also Andrews (1989).

41. Andrews (1988), pp. 168–169.

42. Macklin (1988), pp. 142–143.

43. Ibid., p. 173.

44. Andrews (1988), p. 174.

45. Ibid., pp. 176–178.

46. In full surrogacy, as noted, the parents contracting for the service are the providers of the genetic material, both sperm and egg.

47. See Macklin (1988).

Chapter 6. Artificial Insemination, In Vitro Fertilization, and Surrogacy: Halakhic Analysis

1. Some writers doubted in general whether an artificial insemination procedure could ever be effective. See *Zofnat Paneiaḥ* 138.

2. Those who forbid the practice include *Divrei Malki'el*, part 4, 107–108; *Mishpetei 'Uzi'el*, *'Even Ha-'Ezer* 19; *Yaskil 'Avdi*, part 5, *'Even Ha-'Ezer* 10. R. Waldenberg takes an intermediate position, though tending to forbid the practice; see *Ẓiẓ 'Eli'ezer* 3:27, 9:51, 13:97, 14:98, 15:45, 19:57, 20:58, 22:57. Most other decisors, in contrast, permit artificial insemination with sperm from the husband. See *Maharsham*, part 3, 268, who permits it in exigent circumstances if the husband secures the assent of two eminent rabbis; *Zeqan 'Aharon*, part 2, 97; *Peri Ha-Sadeh*, part 3, 53; *'Emeq Halakhah*, part 1, 68; *Sitri U-Magini* 2:45; *'Aḥi'ezer* 3:24; *Minḥat Shelomoh Tenina* (2–3), 124 (also printed in *No'am* 1, pp. 145–167); *'Iggerot Mosheh*, *'Even Ha-'Ezer*, part 1, 71; part 2, 11, 18; part 4, 32, par. 5; *Seridei 'Eish*, part 3, 5; *Yabi'a 'Omer*, part 2, *'Even Ha-'Ezer* 1; Goren (2001), pp. 163–168; *Minḥat Yiẓḥaq*, part 1, 50 (in part 3, 108, he permits the practice but only after receiving a second opinion); *'Ohel Mosheh*, part 3, 10, sec. 20–24; *Shevet Ha-Levi*, part 8, 251:10, 11 (permitting artificial insemination with sperm from the husband but only until the commandment to procreate has been fulfilled as a matter of biblical law; see also ibid., part 9, *Yoreh De'ah* 209; part 3, 175:2, 176); *'Aparqsata De-'Anya* 1:201. The effort to arrive at results based on the response of R. Jacob Emden suggests that his approach can provide a basis for restrictive and permissive rulings alike. See *She'ilat Ya'aveẓ*, part 1, 4; part 2, 97.

3. *Mishpetei 'Uzi'el* 19.

4. *Sha'arei 'Uzi'el* 2, *sha'ar 41*.

5. *Divrei Malki'el* 4:107.

6. *Yaskil 'Avdi*, *'Even Ha-'Ezer* 5, sec. 10, par. 4.

7. Ibid., par. 8.

8. *Ẓiẓ 'Eli'ezer* 9:51, *sha'ar* 4. Sinclair (2003 Hebrew), p. 16, n. 5, and Breitowitz (2003) include R. Waldenberg among those who forbid AIH, but I do not believe his position is unambiguously negative. In a later responsum, issued in 1997, he expressly writes: "now, what it is possible to permit is injection of the husband's seed directly into the wife's womb, but if the seed is from another man, it is absolutely forbidden" (*Ẓiẓ 'Eli'ezer* 22:57). It certainly is evident in *Ẓiẓ 'Eli'ezer* 15:45 that he qualifies that position substantially, for he writes that everything should be done to avoid the resort to AIH, but even there he does not unambiguously forbid the practice.

9. *Mishpetei 'Uzi'el, 'Even Ha-'Ezer*, part 2, 42.

10. Ibid.

11. It therefore appears that the view of R. Ovadia Hedaya—who believes emission of seed is permissible solely in the natural manner—is more coherent than that of those decisors who permit emission of seed for medical purposes but not for AIH.

12. Only after the fact, of course, for in the view of those who rule strictly, the donor would be violating the prohibition on wasteful emission of seed even if the prohibition did not apply to a husband emitting seed for medical purposes.

13. *Yabi'a 'Omer, 'Even Ha-'Ezer* 2:1.

14. Some infer the prohibition of wasting seed from the prohibition of adultery; and "adultery committed with one's hand" (that is, actively) violates the prohibition even if done for the purpose of fulfilling the commandment to procreate. See *'Iggerot Mosheh, 'Even Ha-'Ezer* 70–71; if there is no alternative, he allows capture of the semen through use of a condom. So, too, *Minḥat Yiẓḥaq* 3:108; *Zeqan 'Aharon* 2:97.

15. There are, of course, a number of obvious ways in which the problem could be resolved. One might allow any one donor to provide sperm for only one recipient; alternatively, one might openly recognize the donor's biological and legal paternity (albeit thereby compromising his anonymity) while seeing the woman's husband as the adoptive father for all purposes. See Zohar (1989), p. 92.

16. See Ross (1998) and her extensive discussion of the exegetical treatment of the verse, of Naḥmanides's comments, and of the decisional literature (pp. 48–53).

17. It may be, however, that she is forbidden to marry the priest because of his elevated degree of sanctity though she herself has committed no sin and certainly has not committed adultery.

18. Rashi on BT Shab. 151a, s.v. "*u-shemu'el 'amar ḥaishinan shema ḥuẓ la-ḥomah.*"

19. Tosafot on BT Ket. 6b, s.v. "*rov beqi'in hen*"; BT Nid. 64b, s.v. "*shani shemu'el de-rav guvreih*"; BT Ḥag. 14b, s.v. "*betulah she-'ibrah ma-hu le-kohen gadol.*"

20. See the suggestion of Firer (1963) that the three passages in Tosafot be reconciled by means of a verbal emendation offered by the *Baḥ* in his annotations to BT *Ḥagigah*.

21. That is the conclusion reached by R. Waldenberg; see *Ẓiẓ 'Eli'ezer* 3:27. *Mishneh La-Melekh* on Maimonides (*Mishneh Torah, Hilkhot 'Issurei Bi'ah* 17:13) believes that Ben Zoma should be understood to mean that if men like Samuel were not unusual, the woman would be permitted to marry the High Priest even though she had had sexual relations inasmuch as the hymen was still intact. That said, *Mishneh La-Melekh* does not believe Ben Zoma's comments represent the halakhah.

22. For a parallel text, see BT Yev. 37b. Goren (2001, pp. 184–186) argues that the

concern about *mamzer*s resulting from sperm donation by a Jew is even more severe because there are men who sell their semen to physicians and there is no way to know who the donor is in any given case (unlike in the case of R. Eliezer b. Jacob, where the list was at least limited). He therefore forbids insemination with sperm from a Jewish donor in all cases.

23. That statement should be qualified and limited to donations from sperm banks. In principle, there could be a direct donation from an identified man.

24. The legend regarding Ben Sira's birth, mentioned in a number of places, tells that his mother was the daughter of the prophet Jeremiah, who was impregnated by her father's seed when she bathed after him in the same tub. See *Sefer Maharil* (*Liqqutim*) 5 and note ibid.; Eisenstein (1952), p. 79. The decisors differ in their views of the legend's authenticity; their views parallel those on whether artificial insemination is permitted. R. Ovadia Yosef (*Yabi'a 'Omer*, part 8, *'Even Ha-'Ezer* 21) believes the legend should not be disregarded; in contrast, R. Waldenberg (*Ẓiẓ 'Eli'ezer* 9:51, *Quntres Refu'ah Ba-Mishpaḥah*, *sha'ar* 4, par. 9) believes there is reason for skepticism. See also *Tashbeẓ* 3:263.

25. This responsum is cited in his annotations to *Sefer Miẓvot Qatan* and quoted in *Baḥ*, *Yoreh De'ah* 195:5. In connection with this version, see also *Beit Shmu'el* on *Shulḥan 'Arukh*, *'Even Ha-'Ezer* 1:10; *Taz* on *Shulḥan 'Arukh*, *Yoreh De'ah* 195:7; *Birkei Yosef*, *'Even Ha-'Ezer* 1:14.

26. That is also the conclusion of *Mishneh La-Melekh* on Maimonides, *Mishneh Torah*, *Hilkhot 'Ishut* 15:4. R. Jonathan Eibeschutz disagrees with *Mishneh La-Melekh* and believes that the cited comment by *Sefer Miẓvot Qatan* does not warrant the inference that insemination by sperm left on a sheet or in a tub by a man other than her husband would be permitted (that is, not result in a *mamzer*). See *Benei 'Ahuvah*, part 1, *Hilkhot 'Ishut* 15:1.

27. Statement by Rabba at BT Yev. 42a.

28. The legend about Ben Sira supports this premise, for Jeremiah was recognized as his father.

29. This concern is pertinent regardless of whether the woman is married or single.

30. Goren (2001) questions that premise, believing that even if paternity were clearly to be attributed to the sperm donor, there still would be doubt about whether he had thereby fulfilled the commandment to procreate, since the pregnancy would not be the direct result of his act.

31. See, e.g., *Divrei Malki'el*, part 4, sec. 107–108.

32. See Corinaldi (1992–94).

33. Part 3, 263.

34. *Birkei Yosef, 'Even Ha-'Ezer* 1:14. See also Ross (1998), p. 57. Goren (2001, p. 165) finds clear proof in Tosafot on BT Yev. 12b, s.v. "*de-'afilu*," that the fetus is considered the child of the sperm donor.

35. M Qid. 4:2.

36. See Ross (1998), pp. 58–59; Sinclair (2003 English), p. 21, n. 41.

37. Almost all agree that artificial insemination with sperm from a Jewish donor is halakhically forbidden. But see the different view, albeit in an unusual case, of R. Saul Yisraeli (in Shafran [1999]), who permitted use of sperm from a Jewish donor on condition that his identity be made known to the couple and that the husband's semen not be mixed with the donor's. See also R. Sharlo, http://www.ypt.co.il/show.asp?id=22400.

38. R. Wosner, for example, permits AIH but believes any penetration of a woman's body by sperm other than her husband's is forbidden as a matter of biblical law (though not a capital offense or one punished by excision, given that the element of intercourse is lacking). See *Shevet Ha-Levi*, part 3, 175, par. 2.

39. Deut. 7:3–4.

40. *'Iggerot Mosheh, 'Even Ha-'Ezer* 1:71.

41. See, e.g., Auerbach (1958), pp. 145–166, who as early as 1958 considered the matter and permitted artificial insemination with sperm from a gentile donor.

42. The letter appears in Friedman (1968), p. 34. There is a reasonable basis, however, for believing it to be a forgery, given that in his responsa he stresses that he did not change his mind. See the discussion below.

43. See above, note 2.

44. Bloch (1965), p. 3.

45. Ibid.

46. Ibid., p. 4. It is worth noting that in his comments here, R. Bloch assumes that the definition of forbidden unions entails childbearing—an assumption close to the one that is to be proven.

47. The Bible allows for *ḥaliẓah*—a ritual involving certain recitations and actions—as a less-favored alternative to *yibbum* (levirate marriage), in which the widow is obligated to marry the surviving brother so as to bear a child who is regarded as continuing her late husband's line. Nowadays, *ḥaliẓah* is primary and *yibbum* rarely if ever takes place—*translator's note.*

48. *Ḥelqat Ya'aqov, 'Even Ha-'Ezer* 14, par. 3. R. Auerbach (1958, p. 162) says the exact opposite.

49. See, e.g., a number of articles published in that journal during 1964 and 1965, especially Sternbuch (1965), who writes: "And in a case where God's Name is desecrated, we do not extend [the customary] honor to a rabbi; on the contrary,

the greatest honor would be to nullify the permissive ruling as something insubstantial."

50. See Amsel (1965), p. 10.

51. See also *'Iggerot Mosheh, 'Even Ha-'Ezer* 3:14.

52. That is how he was understood by R. Ovadia Yosef (*Yabi'a 'Omer*, part 8, *'Even Ha-'Ezer* 21) and by Rabbi Waldenberg (*Ẓiẓ 'Eli'ezer*, part 9, *sha'ar* 4, chap. 5, par. 4), but one might say that the concern is obviated if the husband explicitly consents to use of the procedure. Zohar (1989) and Ross (1998) would assign little value to R. Feinstein's "capitulation letter," as Zohar terms it, inasmuch as R. Feinstein goes on to reiterate emphatically his fundamental position that insemination with sperm from a gentile donor is permitted. That is also the view of Breitowitz (2003).

53. On the status of the child born to a single woman through artificial insemination, see the differing views of Ralbag (2004) and Epstein (2004). R. Ralbag maintains that a child born in this way is entirely fit to marry a Jew (pp. 144–146).

54. He writes explicitly that there is no need for concern here about wasteful emission of seed inasmuch as all the semen is inserted into the woman's womb. See *Ẓiẓ 'Eli'ezer* 15:45.

55. *'Eifer* (dust) is an anagram of *pe'er* (glory).

56. Cf. the comments above of Bloch (1965), p. 305.

57. See Zohar (1989) and Zohar (1997).

58. It may be argued that his reservations about AIH stem from a concern that it might lead to the use of sperm from other donors, but that is uncertain, for the reasons discussed below.

59. With the exception, noted earlier, of R. Yisraeli, who permits it in some extraordinary cases.

60. See also the lenient view of R. Ẓvi Hirsch Grodzinski, who believes use of sperm donated by a gentile is permitted because gentiles are not subject to the commandment to procreate and therefore not bound by any prohibition on wasting their seed. Grodzinski (1988), pp. 153–54.

61. BT Sot. 27a; Maimonides, *Mishneh Torah, Hilkhot 'Issurei Bi'ah* 15:20; *Shulḥan 'Arukh, 'Even Ha-'Ezer* 4:15. Regarding this presumption, see also Schiffman (1989), p. 24; Schereschewsky (1993), pp. 360–366; Green (1995).

62. Shereshevsky (1993), pp. 360–361.

63. On this, see Ben-Refael et al. (1993), pp. 188–190, and, for more detail, Levine and Safran (1995), pp. 28–30.

64. *Yaskil 'Avdi, 'Even Ha-'Ezer* 5:10.

65. By their very nature, the procedures differ in the extent to which they lend themselves to oversight. In artificial insemination, very little time elapses between

the collection of the sperm and its implantation into the woman's body. (The sperm can remain alive for up to forty-eight hours, but the process can be completed as soon as the sperm is emitted by the husband.) In IVF, however, the interval between receiving the sperm and egg and returning the fertilized egg to the woman's body can range between one day and three days, during which the sperm undergoes enhancement processes. The medical literature reports on cases of abuse in this area; see Grazi 2005, pp. 19–23.

66. See *Ẓiẓ 'Eli'ezer* 15:45, 19:40, 20:49.

67. *Ẓiẓ 'Eli'ezer* 20:49.

68. Sternbuch (1987).

69. Ibid., p. 31.

70. Amsel (1978), p. 44.

71. See also, among the leading Ashkenazi decisors who rule permissively, the position of R. Yosef Shalom Elyashiv, cited in Grazi (2005), p. 22.

72. See also *Yabi'a 'Omer*, part 7, *Yoreh De'ah* 24 (par. 5).

73. R. Goren permits the practice under limited conditions meant to ensure that the eggs and sperm that are used are, in fact, exclusively those of the couple. The conditions include a requirement that only one IVF procedure take place at any one time and place and that IVF not be performed at a site where a sperm bank is maintained. See Goren (2001), p. 171.

74. See ibid., pp. 168–172.

75. Ibid., p. 169.

76. Gershuni (1979), p. 21.

77. Breitowitz therefore believes that he permits artificial insemination. See Breitowitz (2003), p. 34, n. 11.

78. *Be-'Ohalah Shel Torah*, pp. 341–348.

79. There could, however, be disagreement over whether to permit IVF after the commandment to procreate has already been fulfilled as a matter of biblical law, given the concern over possible wasteful emission of seed. See Breitowitz (2003), p. 34, n. 11.

80. For the simple reason that sperm donation is more widespread.

81. On the question of the Jewishness of the fetus in cases of surrogacy or egg donation by a gentile woman, see Breitowitz (2003), pp. 65–74.

82. *Nishmat 'Avraham* 4, p. 184.

83. *Nishmat 'Avraham* 4, p. 186.

84. The Israeli Chief Rabbinate assented to surrogacy arrangements subject to a number of conditions. Among others, the surrogate must be unmarried; she must

not be a close relative of the father (that is, one who would be forbidden to marry him); and the egg donor and surrogate must be registered to avoid any possibility of the offspring marrying someone forbidden by reason of family relation. For the full list of conditions, see Breitowitz (2003), pp. 63–64.

85. Schiffman (1989), p. 132.

86. Ibid.

87. It is not entirely clear, however, that this sort of thinking is beyond the halakhic pale. While biological fatherhood remains dominant within the halakhic analysis, biological motherhood is not necessarily the rule; most decisors hold the gestational mother to be the halakhic mother. See in this context the position taken by Zohar (1997), especially his analysis of R. Uziel's views. If one adopts R. Uziel's radical emphasis on human action over genetics—in the absence of intercourse, the child is not halakhically ascribed to its genetic father—it becomes possible to imagine that human actions other than sexual intercourse might be regarded as a basis for parenthood.

88. Goren (2001), p. 177.

89. Ibid., pp. 173–183.

90. Ibid., p. 179.

91. Ibid., p. 183.

92. Ibid.

93. Ibid., p. 184.

94. In this context, Tong (1997, p. 171) reports that current studies show that it is sperm donors who donated anonymously who are interested in finding out if they have become fathers, and many of them are prepared to provide information, both to the recipients of the donation and to the children who resulted from it. It therefore is unclear whether a policy of anonymity in fact works to the donors' benefit.

95. R. Goren may be concerned that disclosing the identity of sperm donors may reduce the size of the donor pool and indirectly diminish the opportunities for artificial insemination or IVF.

96. R. Ariel bases his position on Rashi's understanding of the passage in BT Yev. 98a. See *Be-'Ohalah Shel Torah 'Even Ha'Ezer*, 70.

97. A female who converted to Judaism at the age of three or older may not marry a *kohen*.

98. Feminist criticism has already noted the problematic aspects of using sperm separation technology in a patriarchal society and the harsh consequences that might ensue with regard to favoring the birth of sons over the birth of daughters. See especially Holmes and Hoskins (1987); Rowland (1987), pp. 81–86. Nor is the

Jewish tradition free of that sort of preference; see, for example, Tosafot *had mi-qamai* on BT Yev. 61b, s.v. "*And we learned that the House of Hillel said a male and a female*. But the House of Shammai [say] one fulfills the commandment to procreate by begetting two males, *for males are preferred to females*" (emphasis mine). Nevertheless, it should be noted that the decisors generally do not permit sperm separation in order to determine fetal gender, albeit their rationale is to avoid wastage of seed. See *Nishmat 'Avraham* 4, *'Even Ha-'Ezer*, pp. 179–180.

99. Goldberg (1984a), and compare R. Kilav in Goldberg (1984b). Both of them believe that if both women—the egg donor and the bearer of the pregnancy—are Jews, it is the bearer of the pregnancy who is considered the mother of the offspring. They differ only on whether the child requires conversion in the event the genetic mother is gentile.

100. *Be-'Ohalah Shel Torah*, *'Even Ha-'Ezer* 70, p. 352; Halperin (1999), p. 131. See also Katz (1992).

101. Bick (1986), pp. 267–268.

102. Bick (1997), p. 84.

103. Lev (1989).

104. See *Beit Ha-'Oẓar*, part 1, *ma'arekhet* 1–2, *kelal* 4, s.v. "*avi*."

105. Ibid., p. 28.

106. Halperin (1993), p. 130.

107. *'Even Yeqarah* 29.

108. *'Orlah* refers to fruit that grows during a tree's first three years; biblical law forbids eating it. During the fourth year, the fruit is brought to Jerusalem and eaten there in a state of ritual purity.

109. See Halperin (1993), p. 129, and his halakhic comments on that reasoning.

110. *Ẓiẓ 'Eli'ezer* 19:40, 20:49.

111. "New grain" (*ḥadash*) refers to produce of the new grain harvest. It may not be used until after the time for the *'omer* ceremony.

112. Lev (1989), pp. 153–160.

113. The comparison to a fertilized ovum is not relevant here, for without growth to one-third size, the stalk is considered to be destroyed (cf. Rashi ad loc.).

114. The *'omer* is the grain sacrifice at the start of the barley harvest in the Land of Israel. The time for bringing it is described as "the day after the Sabbath"; according to rabbinic interpretation, this means the day after the first day of Passover, that is, 16 Nisan. Bringing the *'omer* allows use of the *ḥadash*, the new year's harvest of all five species of grain.

115. Lev (1989) reports that R. Auerbach contacted him and said he agreed with

him even though it is difficult to draw a conclusive analogy from a stalk of grain to a living person with a soul.

116. Lichtenstein (1977).

117. It should be noted that R. Yuval Sharlo is among the few to at least recognize the problem and to acknowledge that the halakhah has yet to begin to deal with the complex ethical questions raised by fertility treatments. Regarding the ethical issues related to surrogacy, for example, he writes as follows: "It appears that this question has not yet been examined in depth from the perspective of Judaism." See Sharlo (2009) p. 248. See also the discussion by Grazi and Wolowelsky, who consider the novel ethical issues raised by modern reproductive technologies. Grazi (2005), pp. 409–440.

118. A few writers have noted the illogic of drawing analogies between the question of motherhood and laws pertaining to monetary or agricultural matters. See, for example, Herschler (1980), p. 308; Lev (1989).

119. See Goren (2001), p. 183.

120. It may be argued, however, that the distinction has a logical basis, in that a single sperm donation can easily impregnate numerous women but egg donation, by its very nature (the procedure is an invasive one), is more limited and less subject to wide dispersal of any one woman's genetic material. Accordingly, the concern about tracing a sperm donation is greater than that about tracing an egg donation.

121. R. Waldenberg explicitly says as much: "It seems clear, in my humble opinion, that we look primarily to birthing, and she who bears the infant is the infant's mother . . . and since that is the case, there is no longer any concern that a brother might wind up marrying his sister" (*Ẓiẓ 'Eli'ezer* 20:49).

122. The only book I am aware of that deals comprehensively with reproduction and sees fit to include an article on adoption (by R. Soloveitchik) is Grazi (2005), pp. 101–104. That inclusion stands out prominently against the widespread disregard of attention in the halakhic literature on reproduction to adoption as a legitimate and practical alternative; it is an exception that does not prove the rule.

Afterword. The Gender Project in the Philosophy of Halakhah as an Exercise in Criticism

1. Benjamin (1968).

2. See Ben-Menaḥem (1994).

3. Rusinak (2005), p. 411.

4. Ben-Menahem (1994), p. 128.

5. See Irshai (2010).

6. See Bartlett (1990), pp. 846–847.

7. See Irshai (in press).

8. Cover (1983).

9. On the application of Cover's perspective to a feminist, Jewish-halakhic understanding of law, see Tamar Ross (2001), pp. 731–742; Adler (1998).

10. Ross (1993).

Bibliography

Biographical information for the sections headed "Responsa Literature" and "Primary Sources" is taken for the most part from *Mif'al Ha-Bibliografiyah Ha-'Ivri* (Hebrew Bibliographical Project), sponsored by the Hebrew University, the Israeli Ministry of Education, and E.P.I. Publishers; and from the Bar-Ilan University Responsa Project. Except as otherwise noted, all items in these sections are in Hebrew; translations appearing in the text are by the present translator.

RESPONSA LITERATURE

'Aḥi'ezer Ḥayyim Ozer Grodzinsky (Lithuania, 1863–Vilna, 1940), pub. Ḥayyil, Jerusalem, 1962.

'Amud Ha-Yemini Saul Yisraeli, pub. Makhon Ha-Torah Ve-Ha-Medinah Al Shem Maran Ha-Rav Sha'ul Yisra'eli zaẓal, Jerusalem, 2000.

'Aparqasta De-'Anya David Sperber (Romania, 1875–Israel, 1962), Jerusalem, 1981.

'Aryeh De-Vei 'Ila'ai Aryeh Leivush Lifschitz (Galicia, 1767–1846), Jerusalem, 1990.

'Avnei Nezer Abraham Borenstein (Sochotchov, 1839–1910), pub. Friedman, New York, 1987.

Beit Shelomoh Solomon ben Jacob Drimer (Galicia, 1800–72), Grossman Publications, New York, 1962.

Beit Yehudah Judah Ayyash (Algeria, Jerusalem; d. 1760), pub. Makhon Benei Yissakhar, Jerusalem, 1990.

Beit Yiẓḥaq Isaac Judah Shmelkes (Galicia, 1828–1905), pub. Makhon Ḥatam Sofer, Jerusalem, 1973.

Benei Banim Judah Herzl Henkin, Jerusalem, 1981.

Be-'Ohalah Shel Torah Jacob Ariel (Jerusalem, 1937–Ramat Gan), pub. Makhon Ha-Torah Ve-Ha-'Areẓ, Kefar Darom, 1998.

Binyan Ẓiyyon Jacob Ettlinger (Germany, 1798–1871), pub. Davar Jerusalem–Zikhron Ẓvi, Jerusalem, 2002.

Damaseq 'Eli'ezer Abraham Ẓvi Perlmutter (Poland, 1843–1930), pub. Sifrei Poseqim Rishonim, Brooklyn, 1991.

Divrei Malki'el Zvi Ha-Levi Malkiel (Mutala 1847–Poland 1910), Jerusalem, 1987.

Divrei Yaẓiv Yekutiel Yehudah Halbershtam (Galiẓia 1904–Netanya 1995), Netanya pub. Machon Shefa Ḥaim, 1996–2004.

Divrei Yissakhar Issachar David Berish Graubart (Poland, 1847–1913), pub. Makhon 'Oẓarot Ge'onei Sefarad, Ashdod, 1997.

'Emeq Halakhah Joshua Baumol (Galicia, 1889–New York, 1948), Jerusalem, 1976.

'Emunat Shemu'el Aaron Samuel Kaidenower (Russia, 1614–76), Jerusalem, 1981; pub. Eqed Sefarim, Ramat-Gan, 1997.

'Even Yeqarah Benjamin Aryeh Weiss (Galicia, 1844–Chernowitz, 1912), Mahadurah, telita'ah Drohovitz, 1913.

'Ezrat Kohen Abraham Isaac Ha-Kohen Kook (Latvia, 1865–Jerusalem, 1935), pub. Mosad Ha-Rav Kook, Jerusalem, 1985.

Ge'onei Batra'i *Teshuvat Ha-Ge'onim Batra'i*, in *Shut Ha-Baḥ Ha-Yeshanot* [Old responsa of the *Baḥ*], Jerusalem, 1980.

Ha-Elef Lekha Shelomoh Solomon Kluger (Poland, 1785–Galicia, 1869), pub. Ha-Mosad Le-'Iddud Limmud Ha-Torah, Jerusalem, 1992.

Ha-Noda Bi-Yehudah Ezekiel ben Judah Landau (Poland, 1713–Prague, 1793), pub. Pesaqim, Jerusalem, 1961.

Ḥatam Sofer Moses Sofer (Frankfurt, 1762–Pressburg, 1839), pub. Hod, Jerusalem, 1972.

Ḥatam Sofer Qoveẓ Teshuvot Pub. Makhon Le-Hoẓa'at Sefarim Ve-Ḥeqer Kitvei-Yad 'Al Shem Ha-Ḥatam Sofer zaẓal, Jerusalem, 1973.

Ḥavvot Binyamin *Sefer Ḥavvot Binyamim*, 2, by Saul Yisraeli (Russia, 1909–Jerusalem, 1995), pub. Makhon Ha-Torah Ve-Ha-'Arez, Kefar Darom, 1992.

Ḥavvot Ya'ir Yair Bachrach (Moravia, 1638–Worms, 1702), pub. Makhon Eked Sefarim, Ramat Gan, 1997.

Ḥayyim Sha'al Ḥayyim Joseph David Azulai (Ḥida) (Jerusalem, 1724–Livorno, 1806), pub. Yahadut, Jerusalem, 1986.

Heikhal Yiẓḥaq Isaac Izak Ha-Levi Herzog (Poland, 1887–Jerusalem 1959), pub. 'Agudah Le-Hoẓa'at Kitvei Rosh Ha-Rabbanim Ha-Geri'ah Herzog zaẓal, Jerusalem, 1967.

Ḥelqat Ya'aqov Mordecai Jacob Breish (Poland, 1896–Zurich, 1977), Tel Aviv, 1992.

Ḥemdat Shelomoh Solomon Zalman Lifschitz (Poland, 1765–1839), Brooklyn, 1989).
Hit'orerut Teshuvah Simeon Sofer (Pressburg, 1850–Hungary, 1944), pub. Makhon Le-Hoẓa'at Sefarim Ve-Ḥeqer Kitvei Yad 'Al Shem Ḥatam Sofer zal, Jerusalem, 1990.
'Iggerot Mosheh Moses Feinstein (Russia, 1895–United States, 1986), New York, 1959–Jerusalem, 1996.
Ketav Sofer Abraham Samuel Benjamin Sofer (Pressburg, 1815–71), pub. Makhon Le-Hoẓa'at Sefarim Ve-Ḥeqer Kitvei-Yad 'Al Shem Ha-Ḥatam Sofer zaẓal, Jerusalem, 1960.
Koaḥ Shor Isaac Schor (Galicia, 1700–76), Kalama'a, 1888.
Ma'arkhei Lev Judah Lev Tsirelsohn (Russia, 1859–1941), Israel, 1971.
Maharam Minẓ Moses Ha-Levi Minẓ (Germany, 1415–Poland, 1480), pub. Mif'al Torat Ḥakhmei 'Ashkenaz, Makhon, Jerusalem, 1991.
Maharam Shiq Moses Schick (Hungary, 1807–79), Jerusalem, 1983.
Maharit Joseph Trani (Safed, 1568–Turkey, 1639), pub. Beit Ha-Sefarim, Benei-Beraq, 1994.
Maharsham Shalom Mordecai Ha-Kohen Schwadron (Poland, 1835–1911), pub. Makhon Da'at Torah, Jerusalem, 1992.
Marḥeshet Ḥanokh Henekh Eigesh (Kovno, 1864–Vilna, 1941), Jerusalem, 1989.
Melammed Leho'il David Zvi Hoffmann (Hungary, 1843–Berlin 1921), pub. Frenkel Booksellers, New York, 1954.
Minḥat 'Eliyahu Elijah Kolesniker (Kiev, 1860–?), Brooklyn, 1993.
Minḥat Shelomoh Solomon Zalman Auerbach (Jerusalem, 1910–95), Jerusalem, 2000.
Minḥat Yeḥiel Alter Yeḥiel Nebentsahl (Galicia, 1858–1939), pub. Torah 'Or, Brooklyn, 1992.
Minḥat Yiẓḥaq Isaac Jacob Weiss (Poland, 1902–Jerusalem, 1989), pub. Minḥat Yitzhak, Jerusalem, 1989.
Mishpetei 'Uzi'el Ben-Ẓion Meir Ḥai Uziel (Jerusalem, 1880–1953), pub. Ha-Va'ad Lehoẓa'at Kitvei Maran zaẓal, Jerusalem, 2002.
Naharei 'Afarsemon Jacob Tenenbaum (Hungary, 1832–97), Jerusalem, 1998.
'Ohel Mosheh Moses Jonah Ha-Levi Ẓweig (Galicia, 1909–Antwerp, 1963), Mahadura Telitai, Rio de Janeiro, 1965.
'Or Gadol Judah Perelman (Brisk, 1835–Minsk, 1896), pub. Ha-Mosad Le-'Idud Limmud Ha-Torah, Jerusalem, 1999.
'Or Yisra'el Israel Lifschitz (Germany, 18th century), Brooklyn, 1995.

Peri Ha-Sadeh Eliezer Deutsch (Slovakia, 1850–Hungary, 1915), Brooklyn, 1985.

Rabaz Bezalel Ze'ev Shaffran (Galicia, 1867–Romania, 1929), pub. Feldheim Publishers, Jerusalem, 1992.

Rabbi Akiva Eger Akiva Eger (Eisenstadt, 1761–1837), pub. Makhon Ha-Ma'or, Jerusalem, 2002.

Radbaz David ben Zimra (Spain, 1479–Safed, 1573), Israel, 1972.

Radbaz from ms. *Sefer Shut Ha-Radbaz Mi-Khetav Yad* [Responsa of Radbaz from manuscript], David Ibn Zimra, pub. Et Sofer, Benei-Beraq, 1975.

Rashba Solomon ben Adret (Spain, 1235–1310), pub. Makhon Yerushalayim, Jerusalem, 1997.

Rav Pe'alim Joseph Ḥayyim ben Elijah al-Hakham (author of the Ben Ish Ḥai) (Baghdad, 1834–1909), pub. Siaḥ Yisra'el, Jerusalem, 1994.

Rivash Isaac Bar Sheshet (Barcelona, 1326–Algiers, 1408), pub. Ha-Mosad Le-'Iddud Limmud Ha-Torah, Jerusalem, 1994.

Rosh Mashbir Joseph Samuel Modigliano (Modena) (Salonika, 1714–81), pub. Makhon 'Ozarot Ge'onei Sefarad, Ashdod, 1997.

Seridei 'Eish Jeḥiel Jacob Weinberg (Russia, 1885–Switzerland, 1966), pub. Mosad Ha-Rav Kook, Jerusalem, 2003.

Sha'arei 'Uzi'el Ben-Zion Meir Hai Uziel (Jerusalem, 1880–1953), pub. Ha-Ve'adah Le-Hoẓa'at Kitvei Ha-Rav, Jerusalem, 1991.

She'eilat Ya'aveẓ Jacob Emden (Altona, 1698–1776), Israel, 1978.

Shevet Ha-Levi Samuel Ha-Levi Wosner (Vienna, 1913–Israel), 3rd ed., 2002.

Sitri U-Magini Sinai Schiffer (Hungary, 1853–Germany, 1927), Turnow, 1932.

Tashbeẓ Simeon bar Ẓemaḥ Duran (Majorca, 1361–Algiers, 1444), Tel Aviv, 1990.

Terumat Ha-Deshen Israel Isserlin (Regensburg, 1390–Vienna, 1460), pub. Ha-Mosad Le-'Iddud Limmud Ha-Torah, Jerusalem, 1991.

Teshuvah Sheleimah Ḥayyim Fischel Epstein (Kovno, 1874–St. Louis, 1942), St. Louis, 1941.

Teshuvot Hadashot Le-Rabbi Akiva Eger Akiva Eger, *Sefer Teshuvot Ḥadashot*, Jerusalem, 1978.

Teshuvot Ha-Rosh Asher ben Yeḥiel (Germany, 1250–Spain, 1327), pub. Makhon Yerushalayim, Jerusalem, 1994.

Torat Ḥesed Shneur Zalman Fradkin (Russia, 1830–Jerusalem, 1902), pub. Hod Ve-Hadar, Jerusalem, 1990.

Yabi'a 'Omer Ovadia Yosef (Baghdad, 1920–Israel), Jerusalem, 1954–2004.

Yaḥel Yisra'el Israel Meir Lau (Poland, 1937–Israel), pub. Makhon Masoret, Jerusalem, 1992.

Yaskil 'Avdi Ovadia Hedaya (Syria, 1890–Jerusalem, 1969), Jerusalem, 1958.
Yehudah Ya'aleh Judah Assad (Hungary, 1794–1866), Jerusalem, 2000.
Zekher Yiẓḥaq Isaac Rabinowitz (Poland, 1854–Ponovitch, 1919), Jerusalem, 1967.
Zemaḥ Zedeq Menaḥem Mendel Shneerson (White Russia, 1789–Lubavitch, 1866), pub. Oẓar Ha-Ḥasidim, Brooklyn (Karnei Hod Torah, Kefar Ḥabad), 1984.
Zeqan 'Aharon Aaron Wolkin (Mohilev, 1865–Pinsk, 1942), New York, 1977.
Zikhron Yehonatan Jonathan Abelman (Kovno, 1854–Bialystok, 1903), Jerusalem, 1970.
Ẓiẓ 'Eli'ezer 'Eli'ezer Judah Waldenberg (Jerusalem, 1915–2006), Jerusalem, 1945–98.
Zofnat Pa'aneiaḥ Joseph Rozen (Rogotchov, 1858–Dvinsk, 1936), pub. Ha-Mosad Le-'Iddud Limmud Ha-Torah, Jerusalem, 1995.

PRIMARY SOURCES

Abarbanel *Peirush 'Al Ha-Torah Le-Don Yizhaq 'Abarban'el* [Commentary on the Torah by Don Isaac Abarbanel] (Portugal, 1437–Venice, 1508), pub. Benei Arb'el, Jerusalem, 1964.
'Aqeidat Yiẓḥaq Isaac Aramah (Spain, 15th century), commentary on the Torah, Pressburg, 1849.
'Arukh Ha-Shulḥan Yehiel Mikhel Ha-Levi Epstein (Russia, 1829–1908), pub. Yeẓo Sifrei Kodesh, Tel Aviv, 1976.
'Arukh La-Ner Jacob Ettlinger (Germany, 1798–1871), pub. Sifrei 'Or Ha-Ḥayyim, Benei-Beraq, 2004.
'Avot De-Rabbi Natan Ed. Solomon Schechter, pub. Jewish Theological Seminary of America, New York and Jerusalem, 1967.
'Aẓei 'Arazim Noah Ḥayyim Zvi Berlin (Germany, 18th century), *Sefer 'Aẓei 'Arazim 'Al 'Even Ha-'Ezer*, Jerusalem, 1974.
Babylonian Talmud Pagination per the Vilna Edition.
Bayit Hadash (*Baḥ*) Joel Sirkes (Poland, 1561–1640), commentary on the *'Arba'ah Turim*.
Be'er Heiteiv A commentary on the *Shulḥan 'Arukh*, encompassing various works, most prominently those of Isaiah Bar Abraham (a descendant of the author of *Turei Zahav*) and of Judah Ashkenazi of Ticktin. On the various versions of the work, see the introduction of *Shulḥan 'Arukh, 'Oraḥ Ḥayyim*, pub. Mifal Shulḥan 'Arukh Ha-Shalem, Makhon Yerushalayim, Jerusalem, 1994, p. 77.

Beit Ha-Beḥirah Menaḥem Hameiri (France, 1249–1315), pub. Makhon Ha-Talmud Ha-Yisra'eli Ha-Shalem, Jerusalem, 1967.

Beit Ha-'Oẓar Joseph Engel (Galicia, 1859–Vienna, 1919), Benei-Beraq, 1991.

Beit Me'ir Meir Posner (Posen, 1728?–1807), commentary on *Shulḥan 'Arukh, 'Even Ha-'Ezer*, part 1, pub. Makhon Moreshet Ha-Yeshivot, Jerusalem, 1997.

Beit Shmu'el Samuel Feibush (Poland, 1640–1718), commentary on *Shulḥan 'Arukh, 'Even Ha-'Ezer.*

Benei 'Ahuvah Jonathan Eibeschutz (Poland, 1694?–Germany, 1764), Prague, 1819.

Birkei Yosef Ḥayyim Joseph David Azulai (Ḥida) (Jerusalem, 1724–Livorno, 1806), pub. Ḥ. Wagschal, Jerusalem, 1989.

'Etvan De-'Orayeta Joseph Engel (Galicia, 1859–Vienna, 1919, Benei-Beraq, 1988.

Genesis Rabbah *Midrash Bereshit Rabbah*, ed. Y. Theodor and Ḥ. Albeck, pub. Sifrei Wohrman, Jerusalem, 1965 (2nd ed.).

Ha-Kenesset Ha-Gedolah Ḥayyim Benvenisti (Turkey, 1603–73), pub. Keren Le-Hoza'at Kol Sifrei Kenesset Ha-Gedolah, Jerusalem, 1976.

Halakhot Gedolot Simeon Kayyara (ca. 9th century), pub. Makhon 'Or Ha-Mizraḥ, Makhon Yerushalayim, Jerusalem, 1992.

Ha-Maqneh Pinḥas Ha-Levi Horowitz (Galicia, 1730–Germany, 1805), *Sefer Ha-Maqneh* (part 2 of *Sefer Ha-Fela'ah*), Jerusalem, 1992.

Ha-Rash Mi-Sanz Samson of Sens (Germany, 12th century), *Tosafot Ha-Rashba Mi-Sens 'Al Masekhet Ketubbot*, pub. Makhon HaTalmud Ha-Yisra'eli Ha-Shalem, Jerusalem, 1973.

Ḥasdei David Le-Tosefta David Pardo (Venice, 1718–Jerusalem, 1790), pub. Wagschal, Jerusalem, 1994.

Ḥazon 'Ish Abraham Isaiah Karelitz (Lithuania, 1878–Jerusalem, 1953), *Sefer Hazon 'Ish, 'Even Ha-'Ezer, Nashim*, Benei-Beraq, 1991.

Ḥelqat Meḥoqqeq Moses Lima (Lithuania, early 17th century–Brisk, 1657), *Peirush Le-Shulḥan 'Arukh, 'Even Ha-'Ezer.*

Ḥiddushei Ha-Ramban Moses ben Naḥman (Ramban, Naḥmanides) (Spain, 1194–Land of Israel, 1270), pub. Makhon Ha-Talmud Ha-Yisra'eli Ha-Shalem, Jerusalem, 1970–2002.

Ḥiddushei Ha-Ramban Ha-Shalem *Ḥiddushei Ha-Ramban Ha-Shalem 'Al Masekhet Ketubbot*, ed., and pub. Makhon Ma'arava Le-Meḥqar Torani, Jerusalem, 1994.

Ḥiddushei Ha-Ran Nissim Girondi (Spain, 1320–80), pub. Mosad Ha-Rav Kook, Jerusalem, 1997.

Ḥiddushei Ha-Rashba Solomon ben Adret (Spain, 1235–1310), pub. Mosad Ha-Rav Kook, Jerusalem, 1989, 1990.

Ḥiddushei Ha-Ritva Yom Tov ben Abraham Ishbili (Ritva) (Spain, 1250–1320), pub. Mosad Ha-Rav Kook, Jerusalem, 1975–88.

Ḥiddushei Ḥatam Sofer Le-Hulin Moses Sofer (Frankfurt, 1762–Pressburg, 1839), Vienna, 1893.

Leḥem Mishneh Abraham di Boton (Salonika, 1545–88), commentary on Maimonides's *Mishneh Torah*.

Leviticus Rabbah *Midrash Vayiqra Rabbah*, 3rd. ed., ed. M. Margaliot, pub. Jewish Theological Seminary of America, New York and Jerusalem, 1993.

Magen Avraham Abraham Ha-Levi Gombiner (Gombin, 1637–Kalish, 1683), commentary on the *Shulḥan 'Arukh*.

Maggid Mishneh Vidal di Tolosa (Spain or Provence, 1300–1370), commentary on Maimonides's *Mishneh Torah*.

Mekhilta De-Rashbi *Mekhilta De-Rabbi Shim'on Bar Yoḥai*, ed. Epstein, pub. Mekiẓei Nirdamim, Jerusalem, 1955.

Mekhilta De-Ri *Mekhilta De-Rabbi Yishma'el*, ed. Horowitz and Rabin, pub. Shalem Hafazat Sefarim, Jerusalem, 1998.

Meshekh Ḥokmah Simḥah Meir of Dvinsk (Vilna 1843–Dvinsk 1926), Jerusalem, pub. Feldhaim, 2005.

Minḥat Ḥinukh Joseph ben Moses Babad (Galicia, 1801–74), pub. Makhon Yerushalayim, Jerusalem, 1988.

Mishnah Albeck edition (*Shishah Sidrei Mishnah Meforashim Bi-Yedei Hanokh 'Albeq*), pub. Mosad Bialik, Jerusalem, and Dvir, Tel Aviv, 1989.

Mishneh Torah Moses ben Maimon (Rambam, Maimonides) (Spain, 1138–Egypt 1204). When so noted in the text, English translation per the Yale Judaica Series edition.

Nishmat 'Avraham Abraham Sofer Abraham, *Sefer Nishmat 'Avraham—Hilkhot Holim, Rofe'im U-Refu'ah* [Laws regarding patients, physicians, and medicine], pub. Dr. Falk Schlesinger Institute for Medical Halachic Research at the Shaare Zedek Medical Center, Jerusalem, 1983.

'Or Zaru'a Isaac bar Moses of Vienna (Bohemia, 1180–Vienna, 1250), *Sefer 'Or Zaru'a Ha-Shalem*, pub. Makhon Torani Yeshivat 'Or 'Etzion, Makhon Yerushalayim, Jerusalem, 2001.

'Oẓar Ha-Poseqim *'Oẓar Ha-Poseqim 'Al Shulḥan 'Arukh 'Even Ha-'Ezer*, Jerusalem, 1955–95.

Peirush Ha-Mishnah La-Rambam Maimonides, commentary on the Mishnah, ed. Kafih, pub. Mosad Ha-Rav Kook, Jerusalem, 1965.

Qorban Netan'el Nethanel ben Naphtali Ẓevi Weil (Shtilingen 1687–Rashtat 1769), commentary on Rosh, Babylonian Talmud.

Sedei Ḥemed Ḥayyim Hezekiah Medini (Jerusalem, 1832–Hebron, 1904). *Sedei Ḥemed Ha-Shalem*, pub. Friedman, New York, 1962.

Sefer Ha-Ḥinukh Aaron Ha-Levi of Barcelona (Spain, 13th century), ed. Chavel, pub. Mosad Ha-Rav Kook, Jerusalem, 1962.

Sefer Ha-Yashar *Sefer Ha-Yashar Le-Rabbeinu Tam*, ed. Schlesinger, Jerusalem, 1959.

Sefer Maharil Elazar Zalman ben Jacob (Mainz, 1309–Italy?, 1472) *Sefer Maharil* (*'Az Yaqhel Shelomoh, Sha'al Shelomoh*) (*Ḥeleq Ha-Liqqutim*), pub. Goldenberg Bros., Brooklyn, 2005.

Semag; *Sefer Miẓvot Gadol* Moses ben Jacob of Coucy (France, 13th century), pub. Makhon Yerushalayim, Jerusalem, 2003.

She'iltot De-Rav 'Aḥai Ga'on 'Aḥai Mishivḥa Ga'on (Babylonia, 680–Land of Israel, 752), *She'iltot De-Rav 'Aḥai Ga'on 'Im Bi'ur Ha'ameq She'eilah* (Naftali Zvi Berlin), part 3, Jerusalem, 1978.

Shevet Mi-Yehudah Isser Judah Unterman (Brisk, 1886–Israel, 1976), pub. Mosad Ha-Rav Kook, Jerusalem, 1984.

Shittah Mequbeẓet Beẓalel ben Abraham Ashkenazi (Safed–Jerusalem, d. ca. 1592–95), various editions.

Shulḥan 'Arukh Joseph Karo (Spain, 1488–Safed, 1575), Lemberg 1886 ed., pub. Pe'er Ha-Torah, Jerusalem, 1960.

Sifra *Sifra De-Vei Rav*, ed. Weiss, Vienna, 1862.

Sifrei *Sifrei on Deuteronomy*, ed. Finkelstein, pub. Jewish Theological Seminary of America, New York and Jerusalem, 1963.

Tanḥuma *Midrash Tanḥuma*, pub. Levin-Epstein, Jerusalem, 1969.

Tanḥuma (Buber) *Midrash Tanḥuma*, ed. Buber, Jerusalem, 1964.

Torat Ha-'Adam Moses ben Naḥman (Ramban, Naḥmanides) (Spain, 1194–Land of Israel, 1270), in *Kitvei Ha-Ramban*, vol. 2, ed. Chavel, Jerusalem, 1964.

Tosefta Tosefta, ed. Lieberman, pub. Jewish Theological Seminary of America, New York and Jerusalem, 1993–96.

Tosefta (Zuckermandel) Tosefta, ed. Zuckermandel, with *Tashlum Tosefta* by Saul Lieberman, pub. Sifrei Wahrman, Jerusalem, 1970.

Tosefta Ki-Feshutah Saul Lieberman, *Tosefta Ki-Feshutah*, pub. Jewish Theological Seminary of America, New York and Jerusalem, 1993–96.

Tur Jacob ben Asher (Germany, 1269–Spain, 1343), *'Arba'ah Turim*, pub. El Ha-Meqorot, Jerusalem, 1958.

Turei Zahav (*Taz*) David Ha-Levi (Ludomir, 1586–Lvov, 1667), commentary on the *Shulḥan ʿArukh*.
Yalqut Shimʿoni Simeon Hadarshan of Frankfurt, pub. H. Wagschal, Jerusalem, 2003.
Yam Shel Shelomoh Solomon Luria (Poland, 1510–74), pub. Vaʿad Le-Hoẓa'at Sefarim Neḥuẓim Le-Lomedei Torah, Benei-Beraq, 1959.
Yerushalmi Talmud Yerushalmi [Talmud of the Land of Israel], ms. Scaliger (Or. 3 4720), University of Leiden, with addenda and corrigenda and introduction by Y. Zusman, pub. Academy for the Hebrew Language, Jerusalem, 2001–5.
Yevamot with alt. readings Pub. Makhon Ha-Talmud Ha-Yisraeli Ha-Shalem, Jerusalem, 1996.

SECONDARY SOURCES

English titles of Hebrew secondary sources have been supplied by the present translator. They are meant to allow a Hebrew reader to find the reference and an English-only reader to gain a sense of the content of the source.

Adler (1983) Adler, Rachel. "The Jew Who Wasn't There: Halakha and the Jewish Woman." In S. Heschel (ed.), *On Being a Jewish Feminist: A Reader*, pp. 12–18. New York: Schocken Books, 1983.
Adler (1998) Adler, Rachel. *Engendering Judaism: An Inclusive Theology and Ethics*. Philadelphia: Jewish Publication Society, 1998.
Adler (2001) Adler, Rachel. "Innovation and Authority: A Feminist Reading of the 'Women's Minyan' Responsum." In Walter Jacob and Moshe Zamir (eds.), *Gender Issues in Jewish Law*, pp. 3–32. New York: Berghahn Books, 2001.
Aiken (1992) Aiken, Lisa. *To Be a Jewish Woman*. Northvale, NJ: J. Aronson, 1992.
Amsel (1965) Amsel, Meir. "Clarification Regarding Our Efforts in Recent Months to Promote the Purity and Sanctity of the Family and Eliminate Any Sort of Authorization to Defile It through Insemination with a Donor's Seed" [Hebrew]. *Ha-ma'or* 16 (Adar I 5725), pp. 10–18.
Amsel (1978) Amsel, Meir. "The New Invention of Implanting a Fetus into a Woman's Womb after Fertilization in a Laboratory" [Hebrew]. *Ha-Ma'or* 30/5 (5738), pp. 44–45.
Andrews (1988) Andrews, Lori. B. "Surrogate Motherhood: The Challenge for Feminists." In L. Gostin (ed.), *Surrogate Motherhood: Politics and Privacy*, pp. 167–182. Bloomington and Indianapolis: Indiana University Press, 1988.
Andrews (1989) Andrews, Lori. B. "Alternative Modes of Reproduction." In

S. Cohen and N. Taub (eds.), *Reproductive Laws for the 1990s*, pp. 361–403. New Jersey: Humana Press, 1989.

Antony (1993) Antony, Louise. M. "Ouine as Feminist: The Radical Import of Naturalized Epistemology." In L. M. Antony and C. Witt (eds.), *A Mind of One's Own*, pp. 185–225. Boulder, CO: Westview Press, 1993.

Aptowitzer (1942–43) Aptowitzer, Avigdor. "The Status of the Fetus in Jewish Criminal Law" [Hebrew]. *Sinai* 11 (5702–5703), pp. 9–32.

Ariel (1996) Ariel, Yaakov. "Artificial Insemination and Surrogacy" [Hebrew]. *Teḥumin* 16 (5756), pp. 171–180.

Ariel (2002) Ariel, Yigal. "Intervals between Pregnancies (Halakhic Issues)" [Hebrew]. *Ẓohar* 10 (5762), pp. 223–236.

Ariel (2003–4) Ariel, Yaakov. "The Women's Study Hall" [Hebrew]. In Y. Arzoni (ed.), *Halakhic and Philosophical Issues in Jewish Women's Education* [Hebrew], pp. 205–219. Qiryat 'Arba–Hebron: Makhon Le-Rabbanei Yeshuvim, 2003–4.

Auerbach (1958) Auerbach, Shlomo Zalman. "Artificial Insemination" [Hebrew]. *No'am* 1 (5718), pp. 145–166.

Aviner (1984) Aviner, Shlomo. *Flesh of My Flesh: Bonding in Marriage: Your Children as Olive Shoots; Family Planning and Birth Control* [Hebrew]. Bet-El and Jerusalem, 1984.

Aviner (2001) Aviner, Shlomo. *Aspects of Love—between Man and Wife* [Hebrew]. Bet-'El: Sifriyat Ḥavvah, 2001.

Aviner (2002) Aviner, Shlomo. *My Sister, My Bride: Preparing for Marriage*. Bet-'El: Sifriyat Ḥavvah, 2002.

Bakshi-Doron and Silberstein (2004) Bakshi-Doron, Eliyahu, and Yitzḥak Silberstein. "Chemotherapy for a Pregnant Woman: An Exchange of Letters" [Hebrew]. *Teḥumin* 24 (5764), pp. 117–125.

Bartlett (1990) Bartlett, Katherine T. "Feminist Legal Methods." *Harvard Law Review* 103 (1990), pp. 829–888.

Bartlett and Kennedy (1991) Bartlett, Katherine T. and Rosanne Kennedy (eds.). *Feminist Legal Theory: Readings in Law and Gender*. Boulder, CO: Westview Press, 1991.

Ben-Ḥaim (1994) Ben-Ḥaim. "The Position of Maharit on Abortion" [Hebrew]. In H. Y. Wieder and A. Y. Shmidman (eds.), *Rabbi J. B. Soloveitchik Memorial Volume* [Hebrew], pp. 12–18. New York: Yeshiva University Press, 1994.

Benjamin (1968) Benjamin, Walter. "Theses on the Philosophy of History." In

Walter Benjamin, *Illuminations* (trans. Harry Zohn, ed. Hannah Arendt), pp. 255–266. New York: Schocken Books, 1968.
Ben-Meir (1990) Ben-Meir, Yehoshua. "Legal and Biological Parenthood in Halakhah" [Hebrew]. *'Asiya* 12/3–4 (1990), pp. 80–89.
Ben-Menaḥem (1994) Ben-Menaḥem, Yemima. "History as Therapy: Michel Foucault" [Hebrew]. *'Iyyun* 43 (1994), pp. 123–143.
Ben-Refael et al. (1993) Ben-Refael, Ẓiyon, et al. *The Complete Guide to Fertility* [Hebrew]. Jerusalem and Tel Aviv: Schocken, 1993.
Berg (1995) Berg, Barbara. "Listening to the Voices of the Infertile." In J. C. Callahan (ed.), *Reproduction, Ethics and the Law: Feminist Perspectives*, pp. 80–108. Bloomington: Indiana University Press, 1995.
Berman (1973) Berman, Saul. "The Status of Women in Halakhic Judaism." *Tradition* 14/2 (1973), pp. 5–28.
Biale (1989) Biale, Rachel. "Abortion in Jewish Law." *Tikkun* 4/4 (1989), pp. 26–28.
Bick (1986) Bick, Ezra. "Motherhood of Implanted Fetuses" [Hebrew]. *Teḥumin* 7 (5746), pp. 266–270.
Bick (1997) Bick, Ezra. "Ovum Donations: A Rabbinic Conceptual Model of Maternity." In E. Feldman and J. B. Wolowelsky (eds.), *Jewish Law and the New Reproductive Technologies*, pp. 83–105. Hoboken, NJ: Ktav, 1997.
Bin-Nun (2004) Bin-Nun, Yoel. "Women Will Rule for Themselves" [Hebrew]. *Nequdah* 268 (Shevat 5764), pp. 40–43.
Bloch (1965) Bloch, Moshe Haim Ephraim. "Let Your Camp Be Holy: Statement of Principle against Artificial Insemination" [1965, Hebrew]. In R. Levenbok (ed.), *Collected Responsa and Rulings*, pp. 1–32. Brooklyn, 1994.
Boyarin (1993) Boyarin, Daniel. *Carnal Israel: Reading Sex in Talmudic Culture*. Berkeley: University of California Press, 1993.
Breitowitz (2003) Breitowitz, Yitzchok A. "Halakhic Alternatives in IVF-Pregnancies: A Survey." *Jewish Law Annual* 14 (2003), pp. 29–119.
Broyde (1997) Broyde, Matityahu. "The Obligation of Jews to Promote the Observance by Gentiles of the Seven Noahide Commandments: A Theoretical Overview" [Hebrew]. *Dinei Yisra'el* 19 (1997), pp. 87–111.
Broyde (1999) Broyde, Michael. *Assisted Reproduction and Jewish Law*. Cincinnati: University of Cincinnati, 1999.
Chaudhury (1978) Chaudhury, Rafiqul. H. "Female Status and Fertility Behaviour in a Metropolitan Urban Area of Bangladesh." *Population Studies* 32/2 (1978), pp. 261–273.

Chaves (1997) Chaves, Mark. *Ordaining Women: Culture and Conflict in Religious Organizations*. Cambridge, MA: Harvard University Press, 1997.

Code (1998) Code, Lorraine. "Epistemology." In A. M. Jaggar and I. M. Young (eds.), *A Companion to Feminist Philosophy*, pp. 173–184. Oxford: Blackwell, 1998.

Cohen (1989) Cohen, Jeremy. *"Be Fertile and Increase, Fill the Earth and Master It": The Ancient and Medieval Career of a Biblical Text*. Ithaca, NY, and London: Cornell University Press, 1989.

Cohen (1998) Cohen, Jeremy. "The Commandment to Procreate and Its Place in Religious Controversy" [Hebrew]. In Y. Bartal and Y. Gafni (eds.), *Eros, Marriage, and Prohibitions: Sexuality and Family in History* [Hebrew], pp. 83–96. Jerusalem: Zalman Shazar Center, 1998.

Corea (1985) Corea, Gena. *The Mother Machine: Reproductive Technologies from Artificial Insemination to Artificial Wombs*. New York: Harper & Row, 1985.

Corea (1987) Corea, Gena. "The Reproductive Brothel." In G. Corea et al. (eds.), *Man-Made Women: How New Reproductive Technologies Affect Women*, pp. 38–51. Bloomington and Indianapolis: Indiana University Press, 1987.

Corea (1988) Corea, Gena. "What the King Can Not See." In Baruch E. Hoffman et al. (eds.), *Embryos, Ethics, and Women's Rights: Exploring the New Reproductive Technologies*, pp. 77–93. New York and London: Harrington Park Press, 1988.

Corinaldi (1992–94) Corinaldi, Michael. "The Legal Status of a Child Born through Artificial Insemination from a Sperm Donor or from a Donated Egg" [Hebrew]. *Shenaton Ha-Mishpat Ha-'Ivri* 18–19 (1992–1994), pp. 295–327.

Cover (1983) Cover, Robert M. "The Supreme Court 1982 Term–Foreword: Nomos and Narrative." *Harvard Law Review* 97 (1983), pp. 4–68.

Dalima and Alcoff (1993) Dalima, Vrinda, and Linda Alcoff. "Are 'Old Wives' Tales' Justified?" In L. Alcoff and E. Potter (eds.), *Feminist Epistemologies*, pp. 217–244. New York and London: Routledge, 1993.

Daube (1977) Daube, David. *The Duty of Procreation*. Edinburgh: Edinburgh University Press, 1977.

Daube (1981) Daube, David. "Johanan Ben Broqa and Women's Rights." In M. M. Caspi (ed.), *Jewish Tradition in the Diaspora: Studies in Memory of Professor Walter J. Fischel*, pp. 55–60. Berkeley, CA: Judah L. Magnes Memorial Museum, 1981.

Davis (1991) Davis, Dena. S. "Beyond Rabbi Ḥiyya's Wife: Women's Voices in Jewish Bioethics." *Second Opinion* 16 (March 1991), pp. 11–30.

Davis (1992) Davis, Dena. S. "Abortion in Jewish Thought: A Study in

Casuistry." *Journal of the American Academy of Religion* 60/2 (Spring 1992), pp. 313–324.

De Beauvoir (1953) De Beauvoir, Simone. *The Second Sex*. Translated from the French and edited by H. M. Parshley. New York: Knopf, 1953.

Dorff (1998) Dorff, Elliot. N. *Matters of Life and Death: A Jewish Approach to Modern Medical Ethics*. Philadelphia and Jerusalem: Jewish Publication Society, 1998..

Dreyfuss (2006) Dreyfuss, Yair. "Akdamot Milin" [Hebrew]. In Zohar Ma'or (ed.), *Two Luminaries: A New Jewish Perspective on Family Equality* [Hebrew], pp. 7–33. Efratah: Machon Binah Le-Ittim, 2006.

Dworkin (1983) Dworkin, Andrea. *Right-Wing Women*. New York: G. P. Putnam's Sons, 1983.

Dworkin (1995) Dworkin, Ronald. *Life's Dominion: An Argument about Abortion and Euthanasia*. London: Harper Collins Publishers, 1995.

Eisenstein (1952) Eisenstein, Yehudah D. (ed.). *A Jewish Treasury: An Encyclopedia* [Hebrew]. New York: Pardes, 1952.

Ellenson (1995) Ellenson, David. "Artificial Fertilization and Procreative Autonomy." In J. Walter and M. Zemer (eds.), *The Fetus and Fertility in Jewish Law: Essays and Responsa*, pp. 19–38. Pittsburgh and Tel Aviv: Freehof Institute of Progressive Halakhah, 1995.

Ellinson (1977a) Ellinson, Getsel E. "The Commandment to Procreate" [Hebrew]. *No'am* 19 (1977), pp. 256–262.

Ellinson (1977b) Ellinson, Getsel E. *Family Planning and Birth Control: The Halakhah in Light of Contemporary Medical Developments* [Hebrew]. Tel Aviv: Moreshet, 1977.

Elon (1994) Elon, Menahem. *Jewish Law: History, Sources, Principles*. Translated from the Hebrew by Bernard Auerbach and Melvin J. Sykes. Philadelphia: Jewish Publication Society, 1994.

Epstein (2004) Epstein, Yaakov. "Pedigree of a Child Born of Sperm from a Sperm Bank" [Hebrew]. *Teḥumin* 24 (2004), pp. 147–155.

Feinstein (1978) Feinstein, Moshe. "On the Law of Abortion" [Hebrew]. In Y. A. Buchsbaum (ed.), *Memorial Volume for Rabbi Y. Abramsky* [Hebrew], pp. 461–469. Jerusalem: Moriah, 1978.

Feinstein (1980) Feinstein, Moshe. "Women Jeopardized by Pregnancy and the Halakhah of Neutering of a Woman" [Hebrew]. In M. Hirshler (ed.), *Halakhah and Medicine* 5 [Hebrew], pp. 328–331. Jerusalem and Chicago: Makhon Regensberg, 1980.

Feldman (1986a) Feldman, David M. "The Ethical Implications of New

Reproductive Techniques." In L. Meier (ed.), *Jewish Values in Bioethics*, pp. 174–182. New York: Human Sciences Press, 1986.

Feldman (1986b) Feldman, David. M. *Health and Medicine in the Jewish Tradition, L'ḤAYYIM—to Life*. New York: Crossroad, 1986.

Feldman (1995) Feldman, David. M. *Birth Control in Jewish Law: Marital Relations, Contraception, and Abortion as Set Forth in the Classic Texts of Jewish Law*. 3rd ed. New York: New York University Press, 1995.

Firer (1963) Firer, Benzion. "On Artificial Fertility" [Hebrew]. *No'am* 6 (1963), pp. 295–299.

Firestone (1970) Firestone, Shulamith. *The Dialectic of Sex: The Case for Feminist Revolution*. New York: Morrow, 1970.

Foucault (1984) Foucault, Michel. "Truth and Power." In P. Rabinow (ed.), *The Foucault Reader*, pp. 51–75. New York: Pantheon Books, 1984.

Friedell (1992) Friedell, Steven. F. "The 'Different Voice' in Jewish Law: Some Parallels to a Feminist Jurisprudence." *Indiana Law Journal* 67 (1992), pp. 915–949.

Friedman (1968) Friedman, Zvi. H. *Sefer Ẓevi Ḥemed: Magen Gibborei Koaḥ*. Booklets 41, 42, 43. New York: Shulzinger Brothers, 1968.

Fullam (1975) Fullam, Maryellen. "Half the World." *People* 2/2 (1975), pp. 3–7.

Gafni (1989) Gafni, Isaiah M. "The Institution of Marriage in Rabbinic Times." In D. Kraemer (ed.), *The Jewish Family: Metaphor and Memory*, pp. 13–30. New York: Oxford, 1989.

Gershuni (1979) Gershuni, Yehudah. "The World's First Test-Tube Baby in Light of Halakhah" [Hebrew]. *'Or Ha-Mizraḥ* 27 (1979), pp. 15–21.

Gilligan (1982) Gilligan, Carol. *In a Different Voice: Psychological Theory and Women's Development*. Cambridge, MA: Harvard University Press, 1982.

Goldberg (1984a) Goldberg, Zalman Nehemiah. "Assigning Maternity in Cases of Surrogacy" [Hebrew]. *Teḥumin* 5 (5744), pp. 248–259.

Goldberg (1984b) Goldberg, Zalman Nehemiah (jointly with the editor). "Determining Maternity: Some Afterthoughts" [Hebrew]. *Teḥumin* 5 (5744), pp. 268–274.

Goldberg (1999) Goldberg, Zalman Nehemiah. "On Egg Donation, Surrogacy, Freezing the Sperm of a Bachelor, and Harvesting Sperm from a Deceased" [Hebrew]. *'Asiya* 17/1–2 (1999), pp. 45–49.

Goldstein (1981) Goldstein, Yissaḥar D. *Collected Notes on the Responsa of the Ḥatam Sofer, Yoreh De'ah* [Hebrew]. Vol. 2. Jerusalem: Makhon Lehoẓa'at Sefarim Veḥeqer Kitvei Yad 'Al Shem Ha-Ḥatam Sofer Zal, 1981.

Gordin (2005) Gordin, Harel. "Use of Birth Control: Moral and Halakhic

Considerations" [Hebrew]. In Z. Ma'or (ed.), *Marriage and Family from a New Jewish Perspective* [Hebrew], pp. 72–103. 'Efrata: Makhon Binah La-Itim, 2005.

Goren (2001) Goren, Shlomo. *Halakhic Studies on Medical Issues* [Hebrew]. Jerusalem: Ha-'Idra Rabbah and Mesorah La-'Am, 2001.

Grazi (2005) Richard V. Grazi. *Overcoming Infertility: A Guide for Couples.* New Milford, CT: Toby Press, 2005.

Green (1995) Green, Yossi. *In Vitro Fertilization in Light of the Agreement* [Hebrew]. Tel Aviv: Pearlstein-Ginosar, 1995.

Greenberg (1976) Greenberg, Blu. "Abortion: A Challenge to Halakhah." *Judaism* 25 (1976), pp. 201–208.

Grodzinski (1988) Grodzinski Ẓvi H. "On Artificial Insemination." In M. Herschler (ed.), *Halakhah and Medicine: Collected Essays on Halakhah Related to Medical Matters* [Hebrew], Vol. 5 (1988), pp. 139–154.

Halbertal (1997) Halbertal, Moshe. *Interpretive Revolutions in the Making: Values as Interpretive Considerations in Midrashei Halakhah* [Hebrew]. Jerusalem: Magnes Press, 1997.

Halperin (1993) Halperin, Mordeḥai. "Donation of Genetic Material and Innovative Treatments for Infertility" [Hebrew]. In Y. Katan (ed.), *Gynecology, Fertility, and Births in Light of Halkahah* [Hebrew], pp. 119–137. Jerusalem: The Religious Council, 1993.

Halperin (1999) Halperin, Mordeḥai. "Preserving Information about Biological Parenthood: The Retreat from the Interim Report of the Aloni Committee" [Hebrew]. *'Asiya* 17/1–2 (1999), pp. 83–111.

Halperin-Kaddari (1999) Halperin-Kaddari, Ruth. "Redefining Parenthood." *California Western International Law Journal* 29/2 (1999), pp. 313–337.

Harding (1996) Harding, Sandra. "Rethinking Standpoint Epistemology: What Is 'Strong Objectivity?'" In F. K. Keller and H. E. Longino (eds.), *Feminism and Science*, pp. 235–248. Oxford: Oxford University Press, 1996.

Harkavy (1887) Harkavy, Avraham. E. *Remembrance of the Ancient and the More Recent—Part 1, the Ancients: Fourth Booklet; Remembrance of Some Ge'onim, Especially R. Sherira, His Son R. Hai, and R. Isaac Alfasi* [Hebrew]. Berlin, 1887.

Harris (1990) Harris, Angela P. "Race and Essentialism in Feminist Legal Theory." *Stanford Law Review* 42 (1990), pp. 581–616.

Hartman (2007) Hartman, Tova. *Feminism Encounters Traditional Judaism: Resistance and Accommodation*. Hanover, NH: Brandeis University Press, 2007.

Hawkesworth (1998) Hawkesworth, Mary. "Social Sciences." In A. M. Jaggar and I. M. Young (eds.), *A Companion to Feminist Philosophy*, pp. 204–212. Malden, MA: Blackwell, 1998.

Held (1995) Held, Virginia (ed.). *Justice and Care: Essential Readings in Feminist Ethics*. Boulder, CO: Westview Press, 1995.

Henkin (2003) Henkin, Yehudah Herzl. "Deferring the Commandment to Procreate: A Response to Rabbi Benjamin Lau" [Hebrew]. *Geranot* 3 (2003), pp. 149–152.

Herschler (1980) Herschler, Moshe. "Halakhic Problems Related to Test-Tube Babies" [Hebrew]. In M. Herschler (ed.), *Halakhah and Medicine: Collected Essays on Halakhah Related to Medical Matters* [Hebrew], Vol. 1, 307–320. Jerusalem and Chicago: Machon Regensburg, 1980.

Herschler (1984) Herschler, Moshe. "Test-Tube Babies in Halakhah" [Hebrew]. *Torah She-Be'al Peh* 25 (1984), pp. 124–129.

Heyd (1992) Heyd, David. *Genethics: Moral Issues in the Creation of People*. Berkeley: University of California Press, 1992.

Hibner (1969) Hibner, Shmuel. "Aborting a Fetus to Save the Mother" [Hebrew]. *Ha-Darom* 28 (1969), pp. 31–42.

Himes (1970) Himes, Norman E. *Medical History of Contraception*. New York: Schocken, 1970.

Holmes and Hoskins (1987) Holmes, Helen B., and Betty B. Hoskins. "Prenatal and Preconception Sex Choice Technologies: A Path to Femicide?" In G. Corea et al. (eds.), *Man-Made Women: How New Reproductive Technologies Affect Women*, pp. 15–29. Bloomington and Indianapolis: Indiana University Press, 1987.

Irshai (2006) Irshai, Ronit. "Fertility, Gender and Halakhah: A Feminist Perspective on Modern Responsa Literature (Contraception, Abortion, Artificial Insemination, In Vitro Fertilization and Surrogate Motherhood)" [Hebrew]. Ph.D. diss. Ramat Gan: Bar Ilan University, 2006.

Irshai (2010) Irshai, Ronit. "Toward a Gender Critical Approach to the Philosophy of Jewish Law (Halakhah)." *Journal of Feminist Studies in Religion* 26/2 (2010), pp. 55–77

Irshai (forthcoming) Irshai, Ronit. "The Gap between Public and Private Rulings: A Critical Analysis" (forthcoming).

Irshai (in press) Irshai, Ronit. "Halakhic Discretion and Gender Bias: A Conceptual Analysis." *Democratic Culture* (in press).

Jaggar (1996) Jaggar, Alison. M. "Love and Knowledge: Emotion in Feminist Epistemology." In A. Garry and M. Pearsall (eds.), *Women, Knowledge, and Reality—Explorations in Feminist Philosophy*, pp. 166–190. New York: Routledge, 1996.

Jakobovits (1975) Jakobovits, Immanuel. *Jewish Medical Ethics: A Comparative and Historical Study of the Jewish Religious Attitude to Medicine and Its Practice.* New York: Bloch Publishing Company, 1975.

Jakobovits (2000) Jakobovits, Immanuel. "Jewish Views on Abortion." In Fred Rosner and J. David Bleich (eds.), *Jewish Bioethics*, pp. 139–154. Hoboken, NJ: Ktav, 2000.

Jensen (1995) Jensen, A. "The Status of Women and the Social Context of Reproduction." *Journal of International Development* 7/1 (1995), pp. 61–79.

Jordan (1976) Jordan, Bonnie. C. *The Status of Women and Fertility: Some Implications for Social Work Practice.* Social Work Education and Population Planning Project, University of Michigan, 1976.

Kahn (2000) Kahn, Susan. M. *Reproducing Jews: A Cultural Account of Assisted Conception in Israel.* Durham, NC, and London: Duke University Press, 2000.

Kahn (2002) Kahn, Susan. M. "Rabbis and Reproduction: The Uses of New Reproductive Technologies among Ultraorthodox Jews in Israel." In M. C. Inhorn and F. Van Balen (eds.), *Infertility around the Globe—New Thinking on Childlessness, Gender, and Reproductive Technologies*, pp. 283–297. Berkeley: University of California Press, 2002.

Katan (2003) Katan, Hanna. "Planning the 'Non-family'" [Hebrew]. *Nequdah* 264 (Tammuz 5763), pp. 26–28.

Katan and Harav (2002) Katan, Hanna, and Yoel Harav. "Family Planning in Accord with Halakhah (Response to Dr. Uri Levy)" [Hebrew]. *Ẓohar* 10 (2002), pp. 217–221.

Katz (1992) Katz, 'Aharon. "The Surrogate Mother" [Hebrew]. *Magal—Ḥiddusei Torah Ve-Ma'amarim* 8–9 (1992), pp. 15–18.

Katz (1968) Katz, Jacob. "Toward a Biography of the Ḥatam Sofer" [Hebrew]. In *Studies in Kabbalah and the History of Religions, Presented to Gershom Scholem* [Hebrew], pp. 115–148. Jerusalem: Magnes Press, 1968. Reprinted in Katz (1984), pp. 353–386.

Katz (1984) Katz, Jacob. *Halakhah and Kabbalah: Studies in the History of Judaism* [Hebrew]. Jerusalem: Magnes Press, 1984.

Katz-Rothman (1984) Katz-Rothman, Barbara. "The Meanings of Choice in Reproductive Technology." In R. Arditti et al. (eds.), *Test Tube Women: What Future for Motherhood*, pp. 23–33. London: Pandora Press, 1984.

Katz-Rothman (2000) Katz-Rothman, Barbara. *Recreating Motherhood.* New Brunswick, NJ, and London: Rutgers University Press, 2000.

Kilav (1984) Kilav, Avraham. I. "Who Is the Infant's Mother—the Genetic Parent or the Gestational?" [Hebrew]. *Teḥumin* 5 (1984), pp. 260–267.

Kirschenbaum (1992) Kirschenbaum, Aharon. "Subjectivity in Rabbinic

Decision Making." In M. Z. Sokol (ed.), *Rabbinic Authority and Personal Autonomy*, pp. 61–91. Northvale, NJ: Jason Aronson, 1992.

Knohl (2005) Knohl, Elyashiv. *Man and Woman—If They So Merit, the Divine Presence Is with Them: Manual for Bride and Groom* [Hebrew]. 'Ein Ẓurim: Makhon Shiluvim / Yeshivat Hakibbutz Hadati, 2005.

Korenblith (1999) Korenblith, Hilary. "Distrusting Reason." *Midwest Studies in Philosophy* 23 (1999), pp. 181–196.

Kunstlicher (1993) Kunstlicher, Moshe A. Z. *The Ḥatam Sofer and His Generation: Personalities in Ḥatam Sofer Responses—List of People Who Were Mentioned and Asked with Their Short Bios.* Benei Berak: Makhon Lehotza'at Sefarim–Benei Moshe, 1993.

Landau (1979) Landau, Yehudah. "On Family Planning in Light of Halakhah" [Hebrew]. *Bi-Shevilei Ha-Refu'ah* 1 (1979), pp. 22–26.

Lasker (1988) Lasker, Daniel J. "Kabbalah, Halakhah, and Modern Medicine: The Case of Artificial Insemination." *Modern Judaism* 8 (1988), pp. 1–14.

Lasker and Parmet (1990) Lasker, Judith N., and Harriet L. Parmet. "Rabbinic and Feminist Responses to Reproductive Technology." *Journal of Feminist Studies in Religion* 6/1 (1990), pp. 117–130.

Lau (2003) Lau, Benjamin. "For She Is Your Friend and the Wife of Your Covenant: Two Purposes for the Institution of Marriage" [Hebrew]. *Geranot* 3 (2003), pp. 135–148.

Lau (1992) Lau, Israel M. "Family Planning: A Halakhic Perspective" [Hebrew]. In Y. Katan (ed.), *Gynecology, Fertility, and Births in Light of Halkahah* [Hebrew], pp. 105–118. Jerusalem: The Religious Council, 1992.

LeMoncheck (1996) LeMoncheck, Linda. "Philosophy, Gender Politics, and In Vitro Fertilization: A Feminist Ethics of Reproductive Healthcare." *Journal of Clinical Ethics* 7/2 (1996), pp. 160–176.

Lev (1989) Lev, Ze'ev. "On Motherhood of an Infant Born to a Surrogate Mother" [Hebrew]. *'Or Ha-Mizraḥ* 37/2 (1989), pp. 150–160.

Levine and Safran (1995) Levin, Eybi, and Anat Safran. "In Vitro Fertilization" [Hebrew]. *Asia* 14/3 (1995), pp. 5–41.

Levy (2002) Levy, Uri. "On the Duty to Preserve Health in General and the Health of a Pregnant Woman and Her Children in Particular" [Hebrew]. *Ẓohar* 10 (2002), pp. 205–216.

Lichtenstein (1974) Lichtenstein, 'Aharon. "A Halakhic Opinion" [Hebrew]. *Bri'ut Ha-Ẓibbur* 17/4 (1974), pp. 495–501.

Lichtenstein (1977) Lichtenstein, 'Aharon. "Morality and *Halakhah* in the

Jewish Tradition: Does *Halakhah* Recognize an Ethics Independent of Halakhah?" [Hebrew]. *De'ot* 46 (1977), pp. 5–20.
Lichtenstein (1986) Lichtenstein, 'Aharon. *The Seven Laws of Noah*. 2nd ed. New York: The Rabbi Jacob Joseph School Press, 1986.
Lichtenstein (1988) Lichtenstein, 'Aharon. "Family Planning and Birth Control" [Hebrew]. *'Alon Shevut Le-Bogrei Yeshivat Har 'Eẓiyon* 6 (1988), pp. 19–33.
Lichtenstein (1991) Lichtenstein, 'Aharon. "Abortion: A Halakhic Perspective." *Tradition* 25/4 (1991), pp. 3–12
Lichtenstein (2002) Lichtenstein, 'Aharon. "The Human and Social Factor in Halakha." *Tradition* 36/1 (2002), pp. 1–25.
Lloyd (1996) Lloyd, Genevieve. "The Man of Reason." In A. Garry and M. Pearsall (eds.), *Women, Knowledge, and Reality—Explorations in Feminist Philosophy*, pp. 149–165. New York: Routledge, 1996.
Locke (1988) Locke, John. *Two Treatises of Government*. Student ed. Cambridge: Cambridge University Press, 1988.
Lorber (1988) Lorber, Judith. "In Vitro Fertilization and Gender Politics." In Baruch E. Hoffman et al. (eds.), *Embryos, Ethics, and Women's Rights: Exploring the New Reproductive Technologies*, pp. 117–133. New York and London: Harrington Park Press, 1988.
Lorber (1992) Lorber, Judith. "Gift, or Patriarchal Bargain? Women's Consent to In Vitro Fertilization in Male Infertility." In Holmes H. Bequaert and L. M. Purdy (eds.), *Feminist Perspectives in Medical Ethics*, pp. 169–180. Bloomington and Indianapolis: Indiana University Press, 1992.
Lorberbaum (2004) Lorberbaum, Yair. *The Image of God* [Hebrew]. Jerusalem and Tel Aviv: Schocken, 2004.
MacKinnon (1987) MacKinnon, Catharine A. *Feminism Unmodified: Discourses on Life and Law*. Cambridge, MA, and London: Harvard University Press, 1987.
MacKinnon (1989) MacKinnon, Catherine A. *Toward a Feminist Theory of the State*. Cambridge, MA: Harvard University Press, 1989.
MacKinnon (1990–91) MacKinnon, Catherine A. "Reflections on Sex Equality Under Law." *Yale Law Journal* 100 (1990–91), pp. 1281–1328.
Mackler (2003) Mackler, Aaron L. *Introduction to Jewish and Catholic Bioethics: A Comparative Analysis*. Washington, DC: Georgetown University Press, 2003.
Macklin (1988) Macklin, Ruth. "Is There Anything Wrong with Surrogate Motherhood? An Ethical Analysis." In L. Gostin (ed.), *Surrogate Motherhood—Politics and Privacy*, pp. 136–150. Bloomington and Indianapolis: Indiana University Press, 1988.

Macklin (1991) Macklin, Ruth. "Artificial Means of Reproduction and Our Understanding of the Family." *Hasting Center Report* (January–February 1991), pp. 5–11.

Malakh (1992) Malakh, Daniel. "Issues in Family Planning" [Hebrew]. In Y. Katan (ed.), *Gynecology, Fertility, and Births in Light of Halkahah* [Hebrew], pp. 89–104. Jerusalem: The Religious Council, 1992.

Meacham (2009a) Meacham (leBeit Yoreh), Tirzah. "Abortion." In *Jewish Women: A Comprehensive Historical Encyclopedia*, 2009, http://jwa.org/encyclopedia/article/abortion.

Meacham (2009b) Meacham (leBeit Yoreh), Tirzah. "Contraception." In *Jewish Women: A Comprehensive Historical Encyclopedia*, 2009, http://jwa.org/encyclopedia/article/contraception.

Menkel Meadow (1985) Menkel Meadow, Carrie. "Portia in a Different Voice: Speculations on a Women's Lawyering Process." *Berkeley Women's Law Journal* 1 (1985), pp. 39–63.

Millen (2004) Millen, Rochelle L. *Women, Birth and Death in Jewish Law and Practice*. Hanover, NH: Brandeis University Press, 2004.

Morag-Levine (1994) Morag-Levine, Noga. "Abortion in Israel: Community, Rights, and the Context of Compromise." *Law and Social Inquiry* 19/2 (1994), pp. 313–335.

Nelson (1996) Nelson, Lynn. H. "Who Knows? What Can They Know? And When?" In A. Garry and M. Pearsall (eds.), *Women, Knowledge, and Reality: Explorations in Feminist Philosophy*, pp. 286–297. New York: Routledge, 1996.

Neubart (2002) Neubart, Yehoshua Y. "On Family Planning (Response to articles in *Ẓohar* 10)" [Hebrew]. *Ẓohar* 11 (2002), pp. 135–136.

Noonan (1965) Noonan, John. T. *Contraception: A History of Its Treatment by the Catholic Theologians and Canonists*. Cambridge, MA: Harvard University Press, 1965.

Noonan (1970) Noonan, John T. (ed). *The Morality of Abortion: Legal and Historical Perspectives*. Cambridge, MA: Harvard University Press, 1970.

Novak (1985) Novak, David. "Judaism and Contemporary Bioethics." In D. Novak, *Halakhah in a Theological Dimension*, pp. 82–101. Chico, CA: Scholars Press, 1985.

Oakley (1974) Oakley, Ann. *Woman's Work: The Housewife, Past and Present*. New York: Pantheon Books, 1974.

Oakley (1987) Oakley, Ann. "From Walking Wombs to Test-Tube Babies." In M. Stanworth (ed.), *Reproductive Technologies—Gender, Motherhood and Medicine*, pp. 36–56. Minneapolis: University of Minnesota Press, 1987.

O'Brien (1981) O'Brien, Mary. *The Politics of Reproduction*. Boston: London and Henley, 1981.

Overall (1987) Overall, Christine. *Ethics and Human Reproduction: A Feminist Analysis*. Boston: Allen & Unwin, 1987.

Ozick (1983) Ozick, Cynthia. "Notes toward Finding the Right Question." In S. Heschel (ed.), *On Being a Jewish Feminist: A Reader*, pp. 120–151. New York: Schocken Books, 1983.

Pateman (1988) Pateman, Carole. *The Sexual Contract*. Stanford, CA: Stanford University Press, 1988.

Polatnick (1983) Polatnick, Rivka. M. "Why Men Don't Rear Children: A Power Analysis." In J. Trebilcot (ed.), *Mothering: Essays in Feminist Theory*, pp. 20–40. Totowa, NJ: Rowman & Littlefield Publishers, 1983.

Posner (1998) Posner, Richard A. *Law and Literature*. Cambridge, MA: Harvard University Press, 1998.

Rafael (1976) Rafael, Yiẓḥak. "The Chief Rabbi, Rabbi Isser Yehudah Unterman, Z"L" [Hebrew]. *Sinai* 78 (1976), pp. 1–5.

Rafael (1992) Rafael, Shilo. "Compelling a Patient to Submit to Medical Treatment" [Hebrew]. *Torah She-be'al Peh* 33 (1992), pp. 74–81.

Rappeld (1990) Rappeld, Meir. *The Maharshal and the Yam Shel Shelomoh* [Hebrew]. Ph.D. diss. Ramat-Gan: Bar-Ilan University, 1990.

Rakover (1989) Rakover, Nahum. *The Rule of Law in Israel* [Hebrew]. Jerusalem: Moreshet Ha-Mishpat Be-Yisra'el, 1989.

Rakover (1992) Rakover, Sam S. "Is There Substance to the Feminist Critique of Science?" [Hebrew]. *Psikhologiyah* 3 (1992), pp. 5–12.

Ralbag (2004) Ralbag, Mordeḥai. "Parenthood of an Infant Born through Artificial Insemination" [Hebrew]. *Teḥumin* 24 (2004), pp. 139–146.

Raziel (1981) Raziel, Moshe. "Compelling a Patient to Submit to Medical Treatment" [Hebrew]. *Teḥumin* 2, pp. 325–336.

Reich (1995) Reich, Warren T. (ed). *Encyclopedia of Bioethics*. Vols. 1–5. New York: Simon & Schuster Macmillan, 1995.

Rich (1976) Rich, Adrienne. *Of Woman Born: Motherhood as Experience and Institution*. New York: Norton, 1976.

Robertson (1994) Robertson, John A. *Children of Choice—Freedom and the New Reproductive Technologies*. Princeton, NJ: Princeton University Press, 1994.

Rosenfeld (1997) Rosenfeld, Azriel. "Generation, Gestation, and Judaism." In E. Feldman and J. B. Wolowelsky (eds.), *Jewish Law and the New Reproductive Technologies*, pp. 36–45. Hoboken, NJ: Ktav, 1997.

Rosner (1979a) Rosner, Fred. "Artificial Insemination in Jewish Law" [1979]. In Fred Rosner and J. David Bleich (eds.), *Jewish Bioethics*, pp. 105–117. Hoboken, NJ: Ktav, 2000.

Rosner (1979b) Rosner, Fred. "Contraception in Jewish Law" [1979]. In J. David Bleich and Fred Rosner (eds.), *Jewish Bioethics*, pp. 86–96. Hoboken, NJ: Ktav, 2000.

Rosner (2000) Rosner, Fred. *Encyclopedia of Medicine in the Bible and Talmud.* Northvale, NJ: Jacob Aronson, 2000.

Ross (1998) Ross, Devora. "Artificial Insemination in Single Women" [Hebrew]. In D. Halpern and C. Safrai (eds.), *Jewish Legal Writings by Women*, pp. 45–72. Efrat: Urim Publications, 1998.

Ross (2001) Ross, Tamar. "Between Sodom and Mount Moriah: Some Thoughts Concerning the Halakhic Distress of David Hartman" [Hebrew]. In A. Sagi and Z. Zohar (eds.), *Renewing Jewish Commitment*, Vol. 2 [Hebrew], pp. 709–745. Jerusalem: Shalom Hartman Institute, 2001.

Ross (2004) Ross, Tamar. *Expanding the Palace of Torah: Orthodoxy and Feminism*. Hanover, NH: Brandeis University Press, 2004.

Ross (2011) Ross, Tamar. "The Contribution of Feminism to the Halakhic Discourse: 'A Woman's Voice Is Nakedness' as a Test Case" [Hebrew]. In Avinoam Rosenak (ed.), *Halakhah, Meta-Halakhah and Philosophy: A Multi Disciplinary Perspective*, pp. 35–64. Jerusalem: Van Leer and Magnes, 2011.

Ross (1993) Ross, Thomas. "Despair and Redemption in the Feminist Nomos." *Indiana Law Journal* 69 (1993), pp. 101–136.

Rowland (1987) Rowland, Robyn. "Motherhood, Patriarchal Power, Alienation and the Issue of 'Choice' in Sex Preselection." In G. Corea et al. (eds.), *Man-Made Women: How New Reproductive Technologies Affect Women*, pp. 74–87. Bloomington and Indianapolis: Indiana University Press, 1987.

Rowland (1992) Rowland, Robyn. *Living Laboratories: Women and Reproductive Technologies*. Bloomington: Indiana University Press, 1992.

Ruddick (1989) Ruddick, Sara. *Maternal Thinking: Towards a Politics of Peace.* London and Boston: Women's Press–Beacon Press, 1989.

Rudy (1996) Rudy, Kathy. *Beyond Pro-Life and Pro-Choice: Moral Diversity in the Abortion Debate*. Boston: Beacon Press, 1996.

Rusinak (2005) Rusinak, Sinaya. "Nietzsche: Between Genealogy and Criticism" [Hebrew]. *'Iyyun* 53 (2005), pp. 409–427.

Safrai (1983) Safrai, Shmuel. *The Late Second-Temple Period and the Period of the Mishnah: Essays in Social and Cultural History* [Hebrew]. Jerusalem: Zalman Shazar Center, 1983.

Safrai (1995) Safrai, Shmuel. "Tannaitic Views on Women's Obligations to Observe the Commandments" [Hebrew]. *Bar-Ilan University Jewish Studies and Humanities Annual* 26–27 (1995), pp. 227–236.

Sagi (1998) Sagi, Avi. *Judaism: Between Religion and Morality* [Hebrew]. Tel Aviv: Ha-Kibbutz Ha-Me'uḥad, 1998.

Satlow (2001) Satlow, Michael L. *Jewish Marriage in Antiquity*. Princeton, NJ, and Oxford: Princeton University Press, 2001.

Sawicki (1991) Sawicki, Jana. *Disciplining Foucault: Feminism, Power, and the Body*. New York, London: Routledge, 1991.

Schauer (1988) Schauer, Frederick. "Formalism." *The Yale Law Journal* 97/4 (1988), pp. 509–548.

Schiff (2002) Schiff, Daniel. *Abortion in Judaism*. Cambridge, MA: Cambridge University Press, 2002.

Schiffman (1989) Schiffman, Pinḥas. *Laws of Family in Israel*, Vol. 2. Jerusalem: The Hebrew University Faculty of Law, 1989.

Schremer (2003) Schremer Adiel. *Male and Female He Created Them: Jewish Marriage in the Late Second Temple, Mishnah and Talmud Periods* [Hebrew]. Jerusalem: Zalman Shazar, 2003.

Sered (2000) Sered, Susan S. *What Makes Women Sick: Maternity, Modesty and Militarism in Israeli Society*. Hanover, NH: Brandeis University Press, 2000.

Shafran (1999) Shafran, Yigal. "Sperm Donation by a Jew: The Doctrine of Rabbi Saul Israeli on This Issue and Its Ramifications" [Hebrew]. *Netivei Merḥavim* 6 (1999), pp. 205–210.

Shagar (2006) Rosenberg, Shimshon G. [Shagar]. "Seeing the Voices: Yeshiva Scholarship and the 'Women's Voice' in Torah Study" [Hebrew]. In Zohar Ma'or (ed.), *Two Luminaries: A New Jewish Perspective on Family Equality* [Hebrew], pp. 63–83. Efratah: Machon Binah Le-'Ittim, 2006.

Shalev (1989) Shalev, Carmel. *Birth Power: The Case for Surrogacy*. New Haven and London: Yale University Press, 1989.

Sharlo (2009) Sharlo, Yuval. "Ethical and Halakhic Dilemmas Following Fertility Technology and Its Influence on Marital Life [Hebrew]." In T. Cohen (ed.), *To Be a Jewish Woman*, pp. 239–250. Jerusalem: Kolech–Religious Women Forum, 2009.

Schereschewsky (1993) Schereschewsky, Benzion. *Family Law in Israel* [Hebrew]. Jerusalem: Reuven Mass, 1993.

Sherwin (1987) Sherwin, Susan. "Feminist Ethics and In Vitro Fertilization." In M. Henen and K. Nielsen (eds.), *Science, Morality & Feminist Theory*, pp. 265–284. Calgary, AB: The University of Calgary Press, 1987.

Sherwin (1989) Sherwin, Susan. "Feminist and Medical Ethics: Two Different Approaches to Contextual Ethics." *Hypatia* 4/2, (1989), pp. 57–72.

Sherwin (1992) Sherwin, Susan. *No Longer Patient: Feminist Ethics and Health Care*. Philadelphia: Temple University Press, 1992.

Sinclair (1999) Sinclair, Daniel. "Autonomy and Halakhah in Medicine: Does a Man Have Ownership of His Life?" [Hebrew]. In H. Goldberg (ed.), *A Renewed Examination of the Principles of Religious Zionism and Modern Orthodoxy* [Hebrew], pp. 150–159. Tel Aviv: Modan, 1999.

Sinclair (2003 Hebrew) Sinclair, Daniel. "Artificial Insemination in Jewish Law: Comparative, Methodological, and Moral Aspects" [Hebrew]. *Ha-Mishpat* 16 (2003), pp. 16–26.

Sinclair (2003 English) Sinclair, Daniel. *Jewish Biomedical Law: Legal and Extra-legal Dimensions*. New York: Oxford University Press, 2003.

Singer (1993) Singer, Peter. *Practical Ethics*. 2nd ed. Cambridge: Cambridge University Press, 1993.

Soloveitchik A. H (1998) Soloveitchik, 'Aharon H. "On Saving the Life of a Fetus—the Status of a Fetus in Halakhah" [Hebrew]. *'Asiya* 61–62 (Nisan 5758), pp. 85–94.

Soloveitchik Ḥ. H (1986) Soloveitchik, Ḥaim H. *Novellae of Rabbenu Ḥayyim Ha-Levi: Novellae and Explanations Related to Maimonides* [Hebrew]. Brooklyn: 1986.

Soloveitchik J. B. (1982) Soloveitchik, Joseph B. *Philosophical Essays* (*Divrei Hagut Ve-Ha'arakhah*) [Hebrew]. Jerusalem: World Zionist Organization, 1982.

Soloveitchik J. B. (1983) Soloveitchik, Joseph B. *Halakhic Man*. Translated from the Hebrew by Lawrence Kaplan. Philadelphia: Jewish Publication Society of America, 1983.

Soloveitchik J. B. (1986) Soloveitchik, Joseph B. *The Halakhic Mind: An Essay on Jewish Tradition and Modern Thought*. New York: Seth Press, 1986.

Stanworth (1987) Stanworth, Michelle. *Reproductive Technologies: Gender, Motherhood and Medicine*. Minneapolis: University of Minnesota Press, 1987.

Steinberg (1983) Steinberg, Avraham. "The Jewish General Approach to Birth Control" [Hebrew]. In A. Steinberg (ed.), *Sefer 'Asiya* 4, pp. 139–160. Jerusalem: Reuven Mas, 1983.

Steinberg (2003) Steinberg, Avraham. *Encyclopedia of Jewish Medical Ethics: A Compilation of Jewish Medical Law on All topics of Medical Interest*. 3 vols. Trans. Fred Rosner. Jerusalem: Feldheim, 2003.

Stern (1980) Stern, Michal. *Medicine in Light of Halakhah I: Abortion and In*

Vitro Fertilization [Hebrew]. Jerusalem: Ha-Makhon Le-Ḥeker Ha-Refuah Lefi Ha-Halakhah, 1980.

Sternbuch (1965) Sternbuch, Moshe. "On the Prohibition against Artificial Insemination" [Hebrew]. *Ha-Ma'or* 16 (Adar 1) (1965).

Sternbuch (1987) Sternbuch, Moshe. "Test Tube Baby" [Hebrew]. *Bishvilei Ha-Refuah* 8 (1987), pp. 29–36.

Ta-Shma (2000) Ta-Shma, Israel M. *Talmudic Commentary in Europe and North Afrika—Literary History, Part 2: 1200–1400* [Hebrew]. Jerusalem: Magnes Press, 2000.

Tendler (1979) Tendler, Moshe D. "Population Control: The Jewish View" [1979]. In J. D. Bleich and F. Rosner (eds.), *Jewish Bioethics*, pp. 97–104. Hoboken, NJ: Ktav, 2000.

Thompson (2002) Thompson, Charis M. "Fertile Ground: Feminists Theorize Infertility." In M. C. Inhorn and F. van Balen (eds.), *Infertility around the Globe: New Thinking on Childlessness, Gender, and Reproductive Technologies*, pp. 52–78. Berkeley: University of California Press, 2002.

Thomson (1971) Thomson, Judith J. "A Defense of Abortion" [1971]. In R. M. Baird and S. E. Rosenbaum (eds.), *The Ethics of Abortion: Pro-Life vs. Pro-Choice*, 3rd ed., pp. 241–256. New York: Prometheus Books, 2001.

Tong (1989) Tong, Rosemarie. *Feminist Thought: A Comprehensive Introduction*. Boulder, CO, and San Francisco: Westview Press, 1989.

Tong (1997) Tong, Rosemarie. *Feminist Approaches to Bioethics: Theoretical Reflections and Practical Applications*. Boulder, CO, and Oxford: Westview Press, 1997.

Tooley (1989) Tooley, Michael. "Abortion and Infanticide." In R. M. Baird and S. E. Rosenbaum (eds.), *The Ethics of Abortion: Pro-Life vs. Pro-Choice*, pp. 45–60. Buffalo: Prometheus Books, 1989.

Tzuriel (2005) Tzuriel, Moshe. "Aborting a Fetus with Severe Illness" [Hebrew]. *Teḥumin* 25 (2005), pp. 64–78.

United Nations (1975) United Nations (Helvi Sipilä). *Status of Women and Family Planning: Report of the Special Rapporteur Appointed by the Economic and Social Council under Resolution 1326 (XLIV)*. New York: United Nations, 1975.

Unterman (1952) Unterman, Yehudah. "The Commandment to Save a Life and Its Limitations" [Hebrew]. *Ha-Torah Ve-Ha-Medinah* 4 (1952), pp. 22–29.

Unterman (1963) Unterman, Yehudah. "On Transgressing to Save the Life of a Fetus" [Hebrew]. *No'am* 1 (1963), pp. 145–166.

Urbach (1976) Urbach, Ephraim E. *The Sages: Their Beliefs and Ideas* [Hebrew]. Jerusalem: Magnes, 1976.

Urbach (1980) Urbach, Ephraim E. *The Tosafists: Their History, Writings, and Method* [Hebrew]. 2 vols. Jerusalem: Mosad Bialik, 1980.

Wahrhaftig (1979–80) Wahrhaftig, Zeraḥ. "The Precedent in Jewish Law" [Hebrew].. *Shenaton Ha-Mishpat Ha-'Ivri* 6–7 (1979–80), pp. 105–132.

Walter (1995) Walter, Jacob. "Be Fruitful and Multiply." In J. Walter and M. Zemer (eds.), *The Fetus and Fertility in Jewish Law: Essays and Responsa.* Pittsburgh and Tel Aviv: Freehof Institute of Progressive Halakhah, 1995, pp. 1–17.

Warren (1989) Warren, Mary. A. "On the Moral and Legal Status of Abortion." In R. M. Baird and S. E. Rosenbaum (eds.), *The Ethics of Abortion: Pro-Life vs. Pro-Choice*, pp. 75–92. Buffalo: Prometheus Books, 1989.

Wegner (1988) Wegner, Judith. R. *Chattel or Person? The Status of Women in the Mishnah*. New York: Oxford University Press, 1998.

Weinfeld (1977) Weinfeld, Moshe. "Feticide: The Stance of the Jewish Tradition Compared to That of Other Nations" [Hebrew]. *Zion* 42/1–2 (1977), pp. 129–142.

Weinrib (1988) Weinrib, Ernest. J. "Legal Formalism: On the Immanent Rationality of Law." *Yale Law Journal* 97/6 (1988), pp. 949–1016.

Weiss (1904) Weiss, Isaac H. *Dor Dor Ve-Doreshav: History of the Oral Torah* [Hebrew]. Vilna: Goldenberg Publishers, 1904.

West (1988) West, Robin. "Jurisprudence and Gender." *University of Chicago Law Review* 55/1 (1988), pp. 1–72.

West (1990–91) West, Robin. "Foreword: Taking Freedom Seriously." *Harvard Law Review* 104 (1990–91), pp. 43–106.

West (1993) West, Robin. "Economic Man and Literary Woman: One Contrast." In R. West, *Narrative, Authority and Law*, pp. 251–264. Ann Arbor: University of Michigan Press, 1993.

Westreich (1997) Westreich, Elimelech. "The Commandment to Procreate in Jewish Law in the Ottoman Empire of the Sixteenth Century" [Hebrew]. In M. E. Friedman, ed., *Te'udah 13: Matrimony and Family in Halakhah and Jewish Thought* [Hebrew], pp. 195–240. Tel Aviv: Tel Aviv University Press, 1997.

Westreich (2002) Westreich, Elimelech. *Transitions in the Legal Status of the Wife in Jewish Law: A Journey Among Traditions* [Hebrew]. Jerusalem: Magnes, 2002.

Wolfson (2002) Wolfson, Naomi. "Mother and Children Rejoice (Response to Articles on Family Planning)" [Hebrew]. *Ẓohar* 11 (2002), pp. 137–140.

Yannai (1992) Yannai, Nili. "Toward an Understanding of Feminist Scientific

Research: Response to the Article by Sam S. Rakover" [Hebrew]. *Psikhologiyah* 3 (1992), pp. 13–20.

Yosef (1976) Yosef, Ovadia. "Abortion in Light of *Halakhah*" [Hebrew]. In A. Steinberg (ed.), *Sefer 'Asiya* 1, pp. 78–94. Jerusalem: Dr. Falk Schlesinger Institute for Medical Halachic Research at the Shaare Zedek Medical Center, 1976.

Zevin (1973–2004) Zevin, Shlomo Y. (ed). *Talmudic Encyclopedia* [Hebrew]. [Vols. 1–2 also edited by M. Berlin.] Jerusalem: Talmudic Encyclopedia Publishers, 1973–2004.

Zilberstein and Rothschild (1987) Zilberstein, Yiẓḥak, and Moshe Rothschild. *Torat Ha-Yoledet* [Hebrew]. Bnei Brak: Makhon Halakhah Ve-Refu'ah, 1987.

Zohar (1988) Zohar, Noam. "The Differences between Man and Woman: Editing and Ethics in M Qiddushin, chapter 1" [Hebrew]. *'Et La'asot* 1 (1988), pp. 103–112.

Zohar (1989) Zohar, Noam. "To What Extent Is a Woman 'Acquired' by Her Husband: On the Halakhic Discussion of Artificial Insemination" [Hebrew]. *Shedeimot* 110 (1989), pp. 91–99.

Zohar (1994) Zohar, Noam. "The Human Being as God's Possession: On the Halakhic Opposition to Euthanasia" [Hebrew]. In D. Statman and A. Sagi (eds.), *Between Religion and Morality*, pp. 145–156. Tel Aviv: Ha-Kibbutz Ha-Me'uchad, 1994.

Zohar (1997) Zohar, Noam. *Alternatives in Jewish Bioethics*. New York: State University of New York Press, 1997.

Zohar (1998) Zohar, Noam. "Halakhah, Politics, and Renewal of Torah" [Hebrew]. In M. Roth, ed., *Religious Zionism in New Perspective* [Hebrew], 203–210. Petah Tiqvah: Ne'emanei Torah Ve-Avodah, 1998.

Zohar (2008) Zohar, Noam. "Developing an Halakhic Theory as a Necessary Foundation to the Philosophy of Halakha: A Fundamental Discussion and Three Examples" [Hebrew]. In A. Ravitzki and A. Rosenak (eds.), *New Streams in the Philosophy of Halakhah*, pp. 43–63. Jerusalem: Magnes, 2008

Zohar and Sagi (1995) Zohar, Zvi, and Avi Sagi. *Conversion and Jewish Identity: An Inquiry into the Foundations of the Halakhah* [Hebrew]. Jerusalem: Shalom Hartman Institute and Mosad Bialik, 1995.

Zoloth (2003) Zoloth, Laurie. "'Each One an Entire World': A Jewish Perspective on Family Planning." In Daniel C. Maguire (ed.), *Sacred Rights: The Case for Contraception and Abortion in World Religions*, pp. 21–53. New York: Oxford University Press, 2003.

Zweig (1964) Zweig, Yona H. "On Abortion" [Hebrew]. *No'am* 7 (1964), pp. 36–56.

Index